CLINICAL DOPPLER ECHOCARDIOGRAPHY

Spectral and Color Flow Imaging

NOTICE

Medicine is an ever-changing science. As new research and clinical experience broaden our knowledge, changes in treatment and drug therapy are required. The editors and the publisher of this work have checked with sources believed to be reliable in their efforts to provide information that is complete and generally in accord with the standards accepted at the time of publication. However, in view of the possibility of human error or changes in medical sciences, neither the editors nor the publisher nor any other party who has been involved in the preparation or publication of this work warrants that the information contained herein is in every respect accurate or complete. Readers are encouraged to confirm the information contained herein with other sources. For example and in particular, readers are advised to check the product information sheet included in the package of each drug they plan to administer to be certain that the information contained in this book is accurate and that changes have not been made in the recommended dose or in the contraindications for administration. This recommendation is of particular importance in connection with new or infrequently used drugs.

CLINICAL DOPPLER ECHOCARDIOGRAPHY

Spectral and Color Flow Imaging

José Missri, M.D.

Associate Director, Section of Cardiology
Department of Medicine
Director, Cardiac Catheterization Laboratory
Director, Cardiac Noninvasive Laboratory
Saint Francis Hospital and Medical Center
Associate Professor of Medicine
University of Connecticut School of Medicine
Hartford, Connecticut

McGraw-Hill Information Services Company
HEALTH PROFESSIONS DIVISION

New York St. Louis San Francisco Colorado Springs
Auckland Bogotá Caracas Hamburg Lisbon London Madrid
Mexico Milan Montreal New Delhi Paris
San Juan São Paulo Singapore Sydney Tokyo Toronto

CLINICAL COLOR ECHOCARDIOGRAPHY
Spectral and Color Flow Imaging

12345678910 KGPKGP 89432109

ISBN 0-07-042436-5

This book was set in Novarese Book by York Graphic Services, Inc.
The editors were Avé M. McCracken and Mariapaz Ramos-Englis;
the production supervisor was Robert Laffler;
the text design was done by José Fonfrias;
the cover was designed by Edward R. Schultheis;
the index was prepared by Carl Moxey.
Arcata Graphics/Kingsport was printer and binder.

Library of Congress Cataloging-in-Publication Data

Missri, José, date
Clinical doppler echocardiography : spectral and color flow imaging / José Missri.
p. cm.
Includes bibliographical references.
ISBN 0-07-042436-5
1. Doppler echocardiography. I. Title.
[DNLM: 1. Echocardiography, Doppler. WG 141.5.E2 M678cb]
RC683.5.U5M575 1989
616.1'207543—dc20
DNLM/DLC
for Library of Congress 89-13013
CIP

To Teresa, Esther, Yvette, and Rachael,
and to my loving parents
Moises and Esther

CONTENTS

CHAPTER 11

CHAPTER 12

CHAPTER 13

PREFACE

The introduction of Doppler echocardiography, spectral and color flow imaging, as a supplement to M-mode and two-dimensional techniques has emphasized the need for a comprehensive clinically oriented textbook for the use of all physicians and technologists interested in noninvasive cardiac diagnosis. It was with this need in mind that the idea of writing a textbook that would encompass both spectral (pulsed and continuous-wave Doppler) and color flow imaging was conceived and implemented. It is my hope and expectation that this book will contribute toward fulfilling the needs of the beginning Doppler echocardiographer who already has a working knowledge of both M-mode and two-dimensional techniques and, at the same time, provide thorough coverage of clinical applications for the more experienced ultrasonographer.

The recent development and clinical application of Doppler color flow imaging has enhanced our ability to detect and quantify both congenital and acquired heart disease. This new technique allows a comprehensive study of the direction, velocity, uniformity and timing of intracardiac blood flow, while simultaneously revealing cardiac structures and their movements. By visualizing abnormal flow patterns, we can now more accurately use spectral Doppler techniques to provide quantitative data for making patient-related decisions. A comprehensive Doppler examination is one that, therefore, integrates both spectral and color flow imaging techniques, and the overall interpretation is made in the clinical setting.

This book is organized into 18 chapters. Chapters 1 and 2 explain the basic principles of Doppler echocardiography and instrumentation in spectral and Doppler color flowing imaging. The physics of blood flow is explained in as simple a manner as possible. Mathematical formulas and equations not of practical value to the clinical echocardiographer are excluded. Chapter 3 familiarizes the reader with practical aspects of the Doppler examination, including pulsed, continuous-wave Doppler, and color flow imaging. Chapters 4 to 9 deal with the qualitative and quantitative assessment of various stenotic and regurgitant lesions. Chapter 10 offers a comprehensive discussion of prosthetic valve function. Evaluation of systolic and diastolic cardiac function is discussed in Chapters 11 and 12, respectively. Techniques for determining intracardiac and pulmonary artery pressures are discussed in Chapter 13. Chapter 14 reviews the role of echocardiography and Doppler techniques in evaluating patients with complications of myocardial infarction and in the assessment of patients with suspected ischemic heart disease. Chapter 15 reviews the role of Doppler echocardiography in the evaluation of patients with various forms of cardiomyopathy. Chapter 16 discusses the emerging new field of intraoperative Doppler echocardiography with emphasis on the transesophageal technique. Chapter 17 focuses on the use of Doppler color flow imaging in commonly encountered congenital heart lesions. Chapter 18 illustrates the usefulness of Doppler echocardiography in the format of case studies. Reference is made to the specific chapter(s) relating to each case study. The references listed at the end of each chapter provide background reading material and acknowledge the contributions of numerous workers who have aided in the advancement of Doppler echocardiography.

The illustrations and clinical material were selected from the noninvasive laboratory at Saint Francis Hospital and Medical Center and represent a large accumulated experience over the years. We serve as a referral center for echocardiograhic and Doppler studies and have been able to correlate our findings with that of invasive studies. Thus, I have tried to use material where cardiac catheterization data were available. We were fortunate to have the opportunity to use many Doppler ultrasound systems, including Hewlett-Packard, Aloka, Toshiba, and Acuson in obtaining the illustrations used in this text. This will provide the reader with a greater variety of the systems in use today.

The publication of this textbook will mark my third book in the field of echocardiography and cardiac Doppler. This work has required considerable time and effort above and beyond my clinical, administrative, teaching, and research responsibilities. Yet, it has been an enjoyable and rewarding experience. I hope the reader will find it as enjoyable and rewarding as it has been for me.

JOSÉ MISSRI, M.D.

ACKNOWLEDGMENTS

This work would not have been possible without the support and encouragement from my colleagues in the Section of Cardiology at Saint Francis Hospital and Medical Center. I am especially indebted to Dr. Robert M. Jeresaty, Director of the Section of Cardiology at Saint Francis Hospital and Medical Center, for his encouragement and support. Our medical residents and cardiology fellows provided the academic atmosphere for the development of this book. They served as collaborators and constant sources of stimulation.

Many technicians worked diligently in our noninvasive laboratory, where all the Doppler echocardiographic studies in this book were obtained, but I must give special recognition to Daniel Goodfield.

I am also thankful to Mr. Francis J. Sullo, R.B.P., from our Photography Department, who supervised the reproduction of the Doppler studies. A special note of thanks also goes to the Biomedical Communications at the University of Connecticut Health Center for the highly professional artwork. I extend my appreciation to the staff of The Wilson C. Jainsen Library at Saint Francis Hospital and Medical Center for their help with the bibliographic search. I acknowledge the administrative and leadership support given by Dr. J. David Schnatz, Director of the Department of Medicine at Saint Francis Hospital and Medical Center.

Preparation and typing of this manuscript were undertaken concurrently with all of the other demands made upon my secretary. I am extremely greatful to Mrs. Donna Crowal for doing such a superb job.

I am extremely grateful for the editorial assistance from Ms. Avé McCracken and Ms. Mariapaz Englis of McGraw-Hill. Their support and guidance are deeply appreciated.

Finally, I want to express my gratitude to my family for their patience and support during the many hours of solitude while the book took precedence over all other activities. In large measure they are my most important collaborators.

LIST OF ABBREVIATIONS

Ar	Aortic regurgitation
ASD	Atrial septal defect
AVA	Aortic valve area
CFI	Color flow imaging
CO	Cardiac output
CSA	Cross-section area
CW	Continuous-wave Doppler
2D echo	Two-dimensional echocardiography
FVI	Flow velocity integral
LA	Left atrium
LV	Left ventricle
MR	Mitral regurgitation
PD	Pulsed-wave Doppler
PDA	Patent ductus arteriosus
PFV	Peak flow velocity
PR	Pulmonic regurgitation
PRF	Pulse repetition frequency
RA	Right atrium
RV	Right ventricle
SV	Stroke volume
TEE	Transesophageal echocardiography
TR	Tricuspid regurgitation
VSD	Ventricular septal defect

CLINICAL DOPPLER ECHOCARDIOGRAPHY

Spectral and Color Flow Imaging

CHAPTER 1

Introduction to Doppler Echocardiography

Patients with known or suspected heart disease are often referred for echocardiographic evaluation. M-Mode and two-dimensional (2D) echocardiographic techniques are frequently employed to assess cardiac structure and performance. Both of these noninvasive tests have been extremely useful in patients with valvular heart disease, ischemic heart disease, cardiomyopathies, and congenital disorders.

A major advance in diagnostic applications of ultrasound in heart disease is the development and refinement of Doppler echocardiography. Doppler echocardiography provides direct hemodynamic data that often complement anatomic information derived from conventional echocardiography; and the Doppler examination occasionally provides important diagnostic data that are otherwise unavailable.

During the last 10 years, Doppler echocardiography has been the subject of extensive clinical investigation. Many high-quality, innovative Doppler instruments have been developed as our engineering expertise has progressed and the clinical need for the instruments has been demonstrated.

A direct result of this advanced instrumentation and the clinical research is that the echocardiographic laboratory has moved from the position of a place where disease is identified and qualitative measurements are made into one in which disease can be identified and quantified accurately in many patients. With the ability to quantify disease in the echocardiographic laboratory goes the added responsibility of being certain that the clinical data generated are accurate. Imaging and Doppler data can now be used to make decisions regarding the need for medical or surgical therapy, or the need to perform or avoid cardiac catheterization. Because quantitative information does modify the course of clinical care, examinations must be performed and interpreted by highly skilled and carefully trained individuals. The Doppler data should be checked periodically against other diagnostic standards, such as catheterization, to assure their accuracy. This is especially important if different conclusions arise from clinical versus echocardiographic examinations.

THE DOPPLER PRINCIPLE

Christian Johann Doppler first described the effects of motion on wave patterns for sound and light waves in 1842.[1] If the observer and source (target) are moving toward each other, the frequency of the waves will appear higher. For sound waves, this motion toward the observer produces a shift to a higher pitch or tone, while for light waves this motion toward the observer produces a shift in color to the blue or ultraviolet end of the spectrum. Likewise, when the observer and target are moving away from each other, the measured frequency will appear lower and lead to a lower-pitched sound wave and a shift in the light wave toward the red or infrared end of the color spectrum.

Red blood cells act as ultrasound targets that reflect and shift the frequency of ultrasound in direct proportion to their velocities. The Doppler principle can thus be used to estimate cardiac blood flow velocity (discussed in Chap. 2). Figure 1–1 illustrates this principle. As the red blood cell moves toward the transducer, the reflected ultrasound has less distance to travel. Consequently, the wavelength of the reflected ultrasound diminishes and the frequency increases. Conversely, as the red blood cell moves away from the transducer, the reflected ultrasound has a longer distance to travel, which increases the wavelength and results in a decrease in frequency. Doppler frequency shifts from individual blood cells can be analyzed for velocity, direction, and other characteristics (such as laminar or turbulent blood flow).

DOPPLER ULTRASOUND TECHNIQUES

These Doppler shift principles apply to all wave phenomena and have been used widely throughout science and technology. In the area of cardiovascular ultrasound, the first technology to be developed was continuous-wave Doppler.[2] With this technique, a transmitting transducer continually emits sound waves while a receiving transducer continuously receives the returning sound waves. Since this technology provides very rapid sampling, it can detect very high frequency shifts along the direction of the transducer beam.

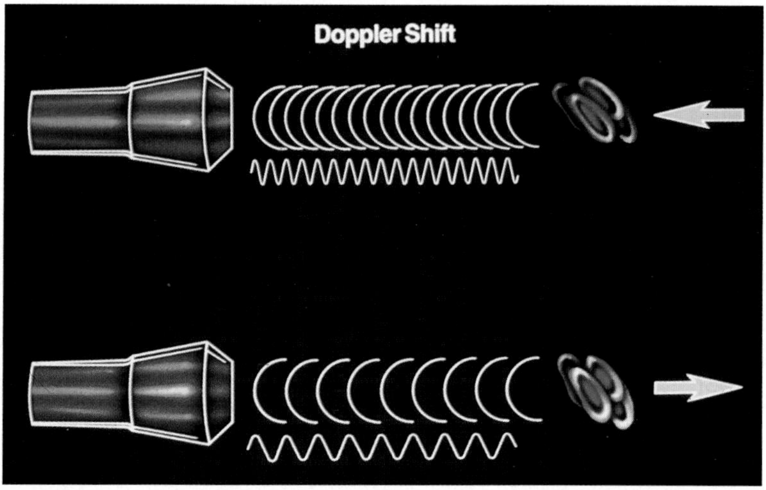

Figure 1–1. The Doppler Principle. For any given transmitted ultrasound frequency, the returned frequency will be higher after encountering red blood cells moving toward the transducer and lower after encountering red cells moving away from the transducer.

Later, a pulsed Doppler (PD) technique was developed that allowed localization of Doppler shifts at different depths within the beam line.[3–6] This technology consisted of a single crystal transducer that both emitted pulses of sound and then received the returning sound waves. The time delay of the returning waves corresponded to the depth of the ultrasound targets. By sampling the returning ultrasound waves at various time delays (range gating), the Doppler shift and corresponding target velocity could be obtained for various depths within the beam. The entire cardiac area could be serially sampled by moving the single sample point throughout the heart.

These standard 2D echocardiographic images were then combined with the single sample point Doppler system (sometimes enhanced with an offline computer) to confirm the sample location site and produce maps of the disturbed flow areas.[7] This point-by-point mapping technique appeared to be useful in a variety of clinical applications, including intracardiac shunts and regurgitation.[8–13]

A technology to sample multiple points simultaneously was also developed. Sampling along an entire beam line yielded more complete velocity information and this information was initially displayed together with the M-mode echo amplitude information on a combined M-mode Doppler image.[14] This technique proved useful in evaluating the timing and depth of flow disturbances in patients with congenital and valvular disease.[15]

The clinical need for additional spatial velocity information led to the development of a system that displayed an entire 2D echo plane of velocity sample points. By sampling from multiple points along the beam line, as well as from multiple beam lines, images could be produced that showed the blood flow from an entire sector plane (color Doppler flow imaging). This technique was first reported using a phased array system approach,[16] and then with a mechanical transducer system approach.[17] Because of inherent limitations in a mechanical flow imaging system, this approach has been abandoned and subsequent developments and clinical reports have been with the phased array flow imaging approach.[18–25]

COLOR DOPPLER FLOW IMAGING

Two-dimensional color Doppler flow imaging (CFI) represents the most recent step in the evolution of Doppler techniques to study cardiovascular phenomena.[20] This new technique enables the simultaneous assessment of the direction and relative velocity of flow at multiple points along multiple beam paths.[26] Accordingly, a visual representation of dynamic flow patterns is achieved within the heart and great vessels that provides topographic and anatomic data comparable to angiography, and familiar not only to the cardiologists but also to colleagues in internal medicine, radiology, surgery, and other disciplines. Doppler flow imaging adds an important degree of certainty to the assessment of cardiovascular disease by ultrasound, provides spatial information about flow disturbances, and in many cases facilitates the examination.

CLINICAL APPLICATIONS OF DOPPLER ECHOCARDIOGRAPHY

Referral of a patient for Doppler evaluation should be considered for a variety of clinical indications. These applications are summarized in Table 1–1. Valvular heart disease and congenital disorders will probably account for the majority of requests for Doppler studies, but Doppler findings may also be helpful with other forms of heart disease.

The recent Doppler echocardiography systems usually have five modes: M-mode, 2D echocardiography, pulsed-wave Doppler, continuous-wave Doppler, and color flow imaging. Table 1–2 summarizes the available modes and clinical applications.

TABLE 1 – 1. Current Applications of Doppler Echocardiography

A. Valvular heart disease
   1. Regurgitation (detect, estimate severity)
   2. Stenosis (detect, localize, estimate severity)
   3. Multiple valve involvement
   4. Prosthetic dysfunction

B. Congenital heart disease
   1. Intracardiac shunts (VSD, ASD)
   2. Extracardiac shunts (PDA)
   3. Great vessel anomalies

C. Quantitation of volume flow

D. Assessment of ventricular performance

NOTE: ASD = atrial septal defect; PDA = patent ductus arteriosus; VSD = ventricular septal defect

TABLE 1 – 2. Doppler Echocardiography Systems: Available Modes and Clinical Applications

Modes	Example of Applications
M-mode echo	Measurement of dimensions
2D echo	Segmental wall motion analysis and valve morphology
Pulsed-wave Doppler	Spectral analysis of aortic, mitral, pulmonic, and tricuspid flows
Continuous-wave Doppler	Measurement of velocity and estimation of pressure gradients across stenotic valves
Color flow imaging	Real-time imaging of regurgitant, stenotic, and shunt flows

REFERENCES

1. Doppler C: Uber das Fabirge der Doppelsterne. Abhandlungen der konglich Bomchen Gessellschaft ab Wisenschaften. 4 to Prog. II:465, 1842.
2. Light LH, Cross G: Cardiovascular data by transcutaneous aorta velography, in Woodcock J(s) (ed): *Blood Flow Measurements*. London, Sector Publishing, 1972.

3. Peronneau P, Deloche A, Bui-Mong-Hung, et al: Debitmetrie ultrasonore: Développements et applications experimentales. *Eur Surg Res* 1:147, 1969.
4. Baker DW: Pulsed ultrasonic Doppler blood-flow sensing. IEEE *Trans* S US SU-17:170, 1970.
5. Peronneau PA, Bugnon A, Bournat JP, et al: Instantaneous bidimensional blood velocity profiles in the major vessels by a pulsed ultrasonic Doppler velocimeter, in de Vlieger M et al (eds): *Ultrasonic in Medicine*. Amsterdam: Excerpta Medica/American Elsevier, 1974 p 259.
6. Baker DW, Rubenstein SA, Lorch GS: Pulsed Doppler echocardiography: Principles and applications. *Am J Med* 63:69, 1977.
7. Bommer W, Mapes R, Miller L, et al: Quantitation of aortic regurgitation with two-dimensional Doppler echocardiography. *Am J Cardiol* 47:412, 1981.
8. Young JB, Quinones MA, Waggoner AD, et al: Diagnosis and quantitation of aortic stenosis with pulsed Doppler echocardiography. *Am J Cardiol* 45:987, 1980.
9. Ciobanu M, Abbasi AS, Allen M, et al: Pulsed Doppler echocardiography in the diagnosis and estimation of severity of aortic insufficiency. *Am J Cardiol* 49:339, 1982.
10. Miyatake K, Kinoshita N, Nagata S, et al: Intracardiac flow pattern in mitral regurgitation studied with a combined use of the ultrasonic pulsed Doppler technique and cross-sectional echocardiography. *J Cardiogr* 9:241, 1979.
11. Asao M, Matsuo H, Kitabatake A, et al: Application of computer-based ultrasonic multigated pulsed Doppler flow mapping in clinical case. *Jpn Soc Ultrason Med, Proc 38th Meeting* 38:13, 1981.
12. Kitabatake K, Inoue M, Asao M, et al: Non-invasive visualization of intracardiac blood flow in human heart using computer-aided pulsed Doppler technique. *Clin Hemorheol* 1:85, 1982.
13. Morita H, Senda S, Matsuo H, et al: Intracardiac flow visualization of regurgitation by a computer-based ultrasound multigated pulsed Doppler flowmeter. *Am J Cardiol* 49:943, 1982.
14. Brandestini MA, Howard EA, Weile EB, et al: The synthesis of echo and Doppler in M-mode and sectorscan. *Proc Annu Meeting* AIUM 125:paper no. 704, 1979.
15. Stevenson G, Kawabori I, Brandestini M: Color-coded Doppler visualization of flow within ventricular septal defects: Implications for peak pulmonary artery pressure. *Am J Cardiol* 49:944, 1982.
16. Bommer W, Miller L: Real-time two-dimensional color-flow Doppler: Enhanced Doppler flow imaging in the diagnosis of cardiovascular disease. *Am J Cardiol* 49:944, 1982.
17. Namekawa K, Kasai C, Tsukamoto M, et al: Imaging of blood flow using autocorrelation. *Ultrasound Med Biol* 8:138, 1982.
18. Omoto R, Yokote Y, Takamoto S, et al: Clinical significance of newly developed real-time intracardiac two-dimensional blood flow imaging system (2-D Doppler). *Jpn Circ J* 47:974, 1983.

19. Omoto R, Yokote Y, Takamoto S, et al: Study on clinical application of real-time intracardiac two-dimensional blood flow imaging system. *Jpn Soc Ultrason Med, Proc 43rd Meeting* 43:655, 1983.

20. Omoto R: *Color Atlas of Real-Time Two-Dimensional Doppler Echocardiography*. Tokyo, Sindan-To-Chiryo Co, 1984.

21. Bommer WJ, Rebeck KF, La Viola S, et al: Real-time two-dimensional flow imaging: Detection and semiquantification of valvular and congenital heart disease. *Circulation* 70:38, 1984.

22. Bommer WJ, White CS, Rozema R, et al: A vortex of the heart: A two-dimensional flow imaging study of diastolic flow eddies in the normal left ventricle. *J Am Coll Cardiol* 5:425, 1985.

23. Bommer WJ, Tam K, Ehret R, et al: 2-D Real-time flow imaging of prosthetic heart valves. *J Am Coll Cardiol* 5:526, 1985.

24. Miyatake K, Izumi S, Okamoto M, et el: Semiquantitative grading of severity of mitral regurgitation by real-time two-dimensional Doppler flow imaging technique. *J Am Coll Cardiol* 7:82, 1986.

25. DeMaria AN, Smith MD, Branco M, et al: Normal and abnormal blood flow patterns by color Doppler flow imaging. *Echocardiography* 3:475, 1986.

26. Bommer WJ: Basic principles of flow imaging. *Echocardiography* 2:501, 1985.

CHAPTER 2

Physical Principles and Instrumentation in Spectral and Color Doppler Flow Imaging

PHYSICAL PRINCIPLES AND THE DOPPLER EFFECT

When ultrasound is propagated in human tissue, it is reflected from each acoustic interface. A stationary interface will result in a reflected ultrasound wave that has the same frequency as the transmitted wave. When the interface is moving (for example, red blood cells), the reflected wave has a frequency that is slightly different from that of the transmitted wave, in accordance with the Doppler effect. Thus, if the flow of blood is toward the transducer, the frequency of the reflected wave will be higher than the transmitted frequency. Conversely, flow of blood away from the transducer will result in a lower frequency of the reflected wave.

The difference between the reflected frequency and the transmitted frequency is the Doppler shift ($\pm\Delta f$), which is expressed in Hertz (Hz). By using the Doppler equation [Eq. (1)], the forward or backward velocity of the blood (moving red blood cells) can be determined.

$$\pm\Delta f = \frac{2f_0 \times \nu \times \cos\Theta}{c} \qquad (1)$$

In this equation, f_0 = the frequency of transmitted sounds (Hz), ν = velocity (cm/s), Θ = the angle between the sound-beam axis and the velocity vector, and c = the velocity of sound in tissue (1560 m/s). Thus, the intracardiac velocity of blood flow can be derived from this equation as follows (Fig. 2–1).

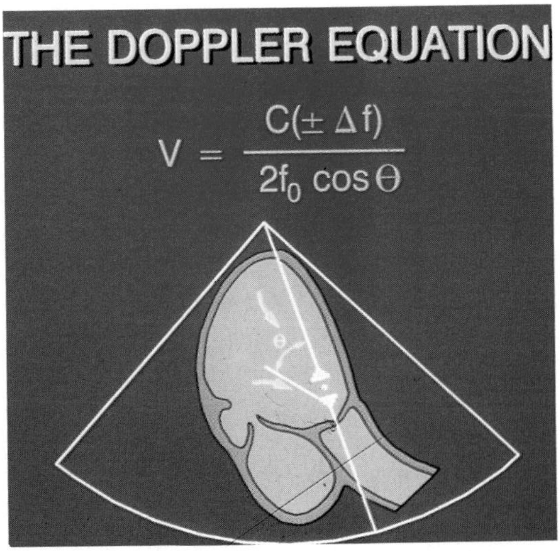

Figure 2–1. The Doppler equation used to calculate blood velocity (V) requires determination of the variables, Doppler frequency shift ($\pm\Delta f$) and the cosine of the Doppler angle ($\cos\Theta$) (the angle between the ultrasound beam and the velocity vector). The constants, the speed of ultrasound in tissue (c) and two times the frequency of transmitted sounds ($2f_0$), are also necessary.

$$V = \frac{c(\pm\Delta f)}{2f_0 \cos\Theta} \qquad (2)$$

From Eq. (2), it is evident that in clinical evaluation the ultrasound beam must be almost parallel to the direction of blood flow (maximal velocity vector) in order to obtain an accurate determination of the velocity of blood flow. The cosine function, however, allows variation between the Doppler beam and the velocity axis to result in minor changes in the calculated velocity. In practice, an angle of up to 20° off the velocity axis will result in only a small (6 percent) underestimation in the true velocity. Intercept angles beyond 20°, however, cause considerable reduction in displayed amplitude.

THE DOPPLER ECHOCARDIOGRAPH SYSTEM DISPLAY

All Doppler echocardiograph systems have an audio output and a graphic display. The changing velocities (frequencies) are converted into audible sounds and, after some processing, are emitted from speakers within the machine. High-pitched sounds result from large Doppler shifts. Flow direction information (relative to the transducer) is provided by a stereophonic audio output in which flow toward the transducer comes out of one speaker and flow away from the transducer comes out of the other.

The audio output also allows the operator to differentiate easily laminar from turbulent flow. Laminar flow produces a smooth audible signal because of the uniform velocities. Turbulent flow, because of the presence of many different velocities, commonly results in a high-pitched and whistling or harsh sound. Experience in interpreting the Doppler audio signals may take weeks to months, and analysis of the audio signal is inherently subjective.

All newer generations of Doppler echocardiography equipment contain sophisticated sound frequency or velocity spectrum analyzers for hard-copy recording. Most commercially available Doppler systems display a spectrum of the various velocities present at any time and are called, therefore, "spectral velocity recordings."

Flow velocity toward the transducer is displayed as a positive, or upward shift in velocities while flow velocity away from the transducer is displayed as a negative, or downward shift in velocities (Fig. 2–2).

The display of the spectrum of the various velocities encountered by the Doppler beam is accomplished by sophisticated microcomputers that are able to decode the returning complex Doppler signal and process it into its various velocity components. The most commonly employed linear method for performing frequency analysis is *fast Fourier transform*.[1] This digital method permits simultaneous analysis of various frequency components within the sample volume by converting received data from the time and amplitude domain to the frequency domain. Another method,

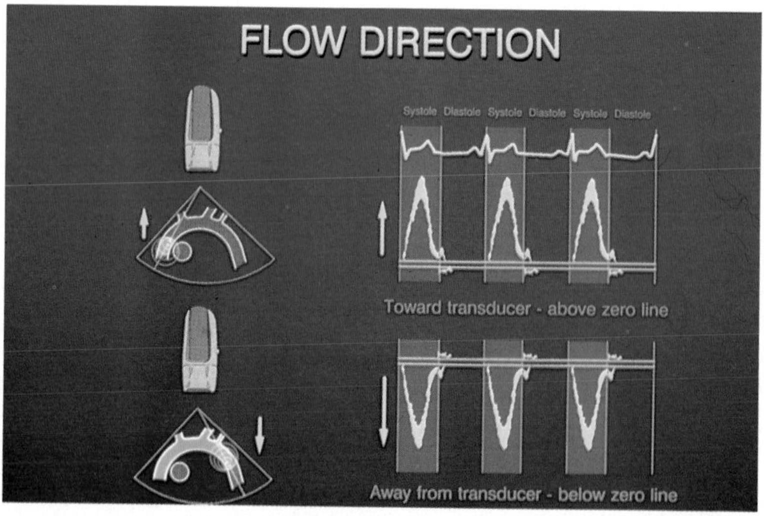

Figure 2–2. Schematic representation of the velocity output of flow. Flow toward the transducer is displayed above the baseline and flow away from the transducer is displayed below the baseline.

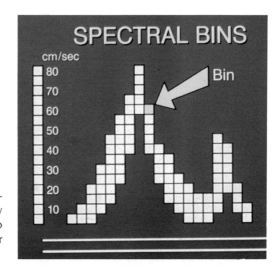

Figure 2–3. The spectral analysis is created by placing the velocity data into bins that are displayed over time.

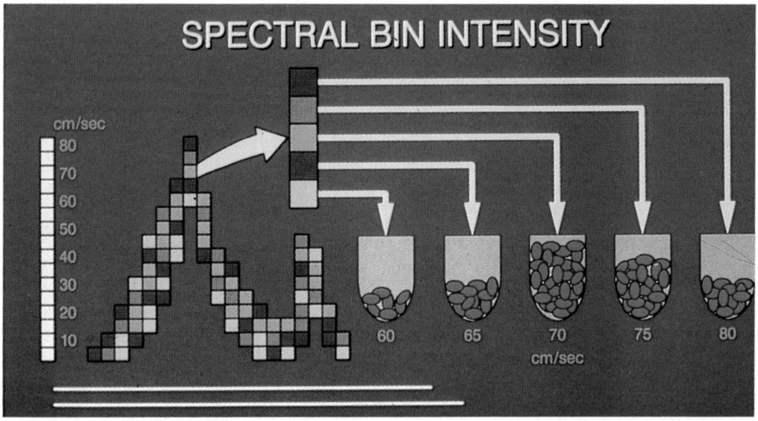

Figure 2–4. The brightness of the signal at any given bin relates to the relative number of red cells detected at that velocity. The term "amplitude" is applied to relative brightness.

Chirp Z analysis, provides approximately similar information with analog techniques.

The spectral recording is made up of a series of "bins" that are recorded over time (Fig. 2–3). At any given point in time, there is a differential speed of movement of red cells, with more red blood cells moving at the velocity of the most intense bin than are moving at the other velocities, which are represented by the less intense bins (Fig. 2–4). The intensity of any bin refers to the "amplitude" or brightness. Thus, the output of Doppler frequency spectrum analysis displays variations in velocity, time, and signal intensity.

BLOOD FLOW PATTERNS

Two basic types of blood flow through the heart and great vessels are distinguished: laminar and nonlaminar.

Laminar Flow

Laminar flow is flow that occurs along smooth parallel lines in a vessel, so that all the red cells in an area are moving at approximately the same speed and in the same direction (Fig. 2–5, *top*). Due to friction, flow is always slightly slower near the walls of a vessel. When blood accelerates, all cells tend to move at the same speed. When blood decelerates, the more densely packed cells at the edges slow down faster than those at the center of the vessel. Flow in most of the cardiovascular system, including the heart and great vessels, is normally laminar and rarely exceeds the maximum velocity of 1.5 m/s.

Nonlaminar Flow

Nonlaminar flow, also referred to as "disturbed flow" or "turbulent flow," is defined as flow which consists of cellular elements moving at different

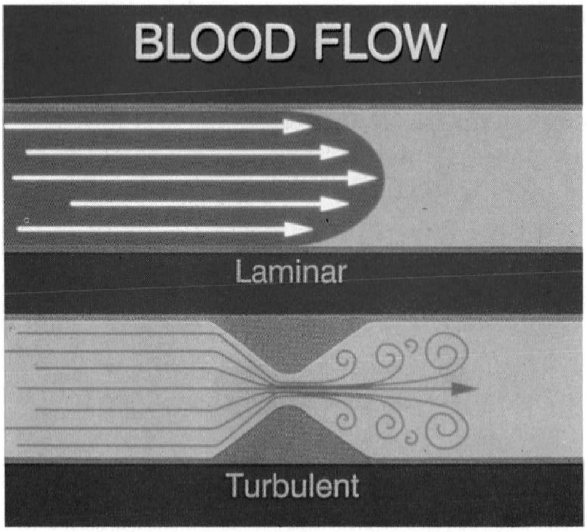

Figure 2–5. Diagrammatic representation of normal laminar flow (*top*) in comparison to nonlaminar or turbulent flow (*bottom*), which results in whirls and eddies of many different velocities.

velocities and/or in different directions (Fig. 2–5, *bottom*). Nonlaminar flow is usually an abnormal finding and is considered indicative of some underlying cardiovascular pathology.

DOPPLER ECHOCARDIOGRAPH MODES

Study of reflections from red blood cells may be accomplished with several types of ultrasonic transmission and processing techniques, including continuous, pulsed wave and high pulse repetition frequency (PRF) Doppler systems. Further, one variant of pulsed Doppler permits color coded velocities to be superimposed on a two-dimensional (2D) image. The following sections will be concerned with the several types of Doppler systems.

Continuous Wave Doppler System

Continuous wave (CW) Doppler uses two crystals, one which continuously sends and one which continuously receives ultrasound (Fig. 2–6, *left*). As a result of frequency, crystal size, and inherent characteristics, CW beams are usually wider than those of pulsed Doppler. Since transmission is continuous, reception is also continuous. Accordingly, information from the full length of the beam is continuously present, a situation that eliminates any possibility of determining the depth from which any given waveform originates. The inability to determine the depth of origin of a waveform is referred to as "range ambiguity." A major advantage of CW over pulsed Doppler is that CW can measure very high velocities (in excess of 7 m/s) because the PRF is very high (continuous).

Two types of CW transducers are available: (1) a small transducer without imaging capabilities (dedicated Doppler transducer),[2–4] and (2) a duplex transducer with capabilities for both 2D and Doppler echocardiography. The smaller nonimaging transducer has been most valuable for assessing valvular lesions. Because of its small size, this transducer can be placed in multiple ultrasonic acoustic "windows," a technique that often cannot be used with a standard larger imaging transducer. Although the use of the dedicated transducer necessitates a blind approach, with experience it becomes easy to use. By adjusting the transducer position and direction, the Doppler ultrasound beam can be placed almost parallel to the maximal velocity vector in most patients solely by using the quality of the audio and spectral signals for guidance. The optimal signal is one with the highest velocity and the clearest spectral envelope.

Pulsed Doppler System

Pulsed Doppler (PD) system uses a single piezoelectric crystal that alternates transmission and reception of reflected ultrasound (Fig. 2–6, *right*). The transducer emits a brief burst of ultrasound, directs it at the heart or great vessels, and then functions in "receive" mode. The ultrasonic burst may encounter one or more regions of moving red cells, which will scatter some of the ultrasonic energy back to the same transducer. The cycle then repeats. Only those backscattered ultrasonic signals that return to the transducer during a brief time window are analyzed for Doppler shifts. If the red cells are moving toward the transducer, the returned frequency will be increased. If the cells are moving away from the transducer, the returned frequency will be decreased. Accordingly, analysis of the Doppler reflected frequency indicates whether the cells are moving toward the transducer or away from it. Although it is possible to provide directional information simultaneously for all tissue depths along the transmitted beam, PD also offers the opportunity to interrogate only a small area at a time.

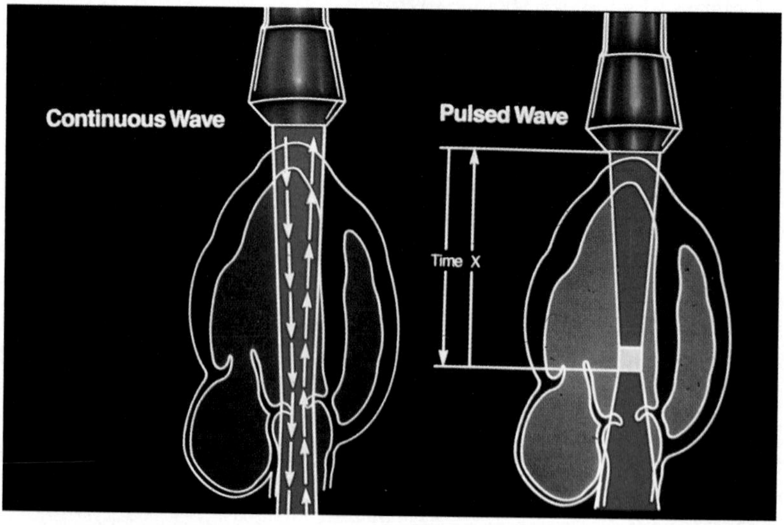

Figure 2–6. Doppler system modes. In continuous-wave Doppler (*left*), the transducer is constantly emitting and receiving ultrasound data. In pulsed-wave Doppler (*right*), the transducer alternately transmits and receives the ultrasound data to a sample volume. This is also know as range-gated Doppler.

Range Gating

Interrogation of one small area along the beam is known as "range gating." Range gating is possible because the speed of ultrasound through tissue is constant at 1560 m/s. Accordingly, it is possible to measure the time required for information from a chosen depth to return to the crystal. Since the velocity and time are known, it becomes simple to solve for the depth of reflection. Analysis of the reflected signal for change in frequency exclusively at a given depth is accomplished by analyzing only for that time interval and totally disregarding reflections from all other depths. The range gate is variable in length usually from 1 to 20 mm. The area encompassed within the range gating is called the "sample volume." The advantages of a variable sample volume length are that its length can be tailored to the anatomy under consideration and longer sample volumes usually improve the signal-to-noise ratio over smaller ones. Sample volume width is always equal to beam width at the sample volume site. Since beam width expands in the far field, sample volume width also expands in this area. Beam width is a function of transducer frequency, aperture size, and sample volume depth.[2]

All PD instruments allow the operator to set the sample volume at various depths along a cursor line within the heart. This is usually accomplished by demonstrating simultaneously the sample volume location and a 2D image of the heart (Fig. 2–7). Thus, the operator can set the sample volume within a cardiac chamber or a great vessel of interest, and then lengthen or shorten the sample volume so that its length fits into the area

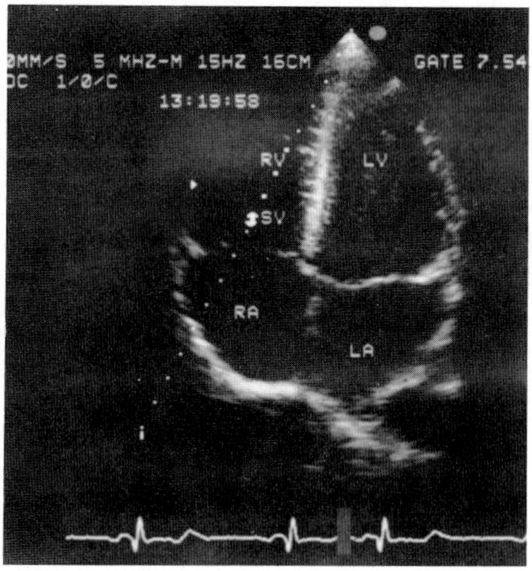

Figure 2–7. Pulsed wave Doppler examination combined with simultaneous 2D echo. The direction of the ultrasound beam and the position of the sample volume (SV) along that beam are superimposed on an apical four chamber view of the heart. RV = right ventricle, LV = left ventricle, RA = right atrium, LA = left atrium.

of interest throughout the entire cardiac cycle. Further, most mechanical and phased array instruments allow the cursor line to be moved right or left within the image.

PD has limited high velocity measurement capability because it permits only a single pulse to be within the examining range at any one time. This pulse may be either traveling toward or reflecting from the target. Since ultrasound travels through tissue at a fixed speed, two factors will determine whether more than one pulse will be in the body at one time: (1) the PRF (i.e., determination of the time interval between pulses) and (2) the distance that the pulse must travel to the farthest target. The user deals with this situation by moving the sample volume to an area of interest. Instruments are programmed to determine depth of the sample volume and for this depth to transmit the maximum possible PRF. The higher the PRF, the greater the velocity that can be recorded. Accordingly, all velocities within the sample volume will be assessed, however, only a certain range of velocities can be determined accurately without ambiguity.

Aliasing

The maximum Doppler frequency shift detectable by a PD system at any given depth of the sample volume depends upon the PRF of the system at that depth. Maximum detectable Doppler shift, or the *Nyquist limit,* as it is sometimes called, is expressed as

$$\Delta f_{max} = \frac{PRF}{2}$$

where Δf_{max} is maximum Doppler shift.

This formula means that the system PRF, which varies with depth setting, must be twice the frequency of the returning Doppler signal. If the Doppler frequency shift exceeds one half the system PRF, or Nyquist limit, then a condition known as aliasing occurs in which the peak Doppler frequencies are displayed on the opposite channel (Fig. 2–8).

It is important to realize that the maximum recordable velocities in any jet relate to the frequency of the transducer used. A lower frequency transducer increases the ability of a PD system to record high velocities at any given range. Thus, aliasing will be encountered at lower velocities with a 5 MHz transducer than with a 2.5 MHz transducer.

Several other approaches to the problem of aliasing are possible. Blood flow could be examined at a steep intercept angle, thereby decreasing the frequency of the Doppler shift corresponding to a given flow

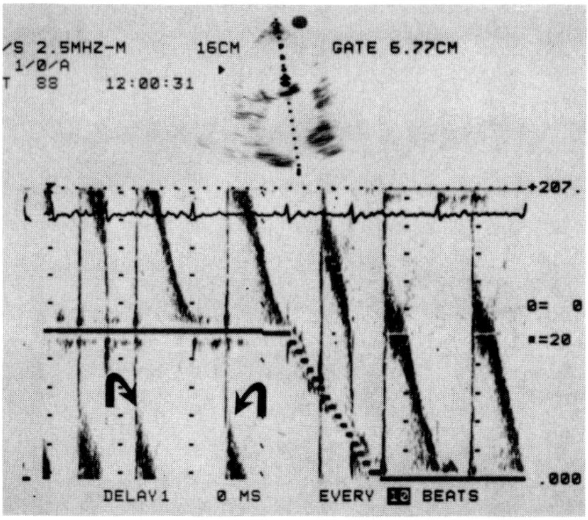

Figure 2-8. Aliasing. The Doppler frequency shift exceeds the maximum frequency limit at that depth setting. Note blunted waveform at the top of the display and the simultaneous appearance of aliased signals at the bottom of the display (arrows). The zero baseline is then moved to the bottom of the display and the maximum frequency limit is doubled. Spectral display of the mitral valve from an apical view from a patient with mitral stenosis. (Scale marks = 20 cm/s.)

velocity. However, this approach would make accurate knowledge of the intercept angle crucial if one wished to use the measured Doppler shift to calculate the actual flow velocity. Another approach would involve placing the Doppler sample volume at the shallowest possible depth in relation to the transducer in order to increase the PRF optimally. Also, many instruments have the capability of shifting the zero line to the bottom or top of the display and the maximum frequency limit is doubled (Fig. 2–9).

High Pulse Repetition Frequency

An intermediate modality, high pulse repetition frequency (high PRF) Doppler, which is a cross between CW and PD, has been developed. The major difference between high PRF Doppler and standard PD is that the listening period for high PRF is too short to allow reflections to return to the crystal from deep structures. In conventional PD, only one pulse is considered to be in the body at any time. In CW Doppler, a continuous waveform is transmitted. In high PRF Doppler, several pulses are in the body simultaneously. Instead of using one sample volume, as is customary in standard PD, two or more pulses are within the heart simultaneously at

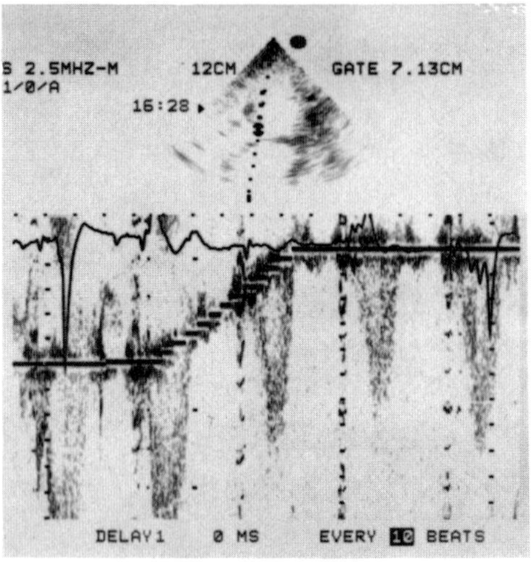

Figure 2–9. Zero-shift display in which the center zero baseline is moved to the top of the display and the maximum frequency limit is doubled. Normal spectral display of the left ventricular outflow tract from an apical view. (Scale marks = 20 cm/s.)

different depths. The logic for this approach is that high velocity resolution is a function of the PRF. Thus, increasing PRF allows resolution of higher velocities, but the depth from which the velocity is reflected is unknown (range ambiguity) because more than one pulse is in the body simultaneously. Velocity measured by high PRF is accurate.

A fundamental reason that high PRF Doppler evolved is that it requires only a single crystal and conventional PD circuitry. The interrogation line can be visualized on the 2D image, and this is a distinct advantage over nonimaging CW but less desirable than imaging combined with CW. High PRF Doppler, however, uses a narrow beam that makes jet detection more difficult than with CW Doppler. Further, the system may not be as sensitive as conventional PD. After initial enthusiasm, high PRF Doppler seems to have diminishing clinical usage.

MAJOR DIFFERENCES BETWEEN CONVENTIONAL DOPPLER MODES

Although all three modes provide generally similar information, at least two important differences exist. Standard single sample volume PD is the only mode that permits velocity to be sampled exclusively from the area of interest, the sample volume. However, the very same principle that permits exclusive interrogation of the sample volume also limits the maximal velocity that can be recorded within the sample volume. CW and high PRF Doppler permit much higher velocities to be sampled, but the point

TABLE 2-1. Comparison of Pulsed and Continuous Wave Techniques

	Pulsed Wave	Continuous Wave
Advantages	Range resolution	Measures high velocity
Disadvantages	Measurement of high velocity is limited	No range resolution

along the line of interrogation from which the velocity is recorded is unknown.

Both CW and PD complement each other during a Doppler echocardiographic examination. PD localizes a specific area of abnormal flow. When accurate measurement of elevated flow velocity is required, CW Doppler should be used. The various differences between CW and PD are summarized in Table 2–1.

COLOR DOPPLER FLOW IMAGING

The basic principles of color flow imaging (CFI) originate with the Doppler effect, that is, sound waves emanating from a source traveling toward a receiver are shifted to a higher frequency, and sound waves from a source traveling away from a receiver are shifted to a lower frequency. In the case of CFI, the reflected ultrasound signal from a standard device is split such that one half forms the conventional black and white 2D echocardiogram and the second half is used to derive the CFI. The black and white image is derived from a plot of the amplitude of ultrasound reflected from a given boundary. The color flow map is derived from the change in frequency of ultrasound reflected from red blood cells.

Color Doppler instruments are all currently based upon PD methods. Conventional PD techniques are range gated. The Doppler sample volume is determined in range by the time it takes for the ultrasound pulse to travel to the area of interest and then back. If the same method was employed in color flow, it would simply take too long to sample over the entire image and there would be serious compromises made in frame rate.

Instead, all color flow systems are multigated. In the illustration in Fig. 2–10, a simple 10-gate system is shown and compared with the conventional PD approach. Here, a burst of ultrasound is sent into the tissue along a given line and then the system rapidly receives frequencies at 10 incremental times. This results in the reception of Doppler data from the closer flow areas first, while the pulse is still continuing into the tissue. Reception of the flow data in the furthest field occurs later.

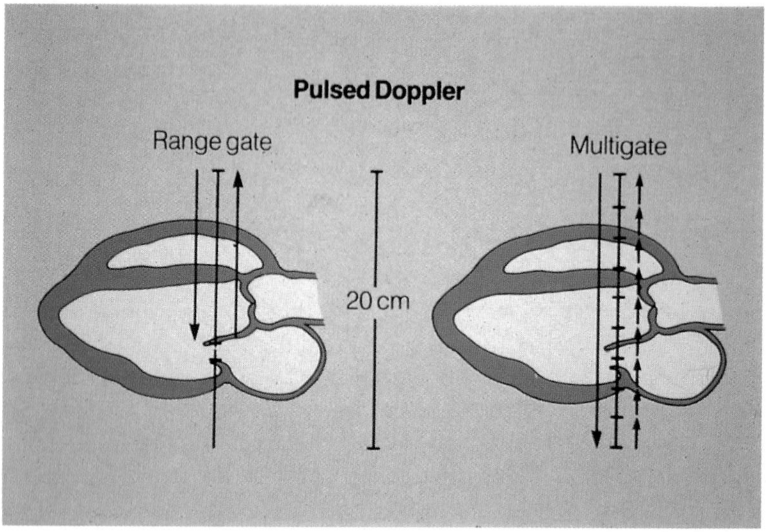

Figure 2–10. Generating color images for Doppler systems uses pulsed-wave Doppler in a multigate, rather than range-rate, format. See text for explanation.

This multigating takes advantage of Doppler information all along the line that is "ignored" in the conventional range gated approach. In reality, each line has many gates that number in the hundreds. Color flow imaging systems collect amplitude and phase shift information at each of the multiple gates and then process the information with color presented in the final display. A typical image can consist of as many as 250 lines depending upon sector size and depth of range (Fig. 2–11).

The first task in creating a color-coded Doppler image is to obtain a cardiac image on which to superimpose color coded velocities. This is done in a manner similar to that used to create any conventional 2D image. The next step, however, requires determining the flow direction and magnitude for each gate within the sector image. Accordingly, many thousands of gates are present and each requires an analysis for each frame. Ordinarily, 15 to 30 frames per second are required to provide the sense of "real-time motion." Clearly, many hundreds of thousands of frequency and directional analyses are needed each second. Determination of flow direction can be performed rapidly by a *quadrature detector* to meet this requirement. However, a fast Fourier transform, the conventional spectral analyzer that is used to determine velocity magnitude, is capable of only hundreds of analyses, at maximum, each second. An *autocorrelation* method for velocity analysis was developed that permitted the number of

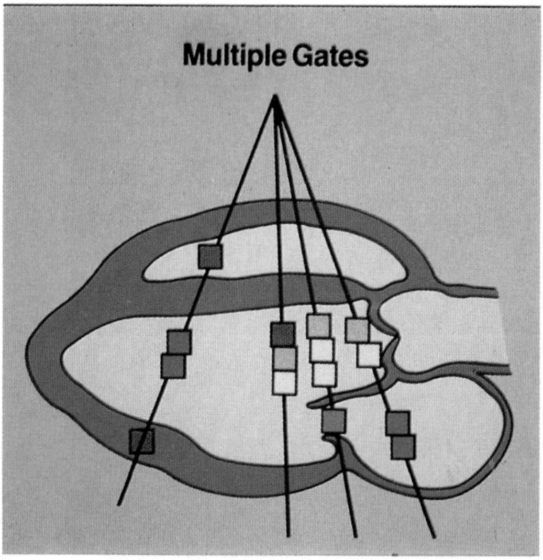

Figure 2–11. Hundreds of gates are present along each line throughout the color flow image. Multiple gates of color flow information are displayed throughout the entire image along each ultrasound line.

analyses required.[5–8] The autocorrelator compares the frequency of the returning signal with that of the original signal and assigns a color value to the difference.

The assignment of color is in accordance with three basic principles: (1) direction of blood flow, (2) mean velocity of blood flow, and (3) variance (nonlaminar flow) of detected frequency shifts.

Color Display

The three colors of red, blue, and green are used in flow mapping and are capable of yielding shades of yellow, white, and cyan. Although contrary to the initial description of motion related frequency shifts presented by Christian Doppler (discussed in Chap. 1), by convention, the color system displays flow *toward* the transducer (direction of flow) in shades of red and flow away from the transducer in shades of blue. In addition, increasing velocity of flow is displayed in the form of shades of color, with brighter hues of red representing higher velocity of flow toward the transducer, and brighter shades of blue representing higher velocities in the opposite direction (Fig. 2–12). Velocities of a magnitude below a certain minimum cutoff are not assigned colors and are represented as black in the image. Accordingly, areas of low flow velocity within the central circulation (such as the cardiac apex) will not be visualized by color flow imaging.

The third color, green, is assigned to nonlaminar blood flow and serves to identify areas of turbulence. Nonlaminar blood flow is identified

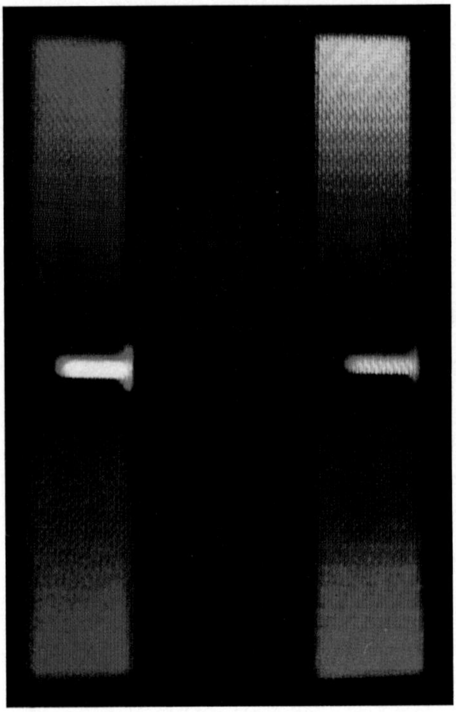

Figure 2–12. Standard color bar (*left*) from a color flow system. When there is no flow, black is displayed (*center*). Flow toward the transducer at the top is red, flow away from the transducer at the bottom is blue. Progressively faster velocities are displayed in brighter shades of red or blue. The bar on the *right* is an enhanced map.

by an algorithm that tests the variation in the frequency shift produced in the returning ultrasound signal of two consecutive transmitted bursts along a given scan line. The greater the deviation, or *variance*, between these two frequency shifts, the higher the turbulence. The color green is then added to red and blue in accordance with the turbulence present in either direction (Fig. 2–13). Forward flow with turbulence would result in yellow. Flow away from the transducer with turbulence results in cyan (blue-green). If multidirectional turbulence could be encountered at the same time, the results of all three colors would be white. The wide range of direction and velocity that results from nomlaminar flow often results in a so-called mosaic pattern consisting of shades of green, red-yellow, blue-cyan, and white, which may have the appearance of confetti.

Advantages of Color Flow Imaging

Efficiency. One of the major advantages of CFI is the speed with which normal and abnormal flow can be identified. The ability to visualize moving cells makes regurgitant lesions or shunts quickly recognizable and

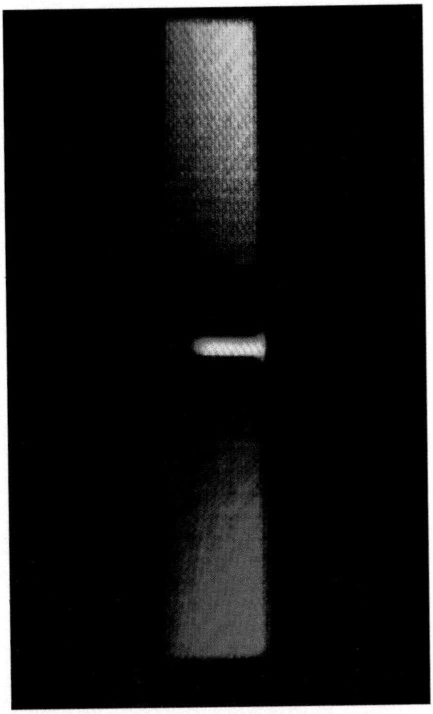

Figure 2–13. Color bar in a variance map. The color green is added to red and blue. Forward flow with turbulence would result in yellow. Backward flow with turbulence results in cyan (blue-green).

facilitates their localization for sampling with conventional PD and CW Doppler systems.

Accuracy. The color display of high velocity jets and regurgitant lesions make it easier to align the Doppler beam with the jet and may improve accuracy as well as efficiency.

Graphic Display. One of the major difficulties of the conventional Doppler system is the need to understand what the tracings mean for appropriate interpretation, making it difficult to convey findings to others who may lack the necessary expertise. Because CFI is similar to other contrast techniques, however, it makes data and spatial orientation easier to comprehend for those without special training.

Problems of Color Flow Imaging

Like all ultrasound systems, particularly conventional Doppler techniques, CFI is limited to available windows and is sensitive to both depth of interrogation and misalignment of beam and flow. Also, the fact that flow mapping is a PD technique imposes some disadvantages such as aliasing.

Aliasing. When the velocity of flow exceeds the Nyquist limit of the system, flow will be depicted as occurring in the opposite direction. This phenomenon, which is presented in spectral techniques as a deflection on the opposite side of the baseline (see Fig. 2–8), appears as a change in color from red to blue or vice versa by flow imaging methods. Thus, flow toward the transducer may appear as blue, while flow away from the transducer may be seen as red. Aliasing occurs at a lower velocity (0.6 m/s) by flow imaging techniques and was originally felt likely to represent a major impediment to this technology. However, flow is typically at its highest velocity in the center of a stream and consists of lower velocities at the periphery. In the absence of turbulence, this velocity distribution results in flow of an appropriate color surrounding a central region of aliased signals of the alternate inappropriate color (Fig. 2–14). In addition, aliased signals often occur only during the period of highest flow, with colors returning to the appropriate designation later in the cardiac cycle.

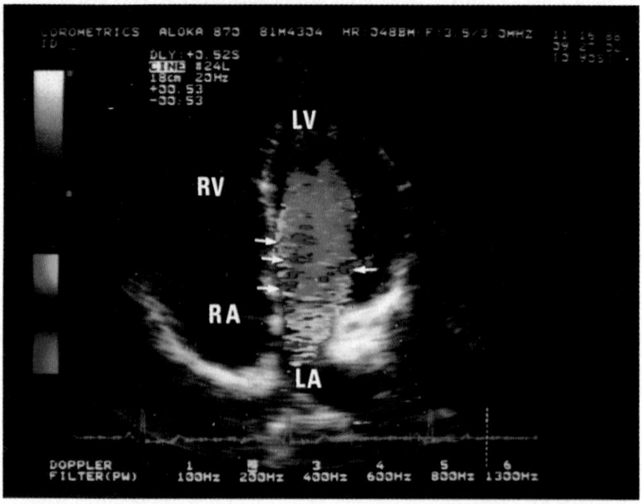

Figure 2–14. Illustration of flow through a normal mitral valve. The flow image demonstrates a classic forward flow jet in which the central portion of the flow is high velocity and therefore aliased (blue) (arrows), whereas the peripheral aspects of the jet are of slower velocity and normally colored for direction (orange-red). RV = right ventricle, RA = right atrium, LV = left ventricle, LA = left atrium.

Wall Motion. Doppler shifts are caused not only by flowing blood but by moving cardiac muscle and valves, which produce stronger returning signals than those from red cells. Various methods are used to reject these unwanted signals, based on echo signal strength, low velocity filters, or a combination of both.

Sensitivity and Gain Dependence. Because of the analysis technique and the volume of information processed, CFI has been less sensitive than conventional Doppler technology to weak signals. The display can be improved by turning up the color gain, but this introduces more noise into the display, which may mask a weak signal. Also, the returning signals may become displayed over a larger area, magnifying the apparent size of a signal source.

Quantitation. All color Doppler machines display increasing flow velocity as gradients of color. However, color difference does not really correlate with difference in speed so that color values themselves can become difficult to differentiate. As a result, quantitation of velocity requires PD and CW Doppler systems.

Frame Rate. The construction of a color flow image takes a great deal of time, dropping the frame rate as low as 10 frames per second. This introduces the disadvantage of temporal ambiguity.

THE BERNOULLI EQUATION

When a constant volume of blood flow passes through a stenotic site in a vessel, blood flow is accelerated. The resultant decrease in pressure across the stenotic area is related to the velocity of the blood flow on the basis of Bernoulli hydrodynamics, as shown in the following equation:

$$P_1 - P_2 = \frac{1}{2}\rho(V_2{}^2 - V_1{}^2) + \rho\int 1^2 \frac{d\vec{v}}{dt} \times d\vec{s} + R(\vec{V})$$

$$\underset{\text{decrease}}{\text{pressure}} = \underset{\text{acceleration}}{\text{convective}} + \underset{\text{acceleration}}{\text{flow}} + \underset{\text{friction}}{\text{viscous}}$$

In this equation, P_1 = pressure before stenosis, P_2 = pressure after stenosis, ρ = mass density of blood, V_1 = velocity of blood before stenosis, V_2 = velocity of blood after stenosis, $d\vec{v}$ = change in velocity during opening of the valve, dt = time for opening of the valve, ds = distance over which the decrease in pressure is measured, R = viscous resistance in a vessel, and $\vec{V}$ = velocity of blood flow. At pressures and flows in clinical practice, the contribution from flow acceleration and viscous friction is negligible.[9] Thus, the equation can be simplified to the following: $P_1 - P_2 = \frac{1}{2}\rho(V_2^2 - V_1^2)$. The square of the velocity of blood upstream to the stenosis (V_1^2) is usually negligible in comparison with the square of the downstream velocity (V_2^2). For blood, $\frac{1}{2}\rho$ is approximately 4; hence, insertion of 4 results in a clinically useful equation that converts velocity in meters per second to pressure decrease (that is, pressure gradient) in millimeters of mercury (mmHg). Thus, in clinical measurements, the following simplified equation can be used to estimate the pressure gradient across a stenotic lesion and across the cardiac chambers.

$$P_1 - P_2 = 4V_2^2 \qquad \text{or} \qquad \Delta P = 4V^2$$

This approach first was suggested as applicable to patients with mitral stenosis by Holen et al[9] and has been subsequently popularized by Hatle and Angelsen[2] in mitral, aortic, and pulmonic stenosis. Numerous other investigators have demonstrated the accuracy and clinical usefulness of the technique.[10–16]

REFERENCES

1. Rabiner LR, Gold B: *Theory and Application of Digital Signal Processing*. Englewood Cliffs, NJ, Prentice-Hall, 1975.
2. Hatle L, Angelsen B: *Doppler Ultrasound in Cardiology*, ed 2. Philadelphia, Lea & Febiger, 1985.
3. Hatle L, Angelsen B, Tromsdal A: Noninvasive assessment of aortic stenosis by Doppler ultrasound. *Br Heart J* 43:284, 1980.
4. Hatle L, Brubakk A, Tromsdal A, et al: Noninvasive assessment of pressure drop in mitral stenosis in Doppler ultrasound. *Br Heart J* 40:131, 1978.
5. Namekawa K, Kasai C, Koyano A: Imaging of blood flow using autocorrelation. *Ultrason Med Biol* 8(suppl 1):138, 1982.
6. Omoto R, Yokote Y, Takamoto S, et al: Clinical significance of newly developed real-time intracardiac two-dimensional blood flow imaging system (2-D Doppler). *Jpn Circ J* 47:974, 1983.
7. Omoto R: *Color Atlas of Real-Time Two-Dimensional Doppler Echocardiography*. Tokyo, Shindan-To-Chiryo Co, 1984.
8. Kasai C, Namekawa K, Koyano A, et al: Real-time two-dimensional blood flow imaging using an autocorrelation technique. IEEE *Trans Sonics Ultrason* SU-32(3):458, 1985.
9. Holen J, Aaslid R, Landmark K, et al: Determination of pressure gradient in mitral stenosis with a non-invasive ultrasound Doppler technique. *Acta Med Scand* 199:455, 1976.
10. Hatle L: Noninvasive assessment and differentiation of left ventricular outflow tract obstruction with Doppler ultrasound. *Circulation* 64:381, 1981.

11. Spencer M, Fujioka K: Doppler spectral analysis in acquired valve disease, in Spencer MR, ed: *Cardiac Doppler Diagnosis*. Boston, Martinus Nijhoff, 1983.

12. Hatle L, Brubakk A, Tromsdal A: Noninvasive assessment of atrioventricular pressure half-time by Doppler ultrasound. *Circulation* 60:1096, 1979.

13. Lima C, Sahn D, Valdes-Cruz L, et al: Noninvasive prediction of transvalvular pressure gradient in patients with pulmonary stenosis by quantitative 2-D echocardiographic Doppler studies. *Circulation* 67:866, 1983.

14. Lima C, Sahn D, Valdes-Cruz L, et al: Prediction of severity of left ventricular outflow tract obstruction by quantitative two-dimensional echo Doppler study. *Circulation* 68:348, 1983.

15. Stamm R, Martin R: Quantification of pressure gradients across stenotic valves by Doppler ultrasound. *J Am Coll Cardiol* 2:707, 1983.

16. Berger M, Berdoff R, Gallerstein P, et al: Evaluation of aortic stenosis by continuous wave Doppler ultrasound. *J Am Coll Cardiol* 3:150, 1984.

CHAPTER 3

Doppler Echocardiograph Examination of the Heart and Great Vessels

Performance of a complete examination requires an echocardiographic system capable of good imaging, PD, and CW Doppler. Since all three modalities are essential, one should not be sacrificed for the other. Color Doppler echocardiography is a newer technology that increases the rapidity of acquisition of certain information by displaying Doppler information as an overlay on the 2D image. However, the color Doppler system has not supplanted standard PD and CW Doppler technologies because of its velocity and recording limitations. Color Doppler echo should, nonetheless, be included in an optimal system.

This chapter will detail a systematic Doppler echocardiographic examination. The normal spectral flow patterns will be described first, followed by the normal blood flow patterns by CFI. An organized approach to a complete examination will expedite the study and maximize the amount of information obtained.

BASIC PRINCIPLES

Optimal Doppler tracings require alignment of the Doppler beam parallel with flow. Patients are examined in the supine position with various degrees of lateral rotation to optimize the acoustic window. Doppler alignment with flow is usually possible and, therefore, correction for beam-flow intercept angles is not only unnecessary, but should be avoided. In most instances, CFI allows proper alignment of the Doppler beam to the exact axis of maximal flow.

When a Doppler examination is being performed, the Doppler audio signal, and not necessarily the spectral display, may provide the best guidance for obtaining an optimal examination. Alignment of the Doppler sample volume or cursor with laminar flow is aided significantly by listening for the highest, "pure" audio signal. Nonlaminar, or disturbed flow, sounds much rougher and contains numerous simultaneous tones (frequencies).

SYSTEMATIC EXAMINATION

The examination begins with standard 2D echo imaging planes in order to display the anatomy and select an acoustic window. Presently, most echocardiographers perform CFI as an integral part of the echocardiographic examination. During 2D imaging, CFI is done in each view prior to moving on to the next transducer position. Color flow mapping is accomplished by pushing a button, on the instrument, and adjusting the transducer angle and gain settings as needed. If desired, the ECG trigger mode could be used to record a 2D map of intracardiac flow from the desired portion of the cardiac cycle. Finally, the color M-mode and spectral frequency analysis could be chosen to investigate flow within specific areas of interest on the flow map. When indicated, CW Doppler is performed for quantitating high velocity jets.

NORMAL SPECTRAL FLOW PATTERNS

Apical Four Chamber Plane

The apical four chamber plane is preferred for interrogation of velocities across the mitral and tricuspid valves. In this plane, velocities are "mapped" anteriorly from the pulmonary veins, through the left atrium and across the mitral valve. Similarly, velocities are mapped anteriorly through the right atrium and across the tricuspid valve. Superior and inferior vena caval blood inflow enters the right atrium nearly perpendicular to the apical four chamber imaging plane and is not studied in this plane.

Mitral Valve

Mitral velocities are obtained by placement of the Doppler sample volume within the valve leaflets just distal to the anulus (Fig. 3–1). The sample volume is aligned parallel to the interventricular septum and then adjusted until optimal waveforms are found. Mitral velocities (Fig. 3–2) are

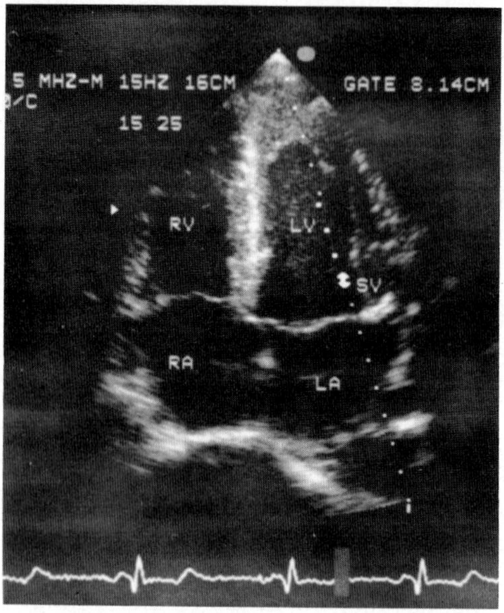

Figure 3 – 1. Apical four chamber view. Note sample volume (SV) location for Doppler interrogation of left ventricular inflow. RV = right ventricle, RA = right atrium, LV = left ventricle, LA = left atrium.

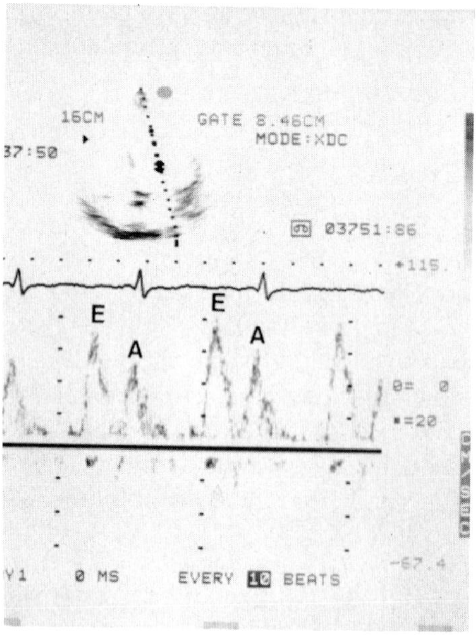

Figure 3 – 2. Transmitral velocities from an apical four chamber view demonstrating the rapid left ventricular filling phase (E) followed by atrial contraction (A) at end diastole. (Scale marks = 20 cm/s.)

TABLE 3–1. Normal Doppler Velocities

Site of Flow	Children* (m/s)	Adults† (m/s)
Mitral diastolic	1.0(0.8–1.3)	0.9(0.6–1.3)
Tricuspid diastolic	0.6(0.5–0.8)	0.5(0.3–0.7)
Right ventricular outflow and pulmonary systolic	0.9(0.7–1.1)	0.8(0.6–0.9)
Left ventricular outflow systolic	1.0(0.7–1.2)	0.9(0.7–1.1)
Aortic systolic	1.5(1.2–1.8)	1.4(1.0–1.7)

*Based on a 5.0 MHz scanhead
†Based on a 3.0 MHz scanhead

characterized by an early diastolic E wave associated with the rapid left ventricular filling phase, followed by an A wave associated with atrial contraction. Table 3–1 lists normal mitral velocities for children and adults. The absolute height, ratio of height, and area under these two time velocity waveforms have been associated with diastolic properties of the left ventricle. These relationships are discussed in Chapter 12. However, characteristics and amplitude of both the E and A waveform may change with slight alterations of the Doppler beam in any plane and with sampling site. Velocities within the anulus area just proximal to the mitral valve are similar to those just distal to the valve. Drinkovic et al[1] demonstrated that the velocities at the tips of the mitral valve leaflets were significantly higher than those at the anulus due to smaller flow area at the leaflet tips. The early diastolic E wave has been shown to decrease with age while the A wave and A/E ratio increase[2,3] (Fig. 3–3). This finding has been attributed to changes in ventricular distensibility. The A wave amplitude has also been shown to increase with heart rate secondary to shortening of the total diastolic filling period.[4] In atrial fibrillation, the A wave is missing, whereas in other atrial arrhythmias, several peaks may be seen, each corresponding to an atrial contraction.

Increased negative systolic velocities of aortic outflow can be simultaneously recorded with mitral velocities when the sample volume is placed medially in the region of the left ventricular outflow tract (Fig. 3–4).

With the use of the CW Doppler mode, the mitral valve flow pattern (Fig. 3–5) can also be easily determined from the same apical approach with the small nonimaging transducer by placing it at the apical impulse and directing the ultrasound beam superiorly, posteriorly, and to the right.

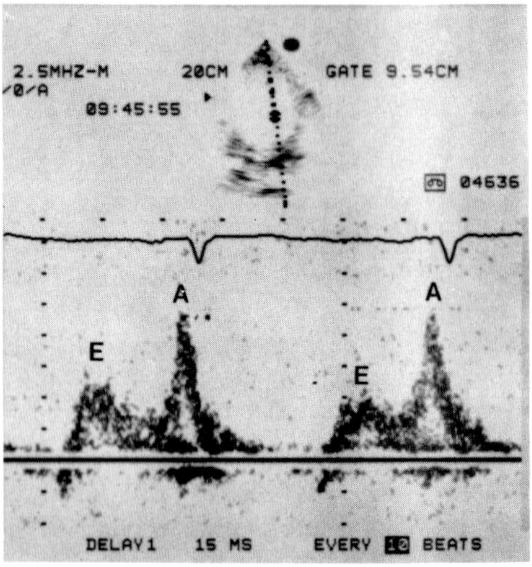

Figure 3–3. Transmitral velocities demonstrating increase of A/E ratio in an 80-year-old patient without clinical heart disease. (Scale marks = 20 cm/s.)

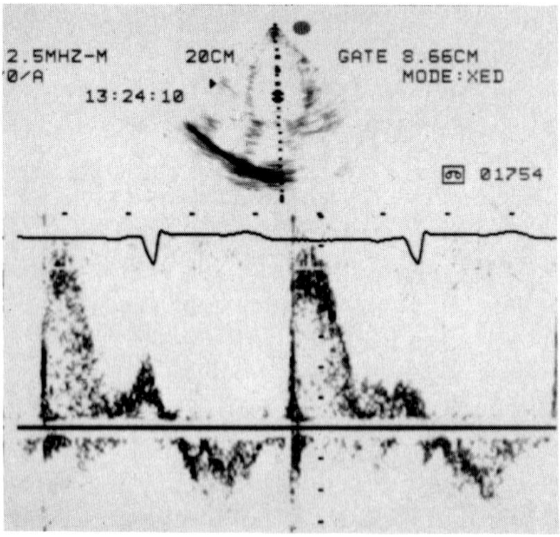

Figure 3–4. Recording from an apical four chamber view in which the sample volume is moved slightly toward the left ventricular outflow tract. Normal mitral velocities are recorded during diastole toward the transducer (above the baseline), and left ventricular outflow velocities are recorded during systole away from the transducer (below the baseline). (Scale marks = 20 cm/s.)

Tricuspid Valve

Tricuspid velocities are obtained by placing the Doppler sample volume within the valve leaflets distal to the anulus. The sample volume is aligned parallel to the interventricular septum and then adjusted until optimal waveforms are found. Tricuspid velocities are similar in configuration to mitral velocities but are generally of lower amplitude. There is an early diastolic E wave associated with the rapid right ventricular filling phase followed by an A wave related to right atrial contraction (Fig. 3–6).

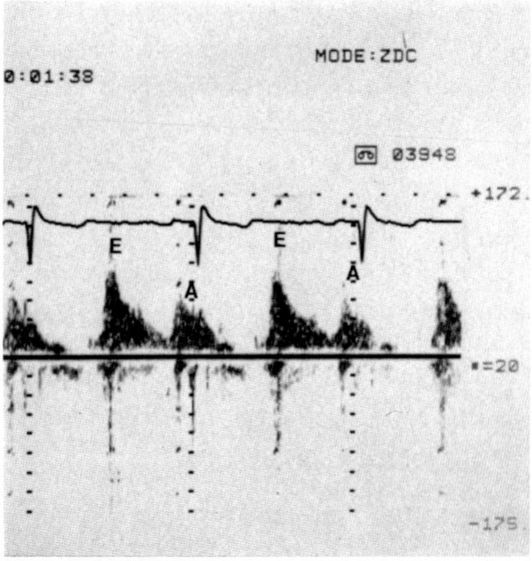

Figure 3–5. Continuous wave Doppler tracing of the left ventricular inflow obtained from the apex. Note the E and A waves.

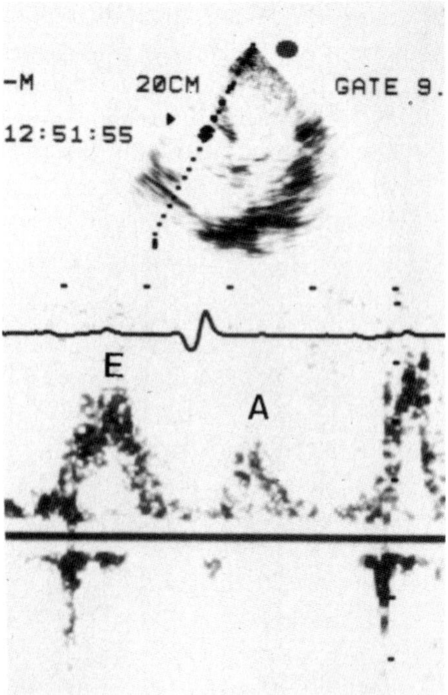

Figure 3–6. Tricuspid velocities from an apical four chamber view demonstrating the E wave of ventricular filling, and A wave associated with atrial contraction. (Scale marks = 20 cm/s.)

The A/E ratio has been associated with diastolic properties of the right ventricle.[5] As diastole shortens, the E and A waves tend to occur close together and in tachycardiac individuals separate peaks may be difficult to differentiate. Tricuspid velocities vary significantly with the respiratory cycle, whereas mitral velocities are influenced minimally. Normal tricuspid valve velocity values are listed in Table 3–1. Peak tricuspid velocities decrease with age,[6] probably related to the increase in tricuspid valve anulus area with age and changes in right ventricular distensibility. In some persons, a flow signal in both systole and diastole can be recorded in the right atrium close to the tricuspid valve, and in the absence of increase flow, this pattern may be caused by coronary sinus flow[7] (Fig. 3–7).

Apical Five Chamber Plane

The apical five chamber plane is optimal for evaluating the left ventricular outflow tract by both PD and CW Doppler echocardiograph. The sample volume is positioned just below the aortic valve (Fig. 3–8). Since flow is away from the transducer, a negative deflection is noted during systole (Fig. 3–9). Low amplitude negative diastolic velocities may be seen. These represent mitral inflow coursing around the anterior leaflet of the mitral valve and into the aortic outflow tract.

When using CW Doppler, the small, nonimaging transducer is placed at the same apical position and directed superiorly, anteriorly, and medi-

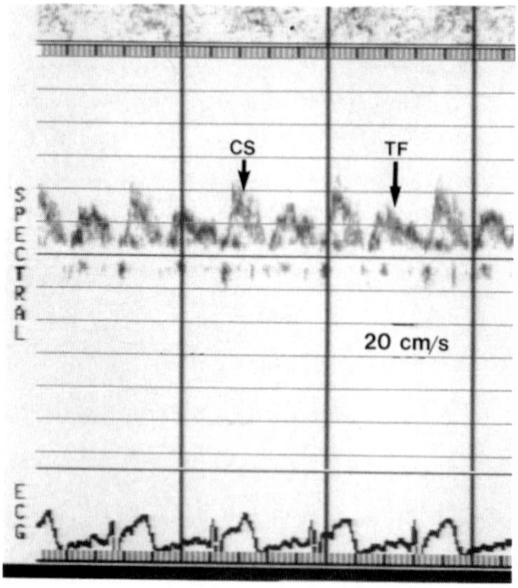

Figure 3–7. Normal tricuspid flow with the sample volume in the right atrium near the tricuspid valve. Flow in systole is caused by coronary sinus flow (CS); tricuspid flow is recorded in diastole (TF).

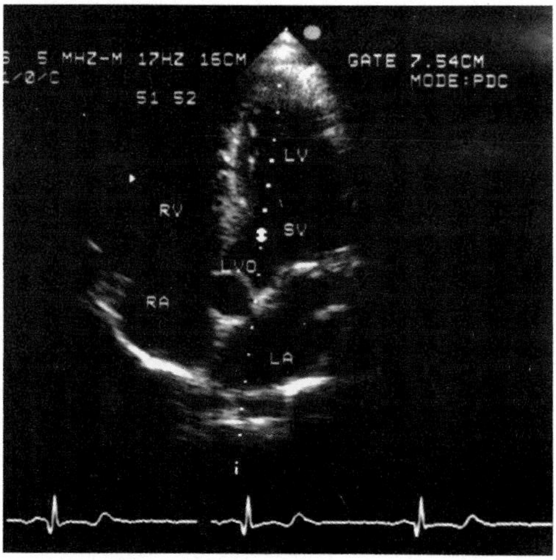

Figure 3–8. Apical five chamber plane. The sample volume (SV) is positioned in the left ventricular outflow (LVO), proximal to the aortic valve. RV = right ventricle, RA = right atrium, LV = left ventricle, LA = left atrium.

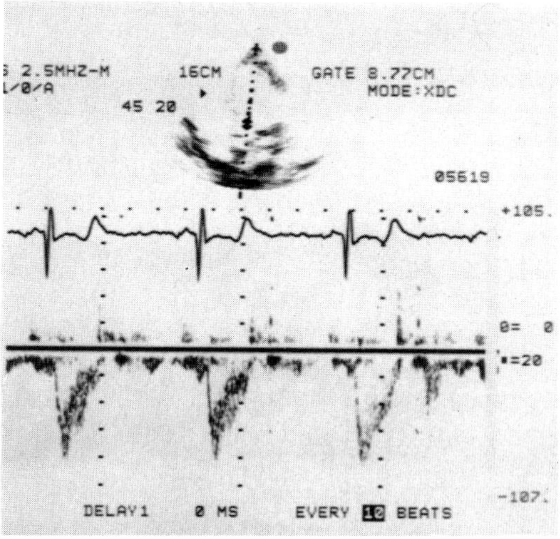

Figure 3–9. Pulsed Doppler velocities from the left ventricular outflow tract obtained from the apical five chamber plane.

ally from the typical M pattern of mitral flow. From this position, a systolic velocity away from the transducer (below the baseline) can be recorded (Fig. 3–10). Normal left ventricular outflow tract velocity values are listed in Table 3–1.

Short Axis Parasternal Plane

The parasternal short axis is the preferred plane for interrogation of pulmonary velocities. Right ventricular outflow tract velocities can also be

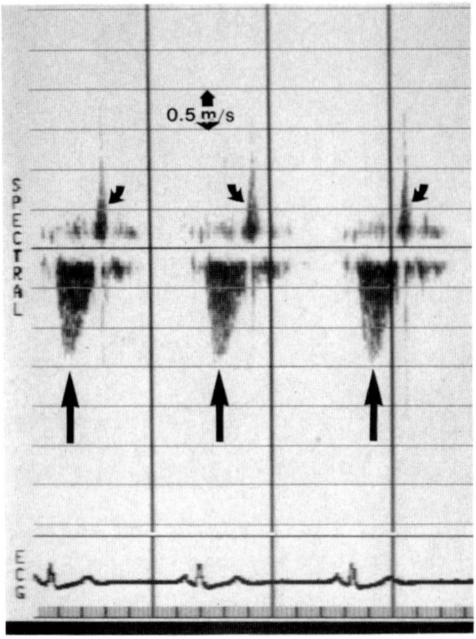

Figure 3–10. Continuous wave Doppler tracing of the left ventricular outflow tract. A nonimaging transducer (2 MHz) is used from the apical position. Normal systolic flow is below the baseline (arrows). Aortic valve closure is recorded (small curved arrows).

interrogated from this same plane. Tricuspid velocities can also be recorded from short axis parasternal planes but alignment with flow across the tricuspid valve is usually best accomplished from the apical four chamber plane.

Pulmonic Valve

Pulmonary velocities are obtained by placing the sample volume at or just distal to the pulmonic valve within the pulmonary artery (Fig. 3–11). The transition from right ventricular outflow tract to pulmonary artery is associated with a slight increase in velocity. Normal flow through the pulmonic valve is directed away from the transducer and displayed below the baseline (Fig. 3–12). Normal pulmonary velocities have a slower upstroke, lower maximal velocity, and later occurring peak than is found for aortic velocities (see Fig. 3–9). The lower pulmonary velocity can be explained, in part, by the difference in vessel cross-sectional areas. Aortic flow equals pulmonary flow in the absence of intracardiac shunting or semi-lunar valve insufficiency. Since the area of the pulmonary artery is usually larger than that of the aorta, pulmonary velocities are lower than aortic velocities.

In normal pulmonary velocity tracings a low amplitude negative diastolic waveform coincident with rapid ventricular filling through the tricuspid valve may be recorded.[8] A second low, negative, late diastolic peak (A

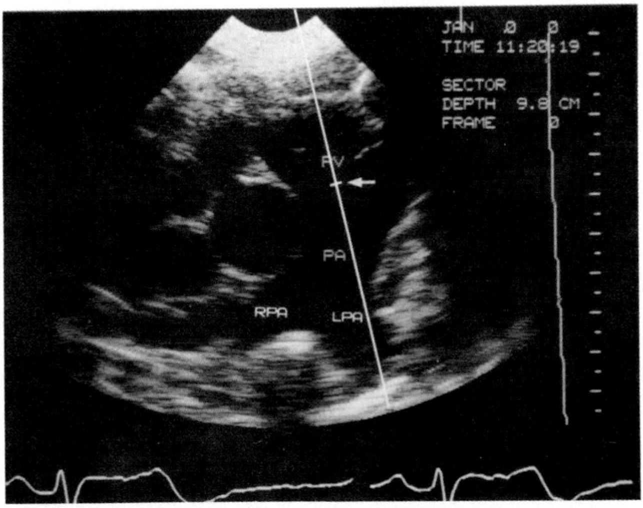

Figure 3-11. Parasternal short axis plane with the sample volume (arrow) at the pulmonic valve (PV). PA = pulmonary artery; RPA = right pulmonary artery, LPA = left pulmonary artery.

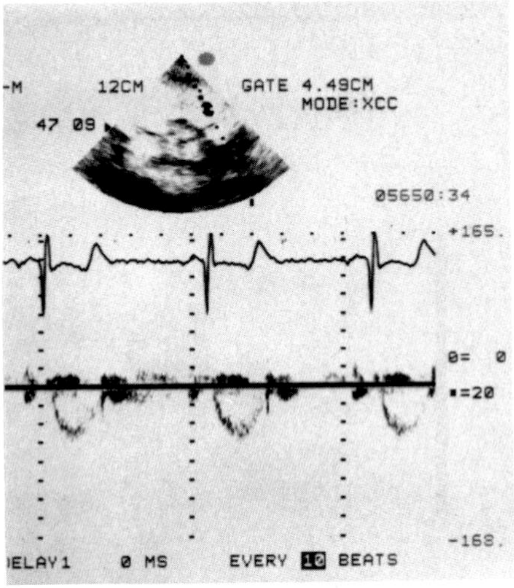

Figure 3-12. Pulmonary velocities from a short axis parasternal view.

wave) immediately precedes the systolic upstroke in patients with normal pulmonary artery pressure and is thought to be related to right atrial contraction. Both diastolic waveforms probably represent minimal diastolic flow through the pulmonary valve. If the sample volume is placed laterally in the main pulmonary artery near the wall, pulmonary velocity decreases in amplitude in late systole and reverses direction in early diastole. It is, therefore, preferable to record pulmonary velocity in the central portion of the vessel. Narrow high velocity spikes of pulmonary valve opening and closure can be seen when the sample volume is near the leaflets (these velocity patterns, which are called valve clicks, can be found for all four valves). Normal pulmonary velocity values are listed in Table 3–1.

Adequate velocity tracings should allow measurement of peak pulmonary velocity, and time to peak velocity (acceleration time) (Fig. 3–13). Peak velocity is measured at the midpoint of the modal velocity. Acceleration time is defined as the interval from onset of the systolic velocity tracing as it leaves baseline, to attainment of peak systolic velocity (Fig. 3–13). In normal subjects ranging in age from 14 days to 35 years, Wilson et al[6] noted a slight decrease in the pulmonary artery peak velocity and a significant increase in the acceleration time with age. These changes are probably related to a decrease in pulmonary artery pressure and increase in vessel area in young subjects. Gardin et al[9] found no significant changes in these parameters in an older population.

Right Ventricular Outflow Tract

Velocity waveforms in the outflow tract are similar in configuration to those in the pulmonary artery but are of lower amplitude and have more velocity spread because the outflow tract has more area than the pulmonary artery. Occasionally, a very short early diastolic reverse flow is recorded above the baseline (Fig. 3–14). This velocity profile probably represents diastolic retrograde flow from the pulmonary artery into the right ventricular outflow

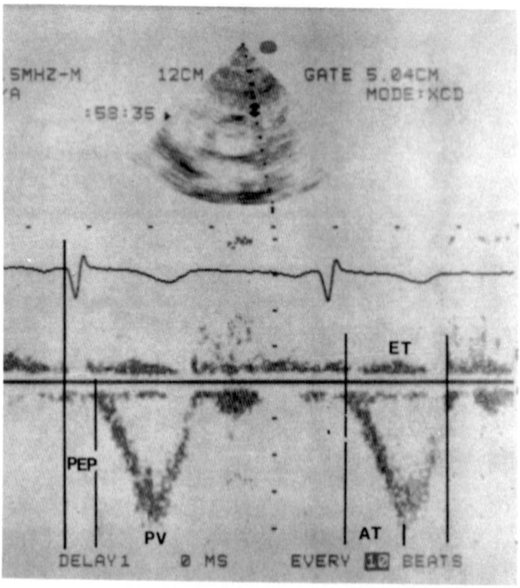

Figure 3–13. Pulmonary artery velocity tracings demonstrating measurement of peak velocity (PV); ejection time (ET); preejection period (PEP); time-to-peak velocity or acceleration time (AT). (Scale marks = 20 cm/s.)

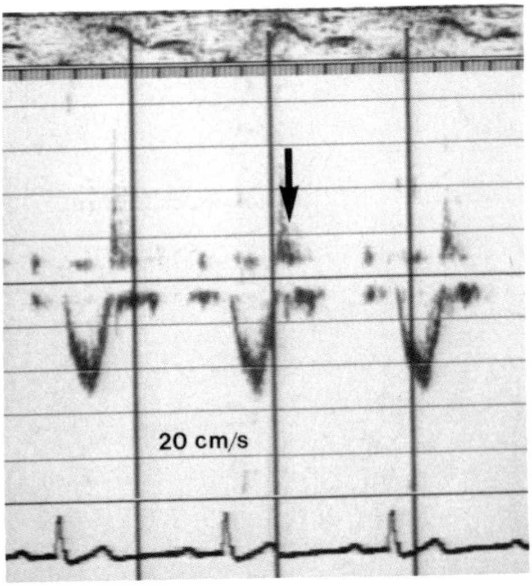

Figure 3–14. Normal right ventricular outflow obtained from a parasternal short axis view. Systolic laminar flow occurs away from the transducer and is displayed below the baseline. Note the early diastolic flow above the baseline (arrow) representing turbulence in the right ventricular outflow, a normal finding.

tract, suggesting that pulmonary regurgitation commonly occurs. This should not be interpreted as pathologic.

Suprasternal Notch Plane

The suprasternal notch is the preferred plane for interrogation of ascending, transverse, and descending aortic velocities. In some patients, improved alignment with flow in the ascending aorta can be obtained by placement of the transducer in the right supraclavicular area. However, ascending aorta velocities may be better obtained from the right upper parasternal region or apical five chamber plane in some larger or older subjects. Therefore, other areas should be interrogated and results compared to those from the suprasternal notch.

When PD mode is used, the sample volume is positioned within the ascending aorta (Fig. 3–15) and maneuvered into the maximum flow jet as close to the aortic valve as possible. Normal flow distal to the aortic valve is normally narrow band, occurs during systole toward the transducer, increases rapidly with the opening of the aortic valve, and decreases at a slower rate in the latter half of systole (Fig. 3–16). Compared with the velocity in the pulmonary artery, velocity in the ascending aorta is higher, peaks earlier in systole, and exhibits a shorter ejection time. Velocity in the ascending aorta varies with different locations of the sample volume. Toward the lateral wall, the velocity curve is similar to the one recorded at valve level, whereas toward the inner curvature, lower velocities are found.[10]

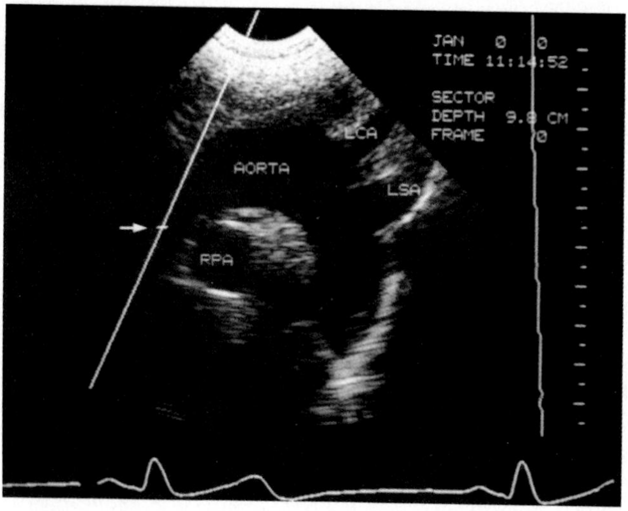

Figure 3–15. Suprasternal long axis view of the aortic arch. The sample volume (arrow) is located in the ascending aorta close to the aortic valve. RPA = right pulmonary artery, LCA = left common carotid artery, LSA = left subclavian artery.

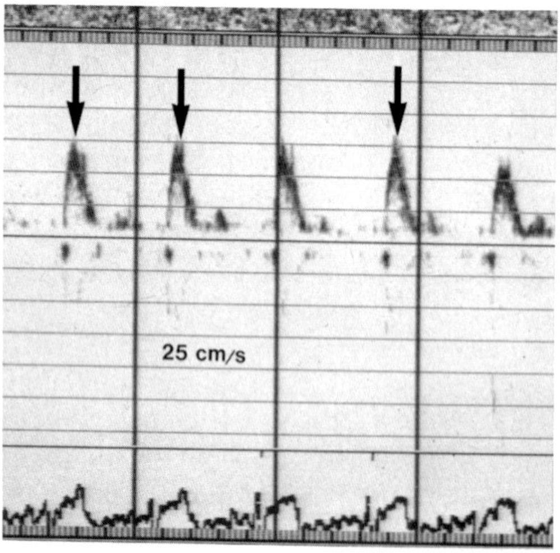

Figure 3–16. Normal ascending aortic flow from a suprasternal long axis view. The spectral display shows rapid systolic flow toward the transducer (arrows), and then deceleration at a slower rate.

Flow in the descending aorta is detected from the suprasternal notch by positioning the sample volume distal to the arch vessels. Flow is away from the transducer and recorded below the baseline (Fig. 3–17). A short period of reverse flow at end-systole is common in both the ascending and descending aorta and may represent the reversal of flow necessary to close the aortic valve.

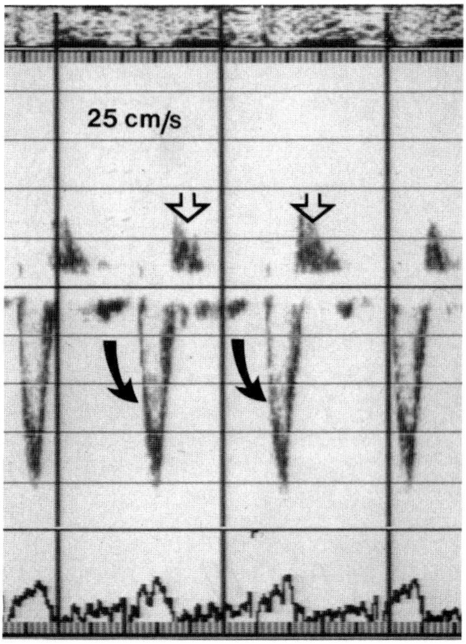

Figure 3–17. Normal descending aortic flow from a suprasternal long axis view. Flow occurs away from the transducer and recorded below the baseline during systole (arrows). Note the short period of reverse flow at end-systole (open arrows).

The CW mode, using a nonimaging transducer from the suprasternal notch, is quicker to use and more comfortable for the patient. Systolic flow is toward the transducer when the ascending aorta is interrogated, and away from the transducer when the descending aorta is interrogated. Normal aorta velocity values are listed in Table 3–1.

Optimal ascending aortic tracings should allow accurate measurement of peak velocity, acceleration time, preejection period and ejection time. Aortic peak velocities decrease with age probably, in part, due to an age related increase in aortic diameter.[9] Peak velocities at age 70 are approximately 60 percent of those found at age 20.[9,11] Aortic acceleration time has been used as an indicator of ventricular performance and is discussed in Chap. 11.

Subcostal Plane

The preferred plane for Doppler interrogation of the atrial and ventricular septum is the subcostal long axis plane. Doppler interrogation of an intact atrial or ventricular septum shows continuous, positive, low amplitude velocities (Fig. 3–18), probably related to wall motion or red blood cell motion impacting the septa.

Interrogation of atrial septal velocities can also be performed in a short axis plane. Perpendicular alignment with the atrial septum can be more easily performed in this plane.

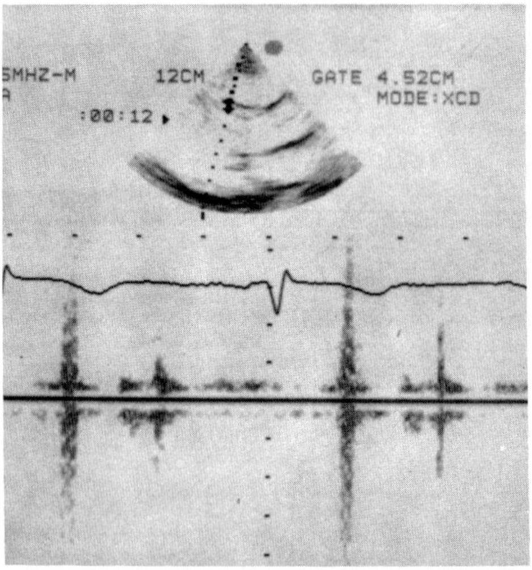

Figure 3–18. Pulsed wave Doppler velocities with the sample volume placed perpendicular to the right ventricular septal surface from a subcostal plane. Note the low amplitude velocities. (Scale marks = 20 cm/s.)

NORMAL PATTERNS BY COLOR DOPPLER FLOW IMAGING

Several phenomena may occur during the performance of a normal CFI examination and result in the assignment of a color that does not seem compatible with the known flow pattern at a given location. The first of these inappropriate color displays is related to the phenomenon of aliasing that is inherent to all PD systems (discussed in Chap. 2).

A second phenomenon that may result in the unusual color representation of flow relates to the all or none assignment of color based on direction of movement. When the ultrasound beam is perpendicular to the direction of flow, red blood cells in one half of the field may be sensed as flowing toward the transducer while red blood cells in the other half of the field are sensed as flowing away from the transducer. For example, when mapping flow in the left ventricular outflow tract from the parasternal long axis view, blood flow in the left hand portion of the field is colored red while flow in the right hand portion of the field is blue despite the consistency of blood movement from left-to-right (Fig. 3–19). This situation should not be confused with an appropriate abrupt change in color such as occurs in the aortic arch when the actual direction of blood flow changes (see Fig. 3–26).

It is often difficult to obtain optimal flow signals while simultaneously recording ideal 2D images. In order to position the Doppler beam in a parallel orientation to flow, an unorthodox position and angle may become necessary. As is true of conventional Doppler techniques, a parallel orientation to the direction of flow will result in the highest velocity re-

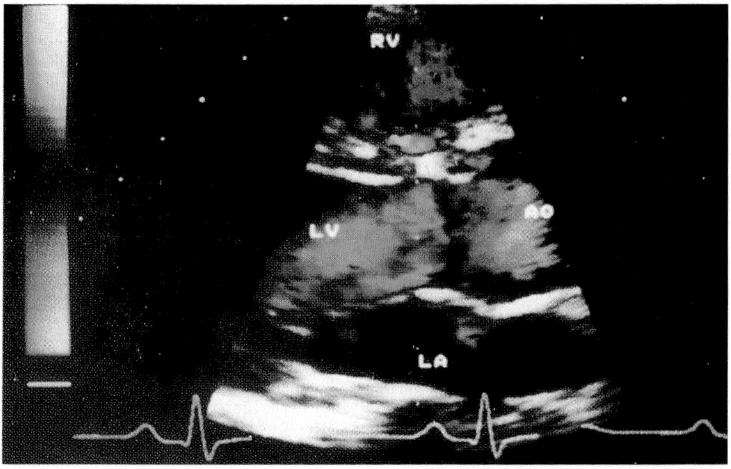

Figure 3–19. Parasternal long axis view of systolic flow in the left ventricle. Due to perpendicular orientation of the Doppler signal, flow in the left-hand portion of the sector is red and flow in the right-hand portion of the sector is blue. This apparent "change in flow direction" is an artifact frequently encountered in color flow mapping.

cordings (i.e., angle θ is $< 20°$). On the other hand, because aliasing is more likely to occur at higher velocities, and since CFI can provide important spectral information from various views, examination of flow from a perpendicular orientation may be advantageous as well.

Long Axis Parasternal Plane

Color flow imaging permits excellent evaluation of the left ventricular inflow and outflow regions in this plane.[12] In the long axis parasternal view (Fig. 3–20), the ultrasonic beam is projected perpendicularly to the greater portion of flow in both systole and diastole. Because of this perpendicular orientation, velocities are generally low. Furthermore, velocities below the threshold of color assignment (which may be machine and operator dependent) will remain black. Thus, in normal patients, in the low parasternal position, diastole is characterized by a broad band of orange-red flow moving through the mitral valve orifice into the left ventricle (Fig. 3–21A). As left ventricular filling proceeds, macrovortices are formed as large eddy currents swirl around the apex and become oriented in the opposite direction. The appearance of blue during diastolic filling is not due, therefore, to abnormal flow but to the same swirling of middiastolic flow that causes the mitral valve to drift partially closed midway

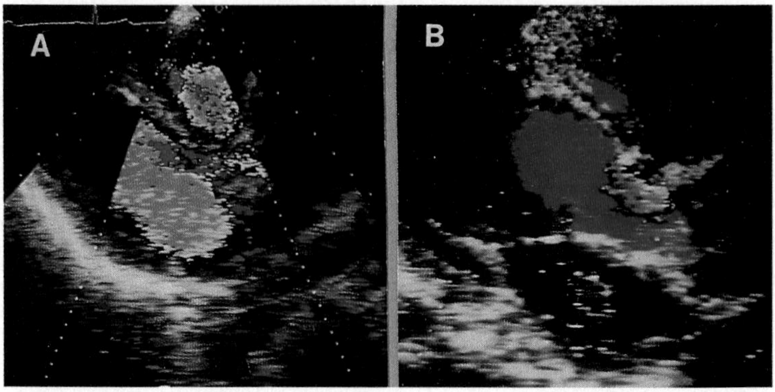

Figure 3–20. Parasternal long axis view of the left ventricle. Diastolic flow across the mitral valve is displayed as red-orange (A), and systolic flow in the left ventricular outflow is displayed in blue (B).

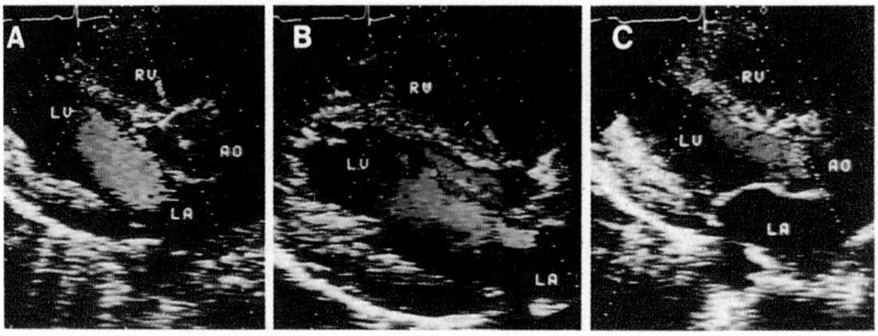

Figure 3–21. Parasternal long axis view showing early diastole (A), mid-to-late diastole (B), and systole (C). The area of blue seen in mid-to-late diastole is due to swirling of diastolic blood flow. LV = left ventricle, LA = left atrium, RV = right ventricle, AO = aorta.

through diastole (Fig. 3–21B). With the onset of systole (Fig. 3–21C), a broad blue stream is seen in the left ventricular outflow tract moving away from the transducer. Also seen from the parasternal window is a portion of the right ventricle (Fig. 3–21A). Red diastolic flow is seen moving toward the transducer through the tricuspid valve into the right ventricle. Imaging from the high parasternal area brings the left ventricular outflow tract and aorta closer to the transducer. This location will usually result in mitral flow passing away from the transducer (coded in blue) and aortic flow being directed toward the transducer (coded in red).

Short Axis Parasternal Plane

In this projection, the aortic valve is seen to be flanked by the tricuspid valve on the left, and by the right ventricular outflow tract and pulmonary artery on the right. In diastole (Fig. 3–22), red flow traverses the tricuspid valve moving toward the transducer. In systole (Fig. 3–23), blue flow is seen moving away from the transducer out the right ventricular outflow tract. Because normal pulmonary artery flow may exceed the Nyquist limit of the instruments, aliasing occurs and the inappropriate color red is seen

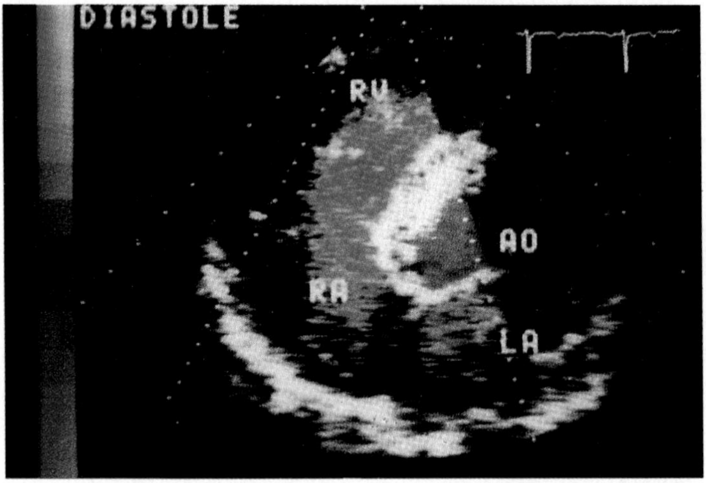

Figure 3–22. Parasternal short axis view of diastolic red flow toward the transducer across the tricuspid valve. RA = right atrium, RV = right ventricle, LA = left atrium, AO = aorta.

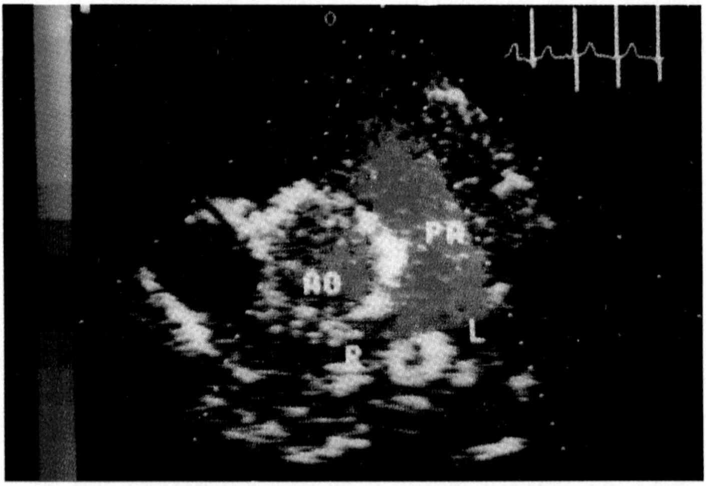

Figure 3–23. Parasternal short axis view of systolic blue flow into the pulmonary artery (PA). AO = aorta, R = right pulmonary artery, L = left pulmonary artery.

in the pulmonary artery. In systole, the flow in the proximal aorta is colored blue as it moves posteriorly, away from the transducer.

Apical Plane

Apical views provide parallel orientation to flow toward and away from the apex of the heart, and thereby allow imaging of maximal flow velocities. With posterior angulation of the four chamber view, red transmitral diastolic flow can be seen to fill the mitral valve orifice and enter the left ventricle in early diastole (Fig. 3–24A). In early diastole, the time of most rapid transmitral flow, areas of blue coloration due to aliasing may be seen near the center of the mitral orifice. This example illustrates how large areas of aliasing may be present in normal subjects. Given the depth of imaging and the small angle of incidence between ultrasound and the course of flow, it is common for such aliasing to occur. As diastole continues (Fig. 3–24B), blood entering the left ventricle strikes the apex creating macrovortices that flow back toward the mitral valve and are appropriately assigned blue coloration. This swirling action, as mentioned previously, also causes partial closure of the mitral valve. Again, flow signals are generally not recorded at the cardiac apex because velocity of flow is below the threshold of color assignment.

With the onset of systole, the mitral valve closes initiating isovolumetric contraction. This short, early period of systole is characterized by lack of flow in normal patients and therefore by the absence of velocity signals. As systole proceeds (Fig. 3–24C), a broad band of blue signals is seen in the left ventricular outflow tract, indicative of systolic flow away from the transducer. Aliasing can be expected and often results in red coloration of the high velocity central aortic jet.

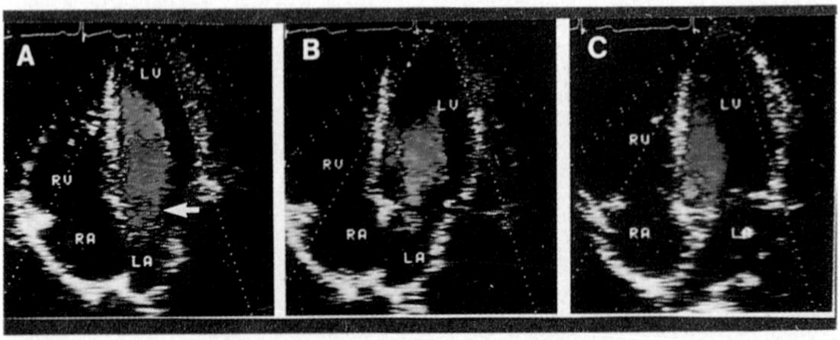

Figure 3–24. Apical four chamber view showing early diastole (A), late diastole (B), and systole (C). Aliasing is seen during early diastole (arrow). RV = right ventricle, RA = right atrium, LV = left ventricle, LA = left atrium.

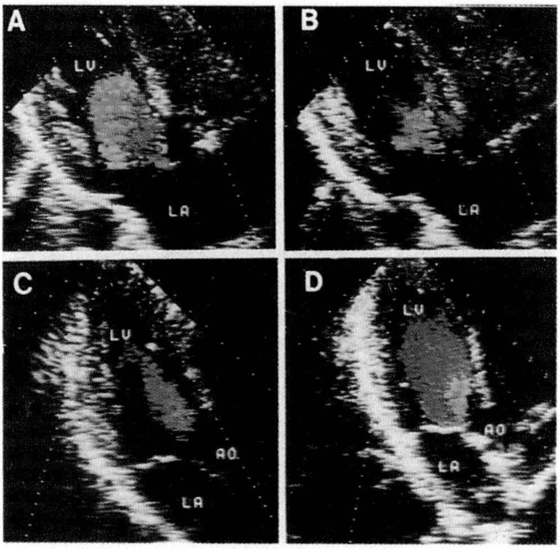

Figure 3–25. Apical long axis view showing early diastole (A), middiastole (B), and systole (C). High velocity flow results in aliasing during systole (D), a common finding in color flow imaging. LV = left ventricle, LA = left atrium, AO = aorta.

A view that frequently enables optimal visualization of flow through both mitral and aortic valves is the apical long axis view. As shown in Fig. 3–25, the aortic valve is seen to the right of the mitral valve. Figure 3–25A shows early diastolic flow moving toward the transducer through the mitral valve. Again, due to the high velocity of flow in early diastole, the parallel orientation of the Doppler signal, and the depth of imaging, aliasing results in areas of blue in the center of the flow map. In middiastole (Fig. 3–25B), red transmitral flow enters the left ventricle moving toward the transducer. Nonturbulent blood flow moving away from the transducer is present below the aortic valve. This represents middiastolic swirling of blood back toward the base of the heart from the apex. With systole (Fig. 3–25C), a broad band of blue is seen in the left ventricular outflow tract. At the center of this flow are lighter shades of blue indicative of higher velocities. In Fig. 3–25D, at the level of the aortic anulus, high velocity flow has exceeded the Nyquist limit and red is inappropriately assigned due to aliasing.

Suprasternal Plane

The suprasternal view allows visualization of the aortic arch. Despite the shallow depth of imaging, aliasing can occur in this high flow velocity area. Not to be confused with aliasing is the expected abrupt change in color assignment as blood flow direction changes from ascending (red) to descending (blue) aorta (Fig. 3–26).

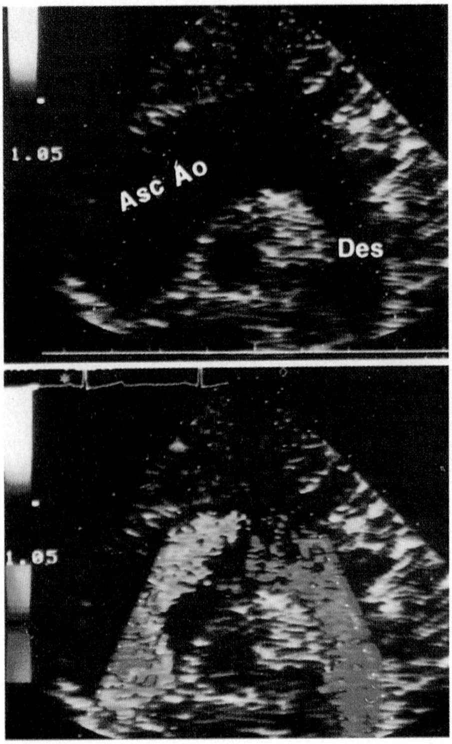

Figure 3–26. *Top*: A 2-D echocardiogram from the suprasternal view of the ascending, transverse, and descending aorta. *Bottom*: Flow in the ascending aorta moves toward the transducer (red) and flow in the descending aorta moves away from the transducer (blue).

Subcostal Plane

Color flow imaging in this plane can be used to investigate flow in the superior vena cava, ascending aorta, and the four cardiac chambers. Velocities across the mitral and tricuspid valves are unlikely to show aliasing from the subcostal plane due to the large beam flow intercept angle.

Color M-Mode Echocardiograph

The major advantage of CFI is its ability to provide spatial information in real time. Additionally, superimposed color coding on an M-mode echocardiograph may yield valuable information in regard to timing of flow events (Fig. 3–27).

REGURGITANT FLOW PATTERNS OF NORMAL VALVES

Multiple studies have reported that the specificity of Doppler echocardiography is not 100 percent in the diagnosis of valvular regurgitation, either

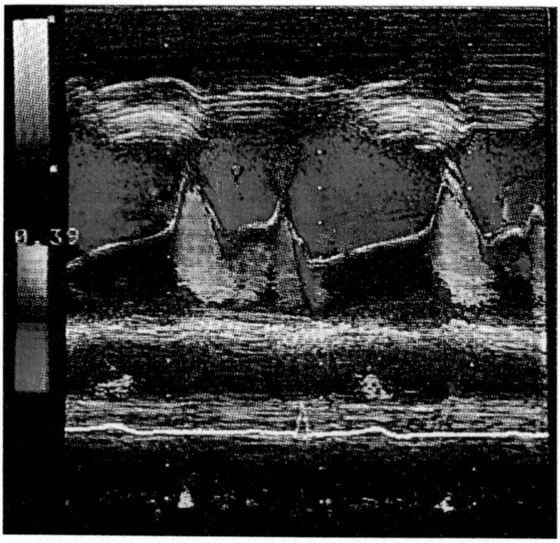

Figure 3-27. Color M-mode echocardiograph of left ventricular inflow and outflow. In diastole, red-orange transmitral flow is seen between the mitral leaflets moving toward the transducer. In systole, blue flow moves away from the transducer in the left ventricular outflow tract.

with PD or CW Doppler echocardiography. False-positive results have been found for the mitral valve,[13,14] aortic valve[15,16] and, even more frequently, for the tricuspid and pulmonic valves.[17,19] A study using CW Doppler in 20 normal subjects showed false-positive rates of 95 percent for the tricuspid valve, 35 percent for the pulmonary valve, 10 percent for the mitral valve and 0 percent for aortic regurgitation.[20] Kostucki et al[21] recently reported a PD echocardiographic study in 25 normal subjects and demonstrated a regurgitant turbulent flow pattern at the pulmonic valve in 23 subjects, and a midsystolic regurgitant flow pattern at the mitral valve in 10 subjects. A similar regurgitant flow was recorded at the tricuspid valve in 11 subjects. An early diastolic regurgitant flow with low maximal velocities and rapid decrease in velocities was recorded at the aortic valve in 8 subjects. In no person could those flows be recorded farther than 1 cm proximal to the valve closure.

Indirect arguments support true valvular regurgitation as an explanation for the regurgitant flow pattern. Injection of intravenous saline solution produces enhancement of the Doppler tricuspid and pulmonic signal amplitude, suggesting that these signals represent right heart flow.[22] Application of Bernoulli's equation to the velocities of these flows, in selected cases with well-defined Doppler signals, can correctly predict transtricuspid and transpulmonic gradient as assessed by catheterization.[22] Moreover, in normal subjects, CFI has shown flow spurting from and proximally to the coaptation of the pulmonic valve during diastole.[23,24]

Whatever the still debated mechanisms of these regurgitant flow patterns in normal subjects is, one should be aware of their existence and characteristics when assessing valvular function by Doppler echocardiograph. In the presence of a structurally normal valve, normal cardiac dimensions, and normal cardiac function, the presence of a mild regurgitant flow pattern should not be considered pathologic and clinical correlation is required.

REFERENCES

1. Drinkovic N, Smith M, Wisenbaugh T, et al: Influence of sampling site upon the ratio of atrial to early diastolic transmitral flow velocities by Doppler (abstr). *J Am Coll Cardiol* 9:16A, 1987.
2. Miyatake K, Okamoto M, Kinoshita N, et al: Augmentation of atrial contribution to left ventricular inflow with aging as assessed by intracardiac Doppler flowmetry. *Am J Cardiol* 53:586, 1984.
3. Gardin J, Rohan M, Davidson D, et al: Doppler transmitral flow velocity parameters: Relationship between age, body surface area, blood pressure and gender in normal subjects. *Am J Noninvas Cardiol* 1:3, 1987.
4. Herzog C, Elsperger K, Manoles M, et al: Effect of atrial pacing on left ventricular diastolic filling measured by pulsed Doppler echocardiography (abstr). *J Am Coll Cardiol* 9:197A, 1987.
5. Fujii J, Yazoki Y, Sawada H, et al: Noninvasive assessment of left and right ventricular filling in myocardial infarction with a two-dimensional Doppler echocardiographic method. *J Am Coll Cardiol* 5:1155, 1985.
6. Wilson N, Goldberg S, Dickinson D, et al: Normal intracardiac and great artery blood velocity measurements by pulsed Doppler echocardiography. *Br Heart J* 53:451, 1985.
7. Hatle L, Angelsen B: *Doppler Ultrasound in Cardiology: Physical Principles and Clinical Applications*, ed 2. Philadelphia, Lea & Febiger, 1985.
8. Gibbs J, Wilson N, Witsenburg M, et al: Diastolic forward blood flow in the pulmonary artery detected by Doppler echocardiography. *J Am Coll Cardiol* 6:1322, 1985.
9. Gardin J, Davidson D, Rohan M, et al: Relationship between age, body size, gender, and blood pressure and Doppler flow measurements in the aorta and pulmonary artery. *Am Heart J* 113:101, 1987.
10. Farthing W, Peronneau P: Flow in the thoracic aorta. *Cardiovasc Res* 13:607, 1979.
11. Mowat D, Haites N, Rawles J: Aortic blood velocity measurement in healthy adults using a simple ultrasound technique. *Cardiovasc Res* 17:75, 1983.
12. Miyatake K, Okamoto M, Kinoshita N, et al: Clinical applications of a new type of real-time two-dimensional Doppler flow imaging system. *Am J Cardiol* 54:857, 1984.
13. Hoffman A, Burckardt D: Evaluation of systolic murmurs by Doppler ultrasonography. *Br Heart J* 50:337, 1983.

14. Robertson J, Krafchek J, Adams D, et al: Reassessment of Doppler ultrasound in minimal aortic and mitral regurgitation (abstr). *Circulation* 70(suppl II):397, 1984.

15. Richards K, Cannon S, Crawford M, et al: Noninvasive diagnosis of aortic and mitral valve disease with pulsed Doppler spectral analysis. *Am J Cardiol* 51:1122, 1983.

16. Bommer W, Rebeck K, Laviola S, et al: Real-time two-dimensional flow imaging: Detection and semiquantification of valvular and congenital heart disease (abstr). *Circulation* 70(suppl II):38, 1984.

17. Waggoner A, Quinones M, Young J, et al: Pulsed Doppler echocardiographic detection of right-sided valve regurgitation. *Am J Cardiol* 47:279, 1981.

18. Patel A, Rowe G, Dhanani S, et al: Pulsed Doppler echocardiography in diagnosis of pulmonary regurgitation: Its value and limitations. *Am J Cardiol* 49:1801, 1982.

19. Yock P, Segal J, Teirstein P, et al: Doppler color flow mapping: Utility in valvular regurgitation (abstr). *Circulation* 70(suppl II): 381, 1984.

20. Yock P, Schnittger I, Popp R: Is continuous wave Doppler too sensitive in diagnosing pathologic valvular regurgitation? (abstr). *Circulation* 70(suppl II): 381, 1984.

21. Kostucki W, Vandenbossche J, Friart A, et al: Pulsed Doppler regurgitant flow patterns of normal valves. *Am J Cardiol* 58:309, 1986.

22. Yock P, Naasz C, Schnittger I, et al: Doppler tricuspid and pulmonic regurgitation in normals: Is it real? (abstr). *Circulation* 70(suppl II):40, 1984.

23. Takao S, Miyatake K, Izumi S, et al: Physiological pulmonary regurgitation detected by the Doppler technique and its differential diagnosis (abstr). *J Am Coll Cardiol* 5:499, 1985.

24. Yoshida K, Yoshikawa J, Shokudo M, et al: Color Doppler evaluation of valvular regurgitation in normal subjects. *Circulation* 78:840, 1988.

CHAPTER 4

Aortic Stenosis

Aortic stenosis is a common form of valvular heart disease, especially in the older population.[1] Nevertheless, the identification and quantification of aortic stenosis remains a significant problem in adults with systolic murmurs. Cardiac catheterization is frequently required to identify patients with significant aortic stenosis and to quantitate its severity by determining mean systolic pressure gradient and valve area. Recent advances in Doppler echocardiography combined with 2D imaging have increased the accuracy of the noninvasive assessment of aortic stenosis. Doppler echocardiography has also provided additional insight into understanding the hemodynamics of this valvular lesion, and in certain instances, challenged the accuracy of measurements at cardiac catheterization.

M-MODE AND TWO-DIMENSIONAL ECHOCARDIOGRAPHY

Echocardiography is a sensitive technique for detecting structural abnormalities of the aortic valve. Valvular calcification or thickening as well as reduced mobility of the aortic valve is best evaluated in the short axis, 2D view.[2] With increasing age and development of calcification, however, recognition of this congenital abnormality is more difficult. With further progression of the severity of aortic stenosis, the cusps become less mobile with a reduced systolic separation. Measurement of cusp separation or visualization of the valve orifice are useful in differentiating the normal or mildly stenotic valve from those with more advanced grades of stenosis.[3,4] Despite improvement in imaging technology, significant overlap still exists in the distinction between moderate and critical stenosis, where a clinical decision as to replacement or balloon valvuloplasty of the aortic valve is needed.

Prior to the application of Doppler ultrasound for the assessment of valvular heart disease, M-mode echocardiography was used to indirectly predict peak left ventricular pressure. Assuming normalization of wall stress by compensatory concentric hypertrophy, measurement of wall thickness and diameter of the left ventricle were performed to predict left ventricular pressure.[5–7] This method was used predominantly in children in whom the quality of M-mode recordings is good. In adult patients, a suboptimal quality M-mode recording or presence of regional dyssynergy, left ventricular dilation, systemic hypertension, or a depressed ejection fraction preclude the use of this concept. This method has been all but abandoned with the recent application of Doppler echocardiography, which provides accurate estimates of instantaneous and mean pressure gradients across the aortic valve.

Doppler echocardiography has had a major impact on increasing the accuracy of the noninvasive assessment of aortic stenosis. Particularly when combined with imaging (including color flow imaging), Doppler echocardiography has improved the accuracy of localizing flow disturbances and differentiating valvular aortic stenosis from other clinically mimicking conditions such as mitral regurgitation and fixed or dynamic subaortic obstruction.[8,9] Recordings of stenotic jet velocity have allowed the determination of instantaneous pressure gradients across the aortic valve using the modified Bernoulli equation (see Chap. 2). More recently, the application of the continuity equation to Doppler recordings combined with 2D echocardiographic imaging, has yielded accurate measurements of valve area.

BLOOD VELOCITY NEAR A REGION OF VASCULAR STENOSIS

An experimental flow model based on concepts developed in models of stenotic lesions and observed in vivo is useful in understanding the velocity patterns near stenotic valves.[10–14] Figure 4–1 illustrates the characteristics of blood velocity near a region of valvular stenosis. Upstream from the region of stenosis at R_1, normal flow is characterized by velocity vectors that have nearly the same speed and direction (laminar flow).

The cross-sectional area of the vessel within the stenosis is small compared with the area of the vessel upstream or downstream from the stenosis. Because volume flow is equal throughout the vessel, blood velocity through the stenosis is elevated. A localized region of high velocity, noted at region R_2, is characterized by very high blood velocities. If the stenosis is symmetric, a high-velocity jet is directed downstream from the stenosis parallel to the long axis of the vessel. If asymmetry is present, the velocity vectors may not be parallel to the long axis of the vessel.

A region of turbulence or nonlaminar flow (R_3) is noted downstream from the high-velocity region. Velocity vectors in the region of turbulence

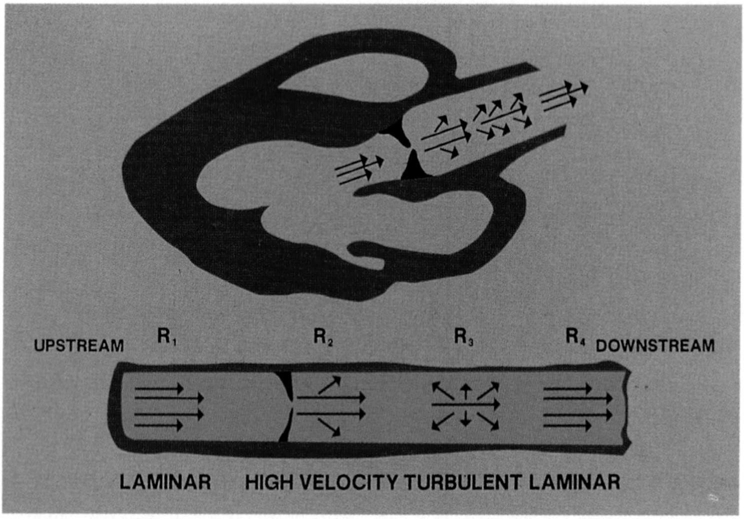

Figure 4–1. A model of blood flow through a region of stenosis shows regions of laminar flow (R_1), high velocity jet (R_2), turbulence (R_3), and reestablishment of laminar flow (R_4). Stenosis can be identified by the presence of high velocity and turbulence.

are characterized by wide differences in direction and speed, even when a small volume of blood is sampled. Within this flow disturbance, red blood cells move in a radial fashion away from the net flow vector, and red blood cell velocities gradually decrease as they move farther away from the jet. Finally, downstream from the region of turbulence, flow again becomes laminar (R_4). Both the velocity of flow in the jet, and the flow disturbance beyond the jet, are useful descriptors of the presence and severity of valvular stenosis.

TRANSDUCER POSITIONS AND SAMPLING SITES

Most Doppler examinations are presently performed by orienting the transducer from multiple available windows to obtain maximal velocity recordings, therefore assuming that the least angle between the ultrasound beam and velocity vector has been obtained. Ignoring the Doppler angle may lead to an underestimation of actual velocities. When actual angles are greater than 20°, the incorrect assumption of a Doppler angle can lead to even larger errors in under or overestimation of the true velocity.[15] The apical, right parasternal, and suprasternal notch positions are most commonly utilized; occasionally in a very difficult patient, the subcostal and left parasternal positions have also proved valuable.

The apical window is the most valuable Doppler transducer location in adults and is particularly useful in patients with emphysema. It should be obtained with the probe placed directly over the cardiac apex and the patient in the left lateral decubitus position. The parasternal approach, with the transducer placed in the second right intercostal space and the patient in the right lateral decubitus position, has also proved quite useful in the elderly. The suprasternal window, performed with the patient supine, may occasionally be useful in adults, but is most valuable in children. Examination from each of these three transducer positions is necessary in every patient for the operator to be sure that the proper jet has been interrogated and the true maximum velocity recorded.

PULSED DOPPLER EVALUATION

With the capability of range-gated resolution (PD) echocardiography can localize precisely the site of disturbed or increased flow velocity associated with valvular stenosis. Because of high velocities through and just distal to the stenosis, aliasing by PD occurs and determination of jet velocity is not possible. Thus, most methods that assess aortic stenosis severity by PD rely on the area or amount of flow disturbance distal to the stenosis and/or on the ejection dynamics proximal to the stenosis. Prior to the application of (CW) Doppler, we used PD to measure the duration of systolic flow disturbance and to quantify the amount of turbulent blood flow distal to the aortic valve.[16] The method was useful in separating patients with valve areas under and above 1 cm^2. Other investigators also have used PD techniques in an attempt to quantify valvular aortic stenosis with varying results.[14,17] With the advent of CW Doppler, these methods now are seldom used.

One recent study evaluated the utility of ejection flow dynamics by PD at the left ventricular outflow tract in 44 patients with aortic stenosis.[18] Among the systolic time intervals tested, a prolonged acceleration time to ejection time ratio of > 0.52, although not sensitive, was 100 percent specific for critical aortic stenosis (valve area < 0.75 cm^2 at catheterization). Thus, a delayed peaking of the systolic velocity proximal to the aortic valve can alert the echocardiographer to the presence of critical aortic stenosis.

In aortic stenosis, the left ventricular ejection time is prolonged but does not correlate well with the severity of the lesion.[19–22] A significant relation between aortic valve area and the degree of prolongation of ejection time in relation to stroke volume at catheterization has been previously reported.[22] This concept has been applied to Doppler echocardiography.[23] Stroke volume was measured by PD at the aortic anulus and ejection time was derived from the Doppler tracing. A predicted ejection time from stroke volume measurements was calculated using a relation described by Harley and coworkers[24] as

$$\text{Predicted ET} = 0.002\,\text{SV} + 0.106$$

where SV = stroke volume in milliliters and ET = ejection time in seconds. An ejection time difference was defined as the measured minus the predicted ejection time. The ejection time difference related significantly to valve area by catheterization ($r = -0.87$). An ejection time difference of >0.060 s was 89 percent accurate for detecting critical aortic stenosis. Because this index is independent of jet velocity measurements, it can be used to corroborate results obtained with the continuity equation (discussed below), particularly in cases where adequate interrogation of the aortic stenosis jet by CW Doppler is in doubt or not feasible.

CONTINUOUS WAVE DOPPLER EVALUATION

With blood flow remaining constant, flow velocity through a valvular stenosis accelerates when compared to the velocity proximal to the stenosis. At present, CW Doppler is the preferred method for measuring the high-velocity jet through the stenotic orifice. From adequate recordings of the jet velocity, hemodynamic assessment of aortic stenosis severity is possible.

Quantitation of Aortic Stenosis

The Bernoulli equation (see Chap. 2) allows the calculation of pressure drop through a stenosis. Initial studies by Hatle and coworkers and several investigations thereafter, in the experimental laboratory and in patients with aortic stenosis, have shown that accurate estimates of instantaneous pressure gradients can be derived with the simplified Bernoulli equation ($P_1 - P_2 = 4\,V^2$) over a wide range of gradients measured hemodynamically.[25–35] The mean systolic gradient can also be calculated from the CW Doppler velocity recordings by determining the mean of multiple systolic instantaneous gradients. The maximal velocity should be measured from multiple points, approximately three to five equally spaced intervals along the spectral envelope, and the gradient calculated at each point using the simplified Bernoulli equation. Adding the sum of the gradients and dividing by the number of points sampled will give a very accurate mean gradient (Fig. 4–2). Comparison between Doppler-derived mean systolic gradients and gradients obtained at cardiac catheterization have

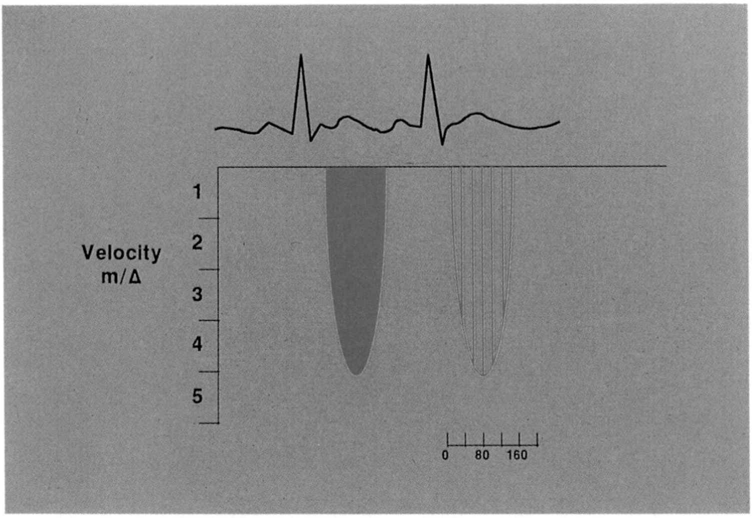

Figure 4–2. Schematic diagram of a patient with severe aortic stenosis. The Doppler spectral envelope shows the maximal instantaneous gradient derived from the highest point on the velocity curve, in meters per second (m/s), using the Bernoulli equation. The mean gradient is the average of the instantaneous gradients.

been performed in experimental animals and in patients with aortic stenosis, with strong correlation between the two techniques.[28,30,31,34,35]

Doppler echocardiography estimates of pressure gradients are those of instantaneous gradients between left ventricle and ascending aorta (Fig. 4–3). Timing of the peak jet velocity by Doppler methods corresponds closely to that of the peak instantaneous gradient between the two chambers. With worsening aortic stenosis, the rate of rise of aortic pressure decreases, resulting in a delayed peak instantaneous gradient into systole. Thus, an inspection of the jet velocity recording by CW Doppler for the contour of the time-velocity curve and for timing of the maximal velocity may be helpful as a qualitative assessment of stenosis severity.[25,34] A symmetric and rounded velocity contour with late peaking of the jet velocity is usually seen in severe aortic stenosis (Fig. 4–4), as opposed to a more asymmetric triangular contour, with early peaking of the jet velocity in mild lesions (Fig. 4–5). One advantage of this simple index is that it is independent of the Doppler angle, and probably is still reliable in the presence of low flow states.

Ideally, measurements of aortic pressure gradients at catheterization should be performed with simultaneous recordings of left ventricular and central aortic pressure. Because of the simplicity of pressure measure-

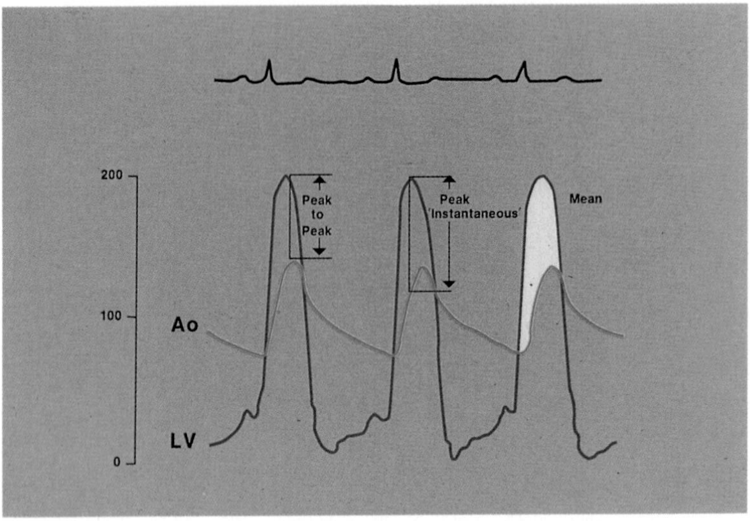

Figure 4–3. The pressure gradient between the aorta (Ao) and left ventricle (LV) reported at cardiac catheterization is the difference between the peak left ventricle and peak aortic pressures (peak to peak) while Doppler techniques measure the peak instantaneous difference. The mean pressure gradient represents the average pressure gradient throughout systole.

ments by catheter pull back from left ventricle to aorta, however, peak-to-peak gradients have been popularized as an index of aortic stenosis severity. As shown in Fig. 4–3, a peak-to-peak catheterization gradient is a nonsimultaneous gradient between ventricle and aorta. The maximal or peak instantaneous gradient during systole, which is the maximal gradient derived by Doppler techniques, is usually higher than peak-to-peak gradient (see Fig. 4–3), especially in mild aortic stenosis. Studies comparing maximal gradients by Doppler tracing with peak-to-peak catheterization gradients have shown, as expected, overall higher values of maximal gradients.[28,31,34,36] Because this catheterization index is not instantaneous, it cannot be directly measured by Doppler methods.

The pressure gradient through a stenotic valve is largely dependent on flow. In patients with hemodynamically significant aortic stenosis (pressure gradients above 50 mmHg) and cardiac output in the normal range, the peak aortic flow velocity usually exceeds 3.5 m/s. Even with critical aortic stenosis, however, the aortic flow velocity may not be very high if left ventricular function is significantly diminished and the cardiac output reduced. Conversely, a high pressure gradient can be found in the absence of severe stenosis in patients with high output states (Fig. 4–6).

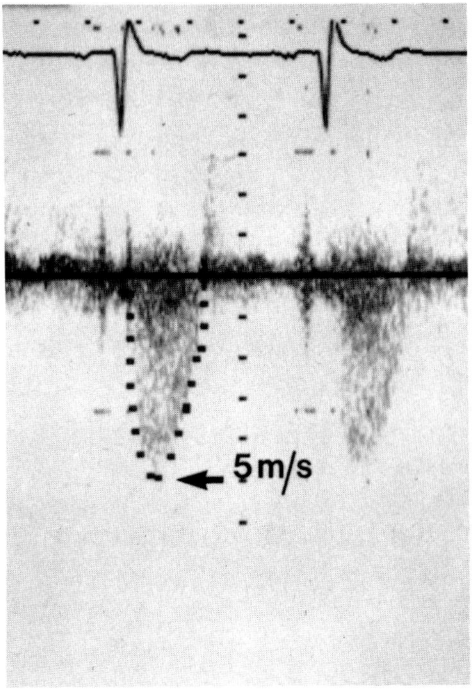

Figure 4–4. Continuous wave Doppler tracing from a patient with severe aortic stenosis. The transducer positioned at the apex records a peak flow velocity of 5 m/s (calculated gradient 100 mmHg). Note the symmetric and rounded velocity contour.

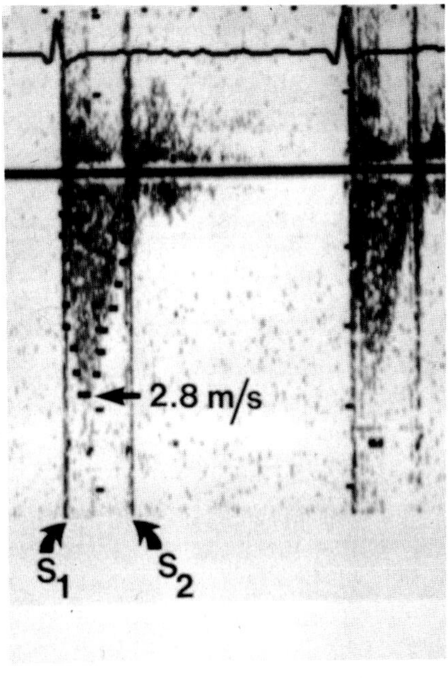

Figure 4–5. Continuous wave Doppler tracing from a patient with insignificant (mild) aortic stenosis. The spectral envelope is asymmetrical, with a very rapid descending limb and a much slower ascending limb. The peak velocity is 2.8 m/s (calculated gradient 31 mmHg). S_1 = first heart sound, S_2 = second heart sound.

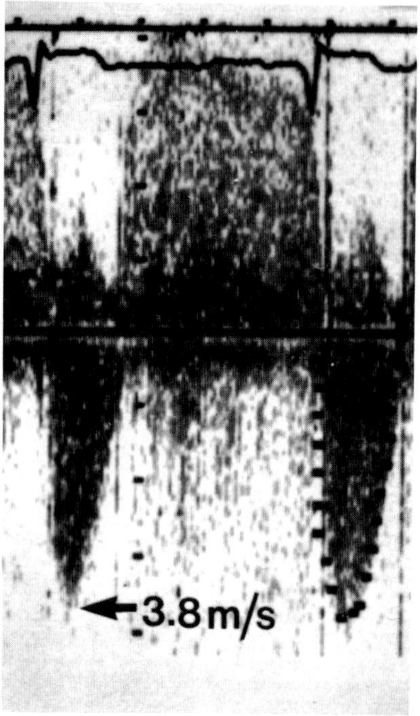

Figure 4–6. Continuous wave Doppler tracing from a patient with mild aortic stenosis and aortic regurgitation. Although the peak velocity is 3.8 m/s (calculated gradient 57 mmHg), at catheterization the peak-to-peak gradient was 10 mmHg. Note the CW spectrum peaks in early systole (arrow).

Thus, a mean pressure gradient of only 25 mmHg may be seen in a patient with severe valvular stenosis and a low cardiac output, whereas a high output state in a patient with a gradient of 50 mmHg may imply only mild to moderate stenosis. In other instances, determination of valve area is important to assess the severity of valvular stenosis.

Differential Diagnosis of the Spectral Envelope

Aortic valvular stenosis, mitral regurgitation, and hypertrophic cardiomyopathy all produce signals from the apical transducer position that are systolic, move in the same direction (away from the transducer and below the baseline), and can be of similar magnitude (Fig. 4–7). Confusion may occur if two of these high velocity signals (e.g., mitral regurgitation and severe aortic stenosis) coexist, or if two left ventricular outflow tract lesions (hypertrophic cardiomyopathy and valvular aortic stenosis) must be differentiated. Notation of beam orientation, analysis of the audio signal, timing of the flow signal, and analysis of the spectral envelope are useful in differentiating these three lesions.

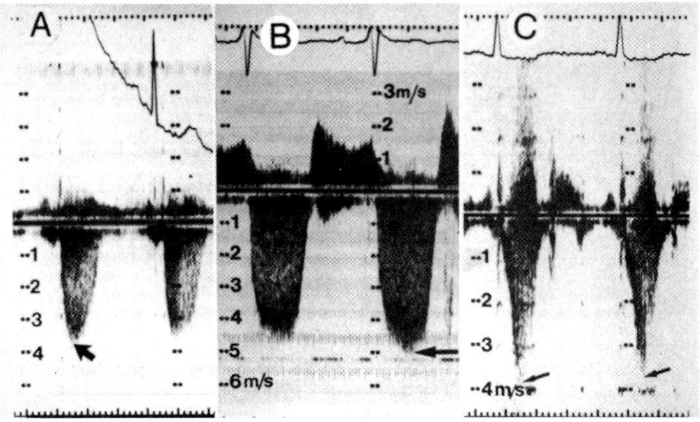

Figure 4 – 7. Continuous wave spectral tracings from three patients with apical systolic murmurs. (A) The relatively narrow band, which begins after the R wave of the electrocardiogram, and increased peak velocity (3.9 m/s) are characteristic of significant aortic stenosis. (B) The wide, clearly defined spectral band that begins with the R wave of the electrocardiogram (holosystolic duration), the markedly increased velocity (5 m/s), and the increased mitral forward flow velocity (2.1 m/s) seen above the baseline are characteristic of severe mitral regurgitation. (C) The mid-to-late systolic peak with the ski-slope appearance and increased peak velocity (3.8 m/s) are characteristic of hypertrophic cardiomyopathy.

The aortic stenosis jet is usually higher pitched, of lower velocity, of shorter duration, and relatively later in onset than is the jet of holosystolic mitral regurgitation. The jet velocity in mitral regurgitation is frequently greater than 4 m/s with peak velocities usually 6 to 7 m/s, whereas the peak velocity of aortic stenosis is directly dependent on the lesion's severity; severe stenosis produces jet velocities above 3.5 m/s, but rarely above 6 m/s. When these lesions coexist, the maximum Doppler velocity of the regurgitant jet is always higher than that of aortic stenosis.

The ejection and regurgitant systolic periods and the relationship of the spectral waveform to the opening and closing of the valve sounds can also be used to differentiate aortic stenosis and mitral regurgitation. The aortic ejection period is usually shorter than the holosystolic mitral regurgitant period; the latter lasts until the mitral valve opens. As aortic stenosis becomes more severe, the ejection time becomes prolonged and the peak velocity is delayed. A major difference, however, is that the maximum velocity of mitral regurgitation almost always is obtained from the apical transducer position, whereas the maximum aortic velocity may be obtained from other acoustic windows (e.g., suprasternal, right parasternal positions).

The shape of the CW spectral envelope is also beneficial in distinguishing hypertrophic cardiomyopathy from valvular aortic stenosis. Hypertrophic cardiomyopathy is characterized by a mid-to-late peaking, ski-slope shaped spectral envelope, whereas valvular or supravalvular stenosis has an early or midspectral peak.

Doppler color flow imaging is also useful in the differential diagnosis of patients with outflow tract murmurs. In addition, PD and CFI can distinguish these three lesions from others that produce systolic murmurs, such as pulmonary stenosis, ventricular septal defect, and tricuspid regurgitation.

DETERMINATION OF VALVE AREA

The pressure gradient across a stenotic valve depends largely on the flow through the area of stenosis, which, in turn, depends on left ventricular performance and the presence of concomitant valvular regurgitation. Thus, to account for the effect of flow, a determination of valve area is necessary. Until recently, cardiac catheterization has been the only definitive means of quantifying aortic stenosis by the determination of stenotic area using the Gorlin equation.[37] Initial noninvasive determination of valve area was demonstrated in young patients with predominant pulmonic stenosis with the use of Doppler-determined velocities and a modification of the Gorlin equation.[38]

More recently, a new noninvasive method has been proposed for estimating aortic valve area by using the continuity equation.[35] The equation is based on a physics principle that states that in the presence of obstruction within a continuous-flow channel, the product of flow area times velocity will remain constant on both sides of the obstruction (Fig. 4–8). Thus, in aortic stenosis, $A_2 \times V_2 = A_1 \times V_1$, where A_2 is the area of the stenotic aortic valve orifice; V_2, the velocity of flow through the orifice; A_1, the area of flow below the obstruction (in the left ventricular outflow tract); and V_1, the velocity of blood flow below the aortic valve (in the outflow tract). By solving for the aortic valve area (A_2), the equation then becomes $A_2 = A_1 \times V_1/V_2$. Recording of the left ventricular outflow velocity (V_1) is performed with PD, using the apical approach, by placing the sample volume within the left ventricular outflow tract proximal to the aortic valve. Peak velocity of flow through the aortic valve (V_2) can similarly be obtained using the CW Doppler technique (Fig. 4–9).

Cross-sectional area of the aortic anulus (A_1) is derived from a diameter (D) measurement assuming a circular geometry as $\pi D^2/4$. The diameter

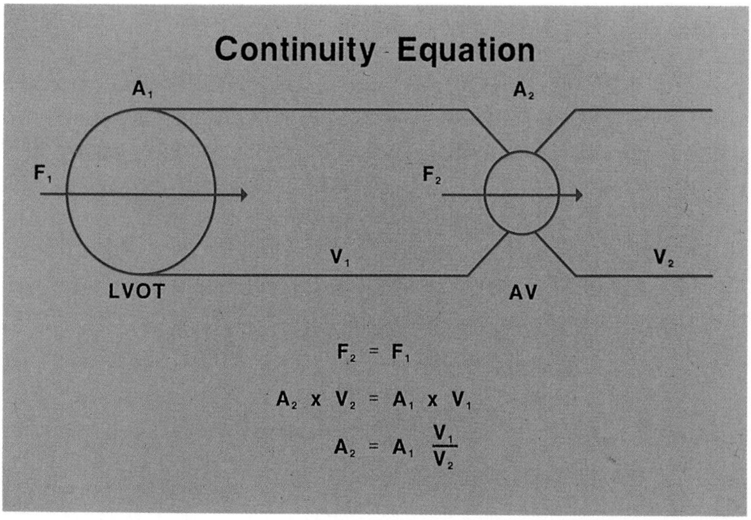

Figure 4-8. Diagram illustrating the principle of the continuity equation for calculating aortic valve area. The continuity principle states that flow (F_1) through the left ventricular outflow tract (LVOT) is equal to flow (F_2) through the aortic valve (AV). The ratio of flow velocity (V_1/V_2) times the LVOT area (A_1) yields the aortic valve area (A_2).

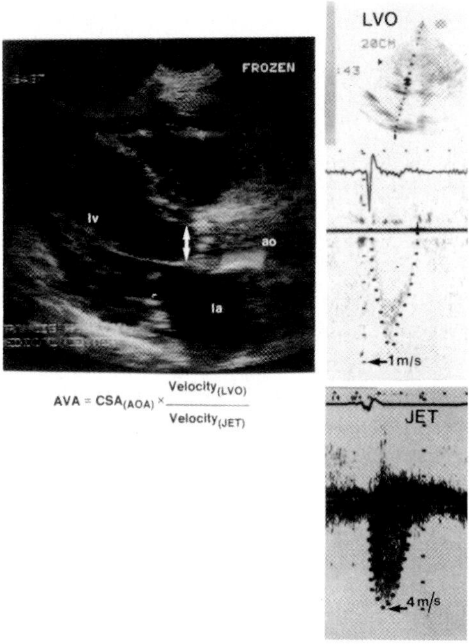

Figure 4-9. Echocardiographic and Doppler recordings needed for aortic valve area (AVA) calculation from the left ventricular outflow approach (LVO), using the continuity equation. *Left*: Echocardiographic freeze frame during early systole in the parasternal long axis view showing the diameter (D) measurement of the aortic anulus (arrow). Cross-sectional area (CSA) of the aortic anulus (AOA) is calculated as $\pi D^2/4$. *Right*: Pulsed Doppler recordings from the apical window in the LVO (upper) and continuous wave recording of jet velocity (lower) from the window providing an adequate recording with the highest peak velocity.

of the aortic anulus is measured during early systole, preferably from a parasternal long-axis view since it involves axial echocardiographic resolution (see Fig. 4–9). The presence of aortic valve calcification usually does not interfere with measurements of the anulus diameter at the insertion of the aortic cusps. Diameter measurements are usually performed from inner echocardiographic edge to inner edge, although some investigators have preferred a leading edge to leading edge method.[35]

Therefore, the simplified continuity equation for determination of aortic valve area (AVA) is

$$AVA = CSA_{AOA} \times \frac{Velocity_{LVO}}{Velocity_{jet}}$$

where CSA_{AOA} is the cross-sectional area of the aortic anulus. This noninvasive approach allows assessment of the severity of aortic stenosis independent of aortic regurgitation and other valve disease. In addition, it is not significantly affected by abnormal left ventricular function.

Multiple reports have validated the use of echo-Doppler techniques to measure aortic valve area by the continuity equation.[35,36,39–45] Most of the reparted discrepancies have been in the range of mild aortic stenosis, where the Gorlin equation probably overestimates valve area as the gradient approaches zero. Furthermore, the Gorlin formula may produce significant errors of up to 20 percent or more by including an empirical constant, the discharge coefficient.[46,47] Additional errors may also arise from measurements of cardiac output and pressure gradients by current catheter techniques.[48,49]

COLOR FLOW IMAGING

Visualization of a discrete jet in aortic stenosis is considerably more difficult than in mitral, tricuspid, or pulmonic stenosis. Comprehensive color flow examination of the aortic valve should be performed along the long axis from high left and right parasternal positions as well as suprasternal notch transducer positions. The apical view is of limited value in adults with aortic stenosis, due to far-field imaging and problems of attenuation of signal strength. When visualized from parasternal and suprasternal notch positions, flow in the ascending aorta is directed toward the transducer and is represented in shades of red. However, the ascending aortic flow velocity frequently exceeds the Nyquist limit in normal patients; therefore, simple aliasing with resultant color reversal is noted in the ascending aorta in early systole (Fig. 4–10). As the velocities diminish in mid and late systole, the flow map assumes a yellow-orange color. In normal

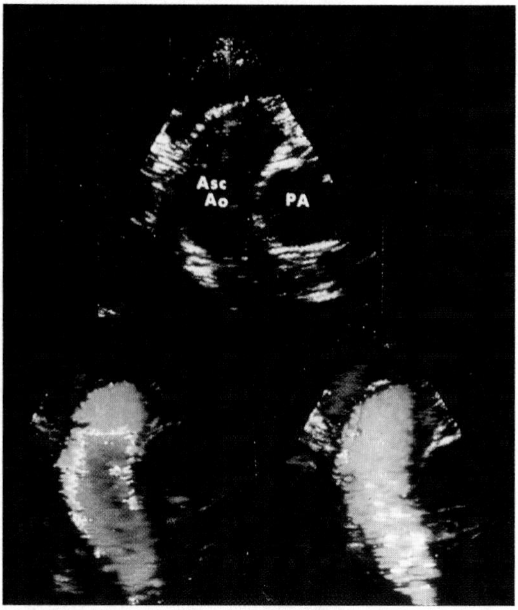

Figure 4–10. Normal ascending aortic flow. *Upper*: Still-frame of 2D echocardiogram from suprasternal position showing the ascending aorta. *Lower left*: Normal aortic flow during early systole. Note the smooth, homogeneous central appearance of blue due to simple color reversal (aliasing). Flow in early systole has a high velocity, resulting in color reversal. Lack of mosaic pattern indicates laminar flow. *Lower right*: Normal aortic flow in midsystole. Note that flow is laminar and returns to red-orange color as velocities decrease to below the Nyquist limit. PA = pulmonary artery, Asc Ao = ascending aorta.

patients, the flow is laminar without turbulence, therefore, mosaic colors are not present.

In aortic stenosis, velocities are high and the flow becomes increasingly turbulent. The color signal becomes aliased and mosaic. A diffuse mosaic pattern in the aortic root and ascending aorta throughout systole typically is seen in patients with severe obstruction. A discrete jet frequently can be recorded in younger patients. Analysis of the jet in early systole is characterized by an area of orange color in the subvalvular region in the left ventricular outflow tract. This turns into blue color (aliasing) as the velocities accelerate immediately below the stenotic orifice. As it emerges through the orifice, the jet assumes a mushroom-like appearance in the ascending aorta and characteristically is composed of mosaic colors due to high velocity turbulent flow. In late systole, due to lowering of velocities, the flow assumes a red-orange color (Fig. 4–11).

The size, direction, shape, and turbulence of the flow jet depend upon the morphology of the stenotic valve, severity of stenosis, and the size of the aortic root. For example, a narrow discrete jet may be seen in young patients with a bicuspid valve while a broad mosaic patterned jet may be seen due to a turbulent flow spray in adult patients with calcific aortic stenosis. The direction of the jet may be central or eccentric. Eccentric jets are often directed toward the right lateral wall of the aortic root, but can be medial, anterior, or posterior.

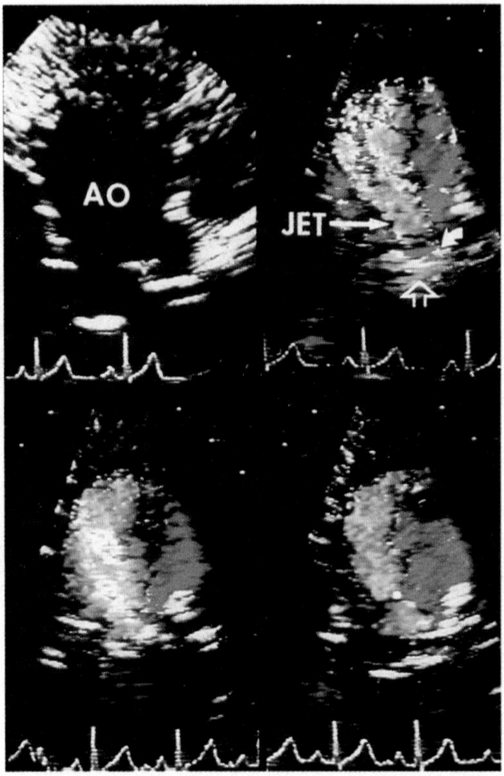

Figure 4–11. Color flow imaging in aortic stenosis. *Upper left*: Still-frame of a 2D echocardiogram of the ascending aorta (AO) from right parasternal position. Note the thickened aortic leaflets. *Upper right*: Jet of aortic stenosis visualized in the ascending aorta in early systole. The jet is shaped like a mushroom and has a mosaic appearance due to high velocity turbulent flow. Also note the surrounding zone of blue due to formation of vortices. Here flow is moving away from the transducer towards the aortic root. In the subvalvular region there is an area of orange (open arrow), signifying normal velocity flow toward the transducer. Just beneath the aortic valve, the color changes to blue (curved, solid arrow) due to color reversal from acceleration of blood flow as it approaches the stenotic orifice. *Lower left*: In midsystole, as the velocities diminish, the flow assumes a candle flame appearance with a central zone of blue from aliasing and color reversal due to velocities exceeding Nyquist limit. The peripheral zone is a mosaic of orange-red representing turbulence. *Lower right*: In late systole, as the velocities diminish further, the flow map becomes orange-red and the jet remains discrete and well defined. The blue color on the periphery represents vortex formation.

In those patients in whom discrete jets are visualized, flow-guided CW Doppler beam can be aligned along the stenosis jet and CW Doppler recordings can be obtained for quantitative analysis[50] (Fig. 4–12). Some investigators have found good correlation between the maximal aortic stenosis jet width and the aortic valve area estimated at catheterization.[51,52] Visualization of aortic stenosis jet has been feasible in up to 60 percent of patients.[51–53] In my experience, however, visualization of a discrete jet has been extremely difficult in older patients with severe calcific aortic stenosis.

Frequently, aortic stenosis is associated with aortic regurgitation. Color flow imaging is valuable in the detection and quantitation of aortic regurgitation (see Chap. 7). If aortic regurgitation is severe, it increases the antegrade flow velocity. This should be taken into account when using the aortic valve gradient as an indicator of the severity of aortic stenosis. De-

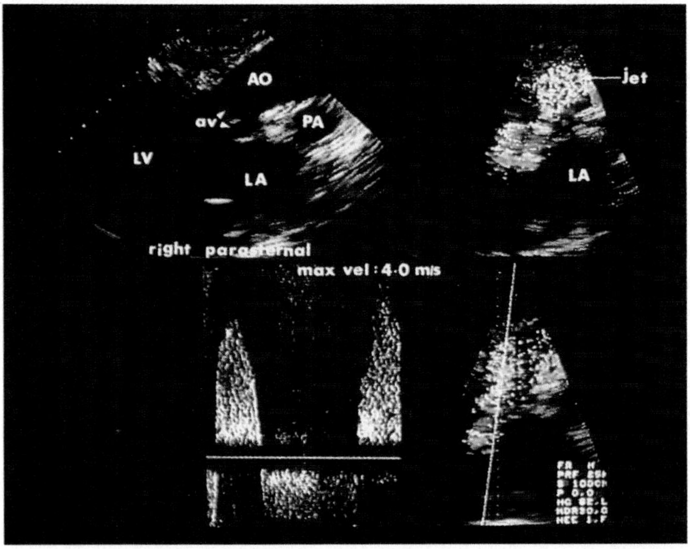

Figure 4–12. Color flow imaging in aortic stenosis. *Upper left*: Still-frame of 2D echocardiogram of the ascending aorta (Ao) from right parasternal position. LV = left ventricle; LA = left atrium; PA = pulmonary artery; av = aortic valve. *Upper right*: Color flow of a systolic frame showing a mushroom-shaped jet of aortic stenosis with a diffuse mosaic pattern, indicating high velocity turbulent flow. Note the area of blue just beneath the valve due to color reversal from aliasing as the flow accelerates in the subvalvular region of the left ventricular outflow tract. *Bottom*: Guided CW Doppler examination of the aortic stenosis jet. Spectral display shows the maximum velocity to be 4.0 m/s. The calculated maximum instantaneous gradient was 64 mmHg.

termination of the extent of aortic regurgitation is also important if a patient with aortic stenosis is considered for balloon valvuloplasty since balloon valvuloplasty would not be favored if valvular regurgitation is severe.[54] When mitral regurgitation coexists with aortic stenosis, the degree of mitral regurgitation can be assessed by color flow imaging (see Chap. 8).

DOPPLER ECHOCARDIOGRAPHIC EVALUATION OF AORTIC BALLOON VALVULOPLASTY

Doppler echocardiography has been used to assess the efficacy of aortic balloon valvuloplasty. There is significant linear correlation between aortic valve area measurements, as derived from continuity equations, and catheterization methods both before valvuloplasty and after valvuloplasty.[55,56] However, one study demonstrated a poorer correlation between catheter-derived and Doppler echo-derived aortic valve areas when taken within 24 h after the valvuloplasty procedure.[55] This has been attributed to a changing hemodynamic milieu in the first few hours immediately after the procedure, which may be related to transient left ventricular dysfunction. This results in significant changes in cardiac output, mean aortic valve gradient, and aortic valve area over a 24-h period after the procedure.[57–59] Therefore, calculation of a Doppler-derived aortic valve area and mean aortic valve gradient performed 24 to 48 h after the procedure would provide a better representation of the immediate results of aortic valvuloplasty.

REFERENCES

1. Selzer A: Changing aspects of the natural history of valvular aortic stenosis. *N Engl J Med* 317:91, 1987.
2. Fowles R, Martin R, Abrams J, et al: Two-dimensional echocardiographic features of bicuspid aortic valve. *Chest* 75:434, 1979.
3. Weyman A, Feigenbaum H, Dillon J, et al: Cross-sectional echocardiography in assessing the severity of valvular aortic stenosis. *Circulation* 52:828, 1975.
4. DeMaria A, Bommer W, Joye J, et al: Value and limitations of cross-sectional echocardiography of the aortic valve in the diagnosis and quantification of valvular aortic stenosis. *Circulation* 62:304, 1980.
5. Bennett D, Evans D, Raj M: Echocardiographic left ventricular dimensions in pressure and volume overload: Their use in assessing aortic stenosis. *Br Heart J* 37:971, 1975.

6. Quinones M, Mokotoff D, Nouri S, et al: Noninvasive quantification of left ventricular wall stress: Validation of method and application to assessment of chronic pressure overload. *Am J Cardiol* 45:782, 1980.

7. Schwartz A, Vignola P, Walker H, et al: Echocardiographic estimation of aortic valve gradient in aortic stenosis. *Ann Intern Med* 89:329, 1978.

8. Hatle L: Noninvasive assessment and differentiation of left ventricular outflow tract obstruction with Doppler ultrasound. *Circulation* 64:381, 1981.

9. Kowaben I, Stevenson J, Dooley T, et al: Evaluation of ejection murmurs by pulsed Doppler echocardiography. *Br Heart J* 43:623, 1980.

10. Clark C: Relationship between pressure difference across the aortic valve and left ventricular outflow. *Cardiovasc Res* 12:276, 1978.

11. Kececioglu-Draelos Z, Goldberg S, Areias J, et al: Verification and clinical demonstration of the echo Doppler series effect and vortex shed distance. *Circulation* 63:1422, 1981.

12. Neren R, Seed W, Wood N: An experimental study of the velocity, distribution and transition to turbulence in the aorta. *J Fluid Mech* 52:137, 1972.

13. Felix W, Sigel B, Gibson R, et al: Pulsed Doppler ultrasound detection of flow disturbances in atherosclerosis. JCU 4:275, 1977.

14. Goldberg S, Kececioglu-Draelos Z, Sahn D, et al: Range gated echo-Doppler velocity and turbulence mapping in patients with valvular aortic stenosis. *Am Heart J* 103:858, 1982.

15. Hatle L, Angelson B: *Doppler Ultrasound in Cardiology*, ed 2. Philadelphia, Lea & Febiger, 1985.

16. Young J, Quinones M, Waggoner A, et al: Diagnosis and quantification of aortic stenosis with pulsed-Doppler echocardiography. *Am J Cardiol* 45:987, 1980.

17. Stevenson J, Kawabori I: Non-invasive determination of pressure gradients in children: Two methods employing pulsed Doppler echocardiography. *J Am Coll Cardiol* 3:179, 1984.

18. Zoghbi W: Echocardiographic and Doppler ultrasonic evaluation of valvular aortic stenosis. *Echocardiography* 5:23, 1988.

19. Benchimol A, Dimond E, Shen Y: Ejection time in aortic stenosis and mitral stenosis: Comparison between the direct and indirect arterial tracings, with special reference to pre- and postoperative findings. *Am J Cardiol* 5:728, 1960.

20. Epstein E, Coulshed N: Assessment of aortic stenosis from the external carotid pulse wave. *Br Heart J* 26:84, 1964.

21. Nesje O: Severity of aortic stenosis assessed by carotid pulse recordings and phonocardiography. *Acta Med Scand* 204:321, 1978.

22. Boche R, Wang Y, Greenfield J Jr: Left ventricular ejection time in valvular aortic stenosis. *Circulation* 47:527, 1973.

23. Zoghbi W, Sterling L, Farmer K, et al: Accurate determination of aortic stenosis severity with pulsed Doppler echocardiography independent of jet velocity (abstr). *Circulation* 72 (suppl III):305, 1985.

24. Harley A, Starmer C, Greenfield J Jr: Pressure-flow studies in man: An evaluation of the duration of the phases of systole. *J Clin Invest* 48:895, 1969.

25. Hatle L, Angelsen B, Tromsdal A: Non-invasive assessment of aortic stenosis by Doppler ultrasound. *Br Heart J* 43:284, 1980.

26. Stamm R, Martin R: Quantification of pressure gradients across stenotic valves by Doppler ultrasound. *J Am Coll Cardiol* 2:707, 1983.

27. Berger M, Bendoff R, Gallerstein P, et al: Evaluation of aortic stenosis by continuous wave Doppler ultrasound. *J Am Coll Cardiol* 3:150, 1984.

28. Currie P, Seward J, Reeder G, et al: Continuous-wave Doppler echocardiographic assessment of severity of calcific aortic stenosis: A simultaneous Doppler-catheter correlative study in 100 adult patients. *Circulation* 6:1162, 1985.

29. Zhang Y, Nitter-Hauge S: Determination of the mean pressure gradient in aortic stenosis by Doppler echocardiography. *Eur Heart J* 6:999, 1985.

30. Callahan M, Tajik A, Su-Fan Q, et al: Validation of instantaneous pressure gradients measured by continuous-wave Doppler in experimentally induced aortic stenosis. *Am J Cardiol* 56:989, 1985.

31. Smith M, Dawson P, Elion J, et al: Correlation of continuous wave Doppler velocities with cardiac catheterization gradients: An experimental model of aortic stenosis. *J Am Coll Cardiol* 6:1306, 1985.

32. Teirstein P, Yock P, Popp R: The accuracy of Doppler ultrasound measurement of pressure gradients across irregular, dual, and tunnel-like obstructions to blood flow. *Circulation* 72:577, 1985.

33. Valdes-Cruz L, Yoganathan A, Tamura T, et al: Studies in vitro of the relationship between ultrasound and Doppler velocimetry and applicability of the simplified Bernoulli relationship. *Circulation* 73:300, 1986.

34. Agatston A, Chengot M, Rao A, et al: Doppler diagnosis of aortic stenosis in patients over 60 years of age. *Am J Cardiol* 56:106, 1985.

35. Skjaerpe T, Hegrenaes L, Hatle L: Noninvasive estimation of valve area in patients with aortic stenosis by Doppler ultrasound and two-dimensional echocardiography. *Circulation* 72:810, 1985.

36. Zoghbi W, Farmer K, Soto J, et al: Accurate noninvasive quantification of stenotic aortic valve area by Doppler echocardiography. *Circulation* 73:452, 1986.

37. Gorlin R, Gorlin S: Hydraulic formula for calculation of the area of the stenotic mitral valve, other cardiac valves, and central circulatory shunts. *Am Heart J* 41:1, 1951.

38. Kosturakis D, Allan H, Goldberg S, et al: Noninvasive quantification of stenotic semilunar valve areas by Doppler echocardiography. *J Am Coll Cardiol* 3:1256, 1984.

39. Warth D, Stewart W, Block P, et al: A new method to calculate aortic valve area without left heart catheterization. *Circulation* 70:978, 1984.

40. Otto C, Pearlman S, Comess K, et al: Determination of the stenotic aortic valve area in adults using Doppler echocardiography. *J Am Coll Cardiol* 7:509, 1986.

41. Teirstein P, Yeager M, Yock P, et al: Doppler echocardiographic measurement of aortic valve area in aortic stenosis: A noninvasive application of the Gorlin formula. *J Am Coll Cardiol* 8:1059, 1986.

42. Richards K, Cannon S, Miller J, et al: Calculation of aortic valve area by Doppler echocardiography: A direct application of the continuity equation. *Circulation* 73:964, 1986.

43. Zhang Y, Myhre E, Nitter-Hauge S: Noninvasive quantification of the aortic valve area in aortic stenosis by Doppler echocardiography. *Eur Heart J* 6:992, 1985.

44. Otto C, Pearlman A, Janko C, et al: Simplification of the Doppler continuity equation for calculating stenotic aortic valve area (abstr). *J Am Coll Cardiol* 9:236A, 1987.

45. Ohlsson J, Wranne B: Noninvasive assessment of valve area in patients with aortic stenosis. *J Am Coll Cardiol* 7:501, 1986.

46. Rodrigo F: Estimation of valve area and "valvular resistance": A critical study of the physical basis of the method employed. *Am Heart J* 45:1, 1953.

47. Cannon S, Richards K, Crawford M: Hydraulic estimation of stenotic orifice area: A correction of the Gorlin formula. *Circulation* 71:1170, 1985.

48. Carabello B: Advances in the hemodynamic assessment of stenotic cardiac valves. *J Am Coll Cardiol* 10:912, 1987.

49. Gorlin R: Calculations of cardiac valve stenosis: Restoring an old concept for advanced applications. *J Am Coll Cardiol* 10:920, 1987.

50. Helmcke F, Perry G, Nanda N: Combined color Doppler and continuous wave Doppler in the evaluation of aortic stenosis (abstr). *J Am Coll Cardiol* 7:101A, 1986.

51. Fan P, Kapur K, Nanda N: Color-guided Doppler echocardiographic assessment of aortic valve stenosis. *J Am Coll Cardiol* 12:441, 1988.

52. Morris A, Roitman D, Nanda N, et al: Color Doppler assessment of stenotic valve area (abstr). *Circulation* 72(suppl III):100, 1985.

53. Grube E, Becher H, Luderitz B: Determination of the severity of aortic valve disease by combined color flow mapping and continuous wave Doppler (abstr). *Circulation* 72(suppl III): 146, 1985.

54. Pandian N, Wang S, McInerney K, et al: Aid of echocardiography in balloon valvuloplasty for aortic stenosis and mitral stenosis (abstr). *J Am Coll Cardiol* 9:217A, 1987.

55. Nishimura R, Holmes D, Reeder G, et al: Doppler evaluation of results of percutaneous aortic balloon valvuloplasty in calcific aortic stenosis. *Circulation* 78:791, 1988.

56. Come P, Riley M, McKay R, et al: Echocardiographic assessment of aortic valve area in elderly patients with aortic stenosis and of changes in valve area after percutaneous balloon valvuloplasty. *J Am Coll Cardiol* 10:115, 1987.

57. Nishimura R, Reeder G, Holmes D, et al: Hemodynamic measurements immediately after percutaneous aortic balloon valvuloplasty may underestimate the resultant valve area (abstr). *Circulation* 76(suppl IV):523, 1987.

58. Borow K, Feldman T, Neumann A, et al: Time-related changes in left ventricular contractility after balloon aortic valvuloplasty (abstr). *Circulation* 76(suppl IV):235A, 1987.

59. Harpole D, Jones R, Bashura T: Serial evaluation of left ventricular function after aortic valvuloplasty utilizing first pass radionuclide angiography (abstr). *Circulation* 76(suppl IV):2076, 1987.

CHAPTER 5

Mitral and Tricuspid Stenosis

MITRAL STENOSIS

One of the most useful applications of the Doppler examination is the quantification of the severity of mitral stenosis. Stenosis of the mitral valve results in a high diastolic velocity (usually exceeding 1.5 m/s) and spectral broadening. The difference in diastolic pressure between the left atrium and left ventricle is increased, and the rapidity of left atrial emptying is reduced in patients with mitral stenosis. This reduced rate of pressure equalization is evident on a Doppler spectral display and appears as a slower decline in the diastolic velocity signal (Fig. 5–1). Mitral stenosis may be identified by using (PD) system to detect abnormal diastolic turbulence downstream from the mitral orifice[1,2] (Fig. 5–2). However, because of aliasing at high velocities, this technique has limitations for the quantitation of the severity of mitral stenosis.

Calculation of Pressure Gradient

Quantitative determination of the transmitral pressure gradient in patients with mitral stenosis has been performed by CW Doppler examination with or without simultaneous imaging.[3–6] This method and the data derived from it appear to yield the most useful clinical information at present. Measurement of the peak diastolic flow velocities is best made from the apical position. Using the modified Bernoulli equation ($\Delta P = 4V^2$), these flow velocities are used to calculate the transmitral pressure change at any point in time during diastole.

Hatle et al[3] and Holen et al[4,7,8] showed that maximal velocity in mitral stenosis is usually obtained after initial opening of the valve. The velocity waveform then decreases slightly and, in sinus rhythm, peaks again following the onset of atrial contraction (Fig. 5–3). In the presence of atrial fibrillation, there is a gradual decrease in velocity from the early diastolic peak; the atrial contraction wave present in normal subjects in late diastole is

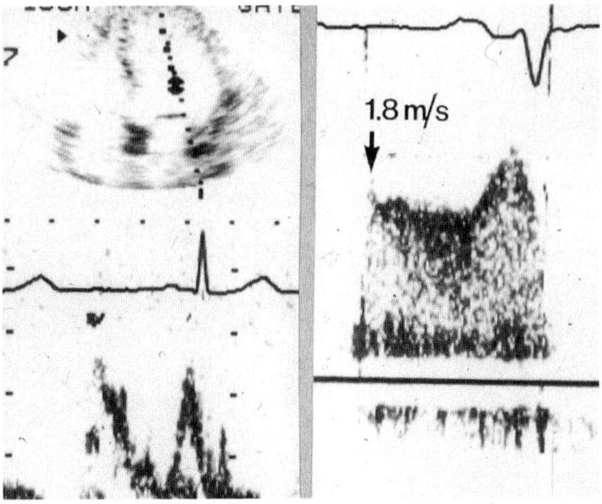

Figure 5–1. Doppler echocardiographic tracings of mitral valve. *Left*: Normal mitral flow pattern (pulsed wave recording). There is low diastolic flow (less than 1.0 m/s), with an early diastolic peak, rapid decline of velocity during middiastole, and end-diastolic peak corresponding to atrial "kick," (Scale marks = 20 cm/s.) *Right*: Mitral stenosis. During diastole, initial velocity is increased (1.8 m/s) and typical M configuration is still evident. This tracing depicts severe mitral stenosis; atrial kick remains as patient is still in normal sinus rhythm. (Scale marks = 1.0 m/s.)

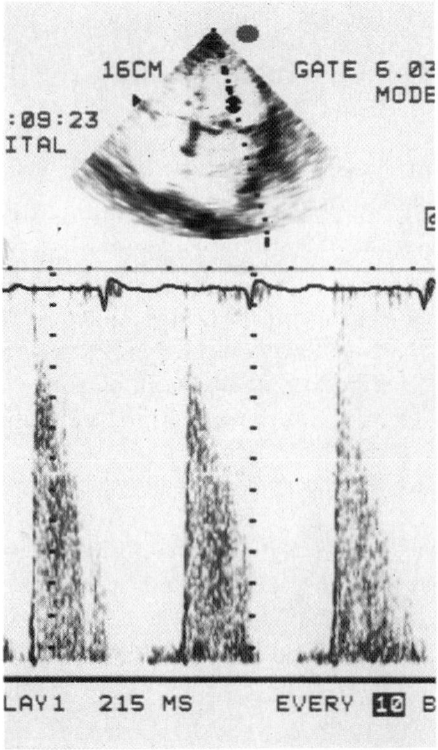

Figure 5–2. Doppler spectral display from a patient with mitral stenosis (pulsed wave recording). Note the diastolic spectral broadening due to turbulence through the stenotic valve. The underlying rhythm is atrial fibrillation. (Scale marks = 20 cm/s.)

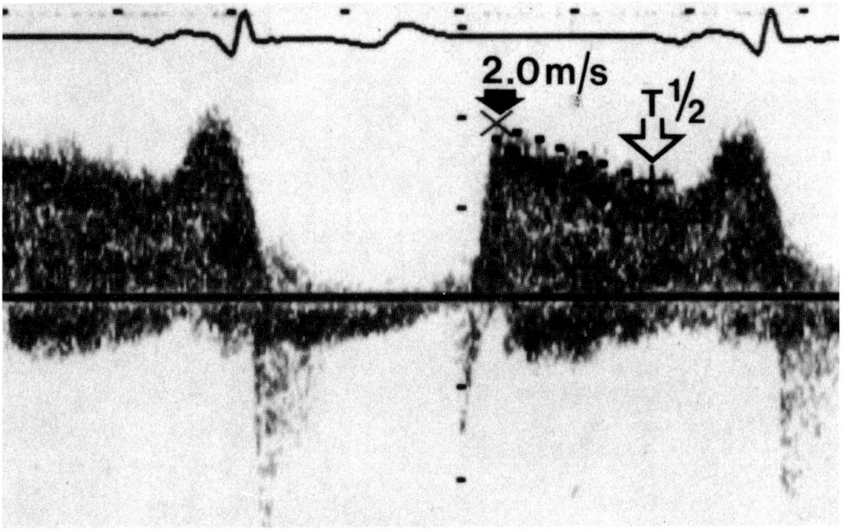

Figure 5-3. Mitral stenosis recorded with continuous wave Doppler. The maximum velocity is 2.0 m/s and the initial gradient (using the modified Bernoulli equation, $\Delta P = 4V^2$) is 16 mmHg. The pressure half-time ($t_{1/2}$) is measured at 235 ms. The estimated valve area is 0.9 cm^2 (see Fig. 5–5 for explanation). Note that after the initial velocity, the waveform velocity decreases slightly and peaks again following the onset of atrial contraction. (Scale marks = 1.0 m/s.)

absent (Fig. 5–4). The rate at which velocity decreases in diastole is inversely proportional to the severity of mitral stenosis.

The mitral pressure gradient measured by CW Doppler method by Holen and Hatle[4,5,7] was virtually identical ($r = 0.92$) to that obtained by simultaneous cardiac catheterization. Other investigators, however, have found that the Doppler technique underestimates the mitral gradient found at catheterization.[9] This inconsistency may be related to an inaccuracy of cardiac catheterization, because the pulmonary wedge pressure may overestimate left atrial pressure, resulting in an artifactually high mitral valve gradient.

Since pressure gradients up to 7 mmHg (velocities up to 1.3 m/s) may be present in normal subjects during early diastole,[3] the calculation of the maximal gradient is not clinically relevant in estimating the severity of mitral stenosis. Attempts to correlate mean mitral gradient with catheterization measurements have also been less successful than those for the aortic valve.[3,5] Limitations in this correlation may be related to (1) errors inherent in measuring relatively small (<20 mmHG) resting gradients that may be present even in severe mitral stenosis, (2) the difficulty in obtain-

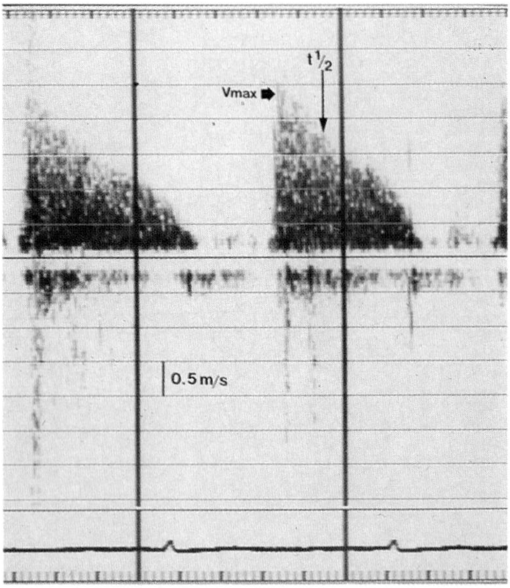

Figure 5–4. Continuous wave Doppler spectral recording from a patient with mitral stenosis. Note absence of atrial contraction due to atrial fibrillation. The maximum velocity (V_{max}) is 2.4 m/s. The pressure half-time ($t_{1/2}$) is measured at 220 ms. The estimated valve area is 1.0 cm^2 (see Fig. 5–5 for explanation).

ing precise left atrial and left ventricular pressure tracings when using standard fluid-filled catheter systems, and (3) the variability of mitral gradient with respect to changes in heart rate, rhythm, and cardiac output.[3]

Use of Pressure Half-Time for Estimating Mitral Valve Area

The sensitivity of the mitral pressure gradient to changes in heart rate and cardiac output clearly makes it an incomplete description of the severity of mitral stenosis. Valve area is generally considered not to vary with changes in cardiac output and is the preferred method for expressing the severity of mitral stenosis.

A method has been described for estimating mitral valve area from Doppler measurements. The approach is based on the measurement of a parameter called the mitral pressure half-time.[6,10,11] The pressure half-time is defined as the time required for the transvalvular gradient to decrease to half its initial value. This measurement is based on the principle that, as the stenosis becomes more severe, the diastolic gradient between the left atrium and the left ventricle is maintained for a longer period and thus results in a slower decline in gradient throughout diastole. When used originally in the cardiac catheterization laboratory, the pressure half-time was shown to be a reasonably accurate measure of the mitral valve area independent of the heart rate or coexistent mitral regurgitation.[10]

Because CW Doppler echocardiography provides an instantaneous recording of pressure drop throughout diastole, the pressure half-time can easily be determined from the Doppler signal (Fig. 5–5). Pressure can be determined from velocity, and, therefore, pressure half-time can be expressed as the time required for the initial velocity to fall to a value equal to the velocity divided by the square root of 2:

$$\text{Pressure half-time} = \frac{\text{Initial velocity (m/s)}}{\sqrt{2}}$$

The normal pressure half-time is 20 to 60 ms. In mitral stenosis, it may range from 100 to 400 ms, depending on the severity of the stenosis. The pressure half-time is inversely proportional to the mitral valve area. An estimate of mitral valve area (in cm^2) can be made by dividing 220 (an empirically derived constant) by the pressure half-time:[9,12]

$$\text{Mitral valve area (cm}^2\text{)} = \frac{220}{\text{Pressure half-time}}$$

These calculations are illustrated in Fig. 5–5. The mitral valve areas obtained using the pressure half-time method have now been shown in several studies to correlate quite well with catheterization measurements.[6,12,13]

The mitral pressure half-time is affected by changes in left atrial and ventricular compliance and initial pressure gradient.[14] Increases in pressure typically decrease atrial and ventricular compliance. For example, in situations of left ventricular hypertrophy or ischemia (with decreased compliance), pressure half-time would be expected to be relatively shortened. Similarly in mitral balloon valvuloplasty, when the dramatic changes in atrial size and pressure greatly affect compliance, the pressure half-time poorly predicts changes in valve area.[15] Furthermore, pressure half-time should not be calculated in patients with atrial tachycardia, prolonged P-R interval, or coexistent severe aortic regurgitation.

Combining the peak velocity and pressure half-time makes deductions about mitral flow possible to some degree. For example, with a long pressure half-time, a high velocity would indicate severe stenosis with maintained or increased flow, and a low velocity would indicate reduced flow across the mitral valve. In a patient with mitral stenosis, an increase in pressure half-time would indicate progressive stenosis, whereas a reduction in velocity would indicate a decrease in mitral flow and cardiac output. When pressure half-time is short, a high velocity would indicate increased flow and in combined mitral stenosis and regurgitation, a high velocity in relation to the pressure half-time would indicate that the regurgitation was significant.

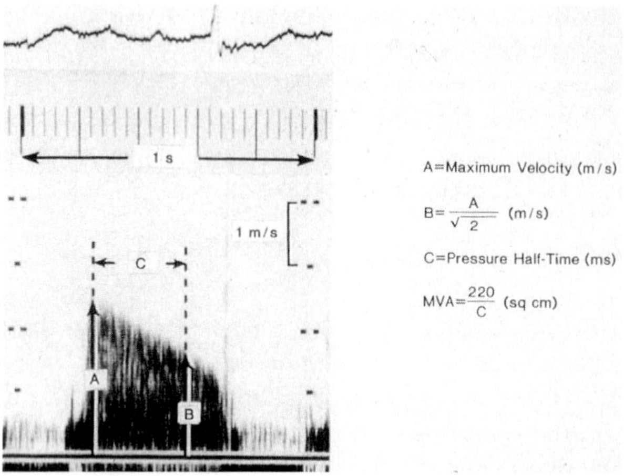

Figure 5–5. Continuous wave Doppler tracing from patient with mitral stenosis and atrial fibrillation demonstrates pressure half-time method for estimating mitral valve area. Point A is highest velocity achieved in early diastole. Point B represents point at which pressure gradient has fallen to half its highest value and is obtained by dividing velocity obtained at point A by square root of 2. Point C represents time (in milliseconds) required for pressure to fall from A to B, or pressure half-time. Mitral valve area (MVA) (in square centimeters) is then calculated by dividing an empirically derived constant by pressure half-time C.

Color Flow Imaging

In mitral stenosis, the broad inflow is replaced by a narrow jet consisting of various colors CFI. The colors are dependent on the flow velocity profile during diastole as well as the magnitude of turbulence (variance). Mitral flow abnormalities in mitral stenosis can be seen in all echocardiographic views such as parasternal long axis, short axis, apical long axis, and apical four chamber views. Apical views are the ideal views to image the mitral flow and to obtain quantitative information.

The characteristic jet of mitral stenosis is comprised of a central blue zone (due to aliasing form high velocities) surrounded by hues of yellow and red (representing lower velocity turbulent flow) (Fig. 5–6). The appearance has been likened to that of a candle flame.[16] In mitral stenosis, there are temporal changes in the color display of the jet since the velocity changes in diastole. During the isovolumic relaxation phase of diastole (mitral valve and aortic valve in the closed position), a trace of red is noted on the atrial side of the mitral valve leaflets. With the onset of the opening of the mitral valve leaflets, the color becomes bright red on the

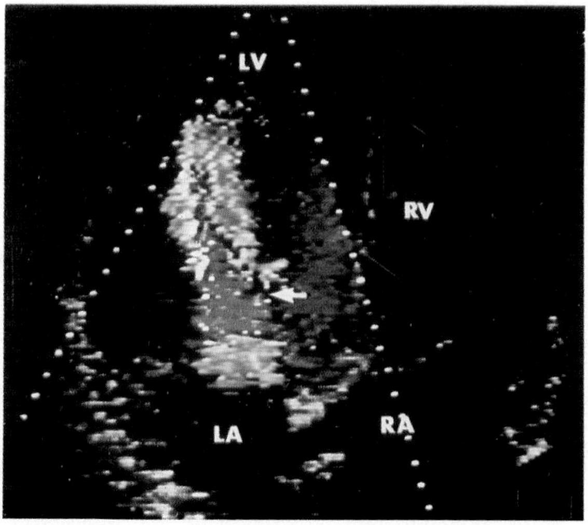

Figure 5–6. Color flow imaging in mitral stenosis. Apical view in diastole showing the characteristic candle flame appearance of the jet in mitral stenosis. The jet has a central blue zone due to color reversal from aliasing of high velocities (arrow). The peripheral zone is orange-yellow representing turbulence. LA = left atrium, RA = right atrium, LV = left ventricle, RV = right ventricle.

atrial side, changing to blue (aliasing and color reversal) in the mitral valve funnel as blood enters the left ventricle. With progression into diastole, the central blue zone becomes surrounded by a yellow-orange color ("candle flame"), representing turbulent flow toward the transducer. In middiastole, as the pressure gradient diminishes, the flow velocity also correspondingly decreases and, therefore, the jet assumes a homogeneous yellow-orange appearance. At end-diastole, in patients with normal sinus rhythm, the jet again assumes the candle flame appearance due to the increase in pressure gradient and velocity after atrial contraction. In severe mitral stenosis where there is a high gradient throughout diastole, the aliasing pattern or the mosaic appearance may persist throughout diastole. The flow jet in mitral stenosis is usually single but occasionally there may be two simultaneous jets.

Various direction and jet configurations are seen in patients with mitral stenosis[3] (Figs. 5–7 and 5–8). In the majority of cases, the jets are central and apically directed and have different shapes (e.g., sickle shaped or a mushroom appearance). A small number of patients have eccentric jets. There appears to be no correlation between jet configuration and severity of stenosis. However, it has been suggested that the

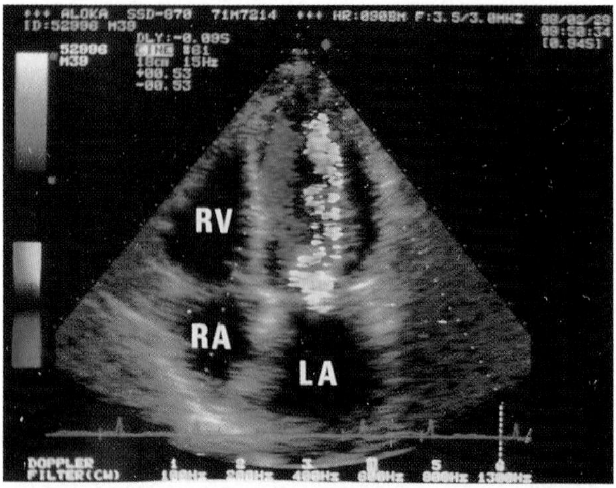

Figure 5 – 7. Color flow imaging in mitral stenosis. The flow jet is central. The central portion of the flow has high velocity and is therefore aliased (blue), whereas the peripheral and apical aspects of the jet are of slower velocity and are turbulent (orange-yellow). A prominent flow stream that has been reflected from the cardiac apex backward can be seen in the medial aspect of the left ventricle in blue. RV = right ventricle, RA = right atrium, LA = left atrium.

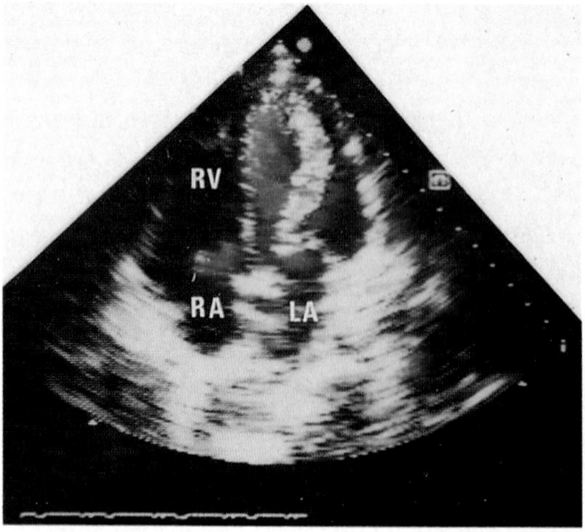

Figure 5 – 8. Color flow imaging in mitral stenosis. Image recorded from apical view portrays a sickle-shaped jet, directed toward the lateral free wall in its proximal-medial portion and deviating toward the apex in its distal portion. Note the mosaic appearance of the jet due to turbulence. RV = right ventricle, RA = right atrium, LA = left atrium.

width of the mitral stenosis jet at the level of the valve correlates with the severity of mitral stenosis and thus may be useful in assessing the valve area.[17] Although this may be true, it warrants further systematic studies. In most patients with mitral stenosis, jet characterization permits accurate guided CW Doppler interrogation, which provides confident determination of pressure gradients, pressure half-time, and valve area (Fig. 5–9).

In many instances, mitral stenosis may be associated with aortic regurgitation. Both jets are then roughly in the same direction and exhibit a mosaic pattern but often have a slight difference in their mix of colors (Fig. 5–10). Furthermore, the aortic regurgitation jet starts earlier, before the mitral valve opens.

Mitral stenosis may be often associated with mitral regurgitation (Fig. 5–11). Color flow imaging allows identification and quantification of the regurgitant flow. Mitral regurgitation, when severe, increases the antegrade diastole flow velocity and may cause overestimation of the mitral valve gradient.

TRICUSPID STENOSIS

The basic principles used to evaluate mitral stenosis should apply in the evaluation of tricuspid stenosis. The left parasternal short axis and apical windows are usually used and the ultrasound beam is aimed to include

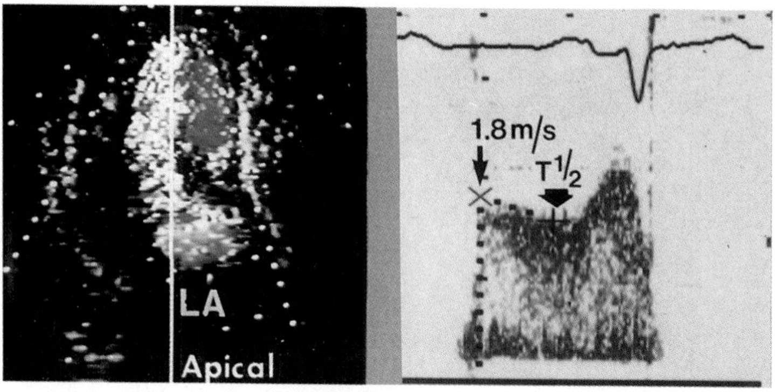

Figure 5–9. Guided continuous wave Doppler examination in mitral stenosis. *Left*: Apical view in diastole showing a mosaic color jet of mitral stenosis. Note that the CW Doppler beam is aligned parallel to the jet. The jet has a mosaic pattern indicating turbulent flow. LA = left atrium. *Right*: Spectral display of CW Doppler interrogation. The peak velocity is 1.8 m/s (maximal gradient = 13 mmHG). The pressure half-time ($t_{1/2}$) is 384 ms, and the valve area is calculated to be 0.6 cm^2.

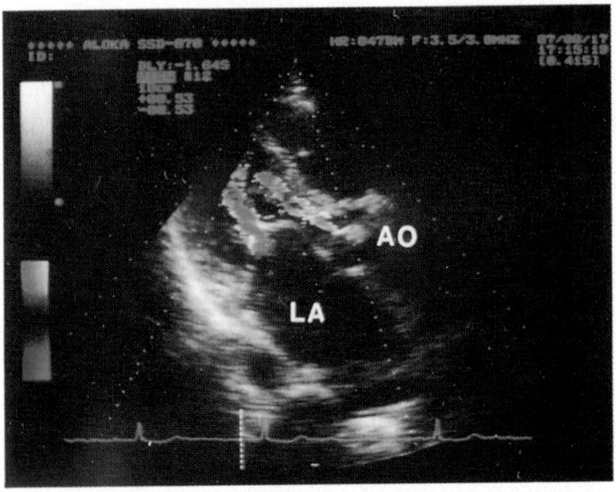

Figure 5–10. Mitral stenosis and aortic regurgitation. Parasternal long axis view depicting the left ventricular inflow jet of mitral stenosis and aortic regurgitant flow in the left ventricular outflow tract. AO = aorta, LA = left atrium.

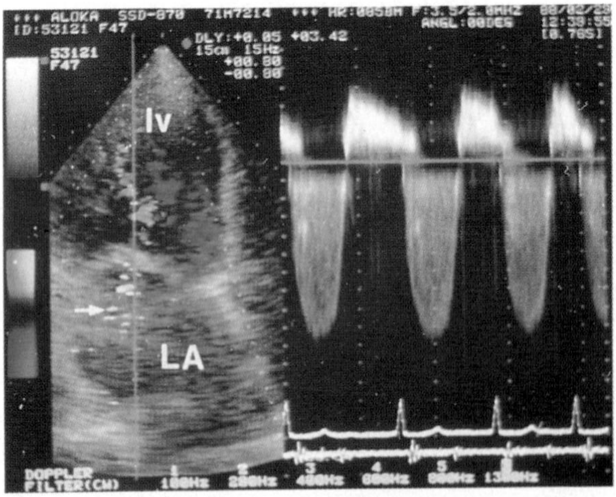

Figure 5–11. Mitral stenosis associated with mitral regurgitation recorded from apical view. *Left*: Mitral regurgitant flow is shown in blue (arrow) during systole. *Right*: Using color flow guided continuous wave Doppler technique the velocity of mitral stenosis and regurgitant jet can be reliably determined. LV = left ventricle, LA = left atrium.

the high velocity region; parallel alignment of the beam and velocity vectors is important. Since the pressure gradients are low even when tricuspid stenosis is clinically significant, the corresponding flow velocities should also be low and within the range detectable using conventional PD. CW Doppler examination provides similar information. One aspect that may cause confusion when using nonimaging CW Doppler is that patients with tricuspid stenosis frequently have mitral stenosis as well. Location, velocity amplitude and variation with respiration, and timing may help separate the two.

Tricuspid stenosis causes abnormal turbulence, an increase in velocity downstream from the tricuspid valve, and a decrease in the rate of decline in the velocity[18] (Fig. 5–12). A more severe stenosis causes a higher velocity and a slower diastolic slope. Increase in velocities with inspiration are more pronounced than in normal subjects. Significant tricuspid regurgitation will also increase forward tricuspid flow velocity, but the increase is of shorter duration and the diastolic slope steeper. In preliminary data from a series of 18 patients, the pressure half-time was significantly longer in patients with stenosis, compared with normal subjects.[18] However, no comparison with catheterization-derived pressure gradients or Doppler technique estimates of tricuspid valve area have been published to date.

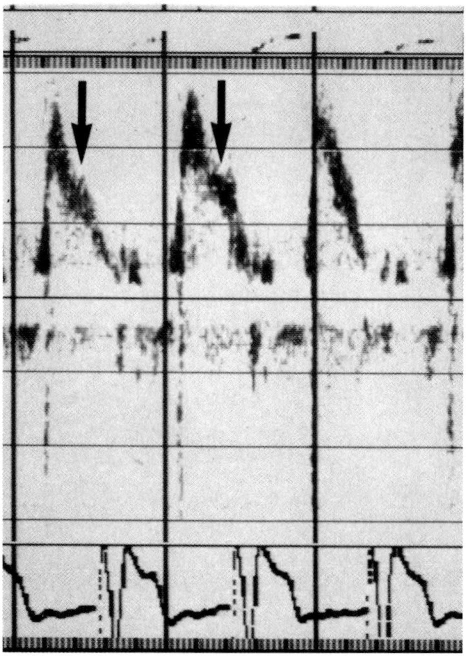

Figure 5–12. Pulse Doppler recording of a patient with rheumatic tricuspid stenosis. Initial velocities are increased (1.4 m/s), and they decrease slowly during diastole (arrows). The underlying rhythm is atrial fibrillation and ventricular pacing. (Scale marks = 0.5 m/s.)

Color Flow Imaging

Color flow examination of the tricuspid valve is also best performed using an apical position for the transducer. Occasionally, a low parasternal inflow view can be used to assess the jet as well as any associated tricuspid valve regurgitation. The color flow pattern is similar in appearance to that of mitral stenosis. When there is tricuspid stenosis, the increased velocity and turbulence result in excessive frequency aliasing and velocity variance. This is seen on color flow as increased brightness, or color reversal with a blue colored jet surrounded by red color, or as a mosaic pattern (Figs. 5–13 and 5–14).

Similar to mitral stenosis, flow jets in tricuspid stenosis also can exhibit various sizes, shapes, and directions. Depending on the severity of tricuspid stenosis, the jet may be wide or narrow, and may be central or eccentric. Using CFI guidance, CW Doppler examination is performed to obtain quantitative velocity recordings (see Fig. 5–14). CFI is useful when mitral stenosis and tricuspid stenosis coexist, as in rheumatic valvular disease. Tricuspid regurgitation may frequently be associated with tricuspid stenosis (see Fig. 5–14). If significant tricuspid regurgitation is present, the antegrade diastolic flow velocity across the stenotic valve would be increased further. Severity of tricuspid regurgitation can be easily assessed by CFI and this can then be taken into consideration when evaluating the severity of tricuspid stenosis.

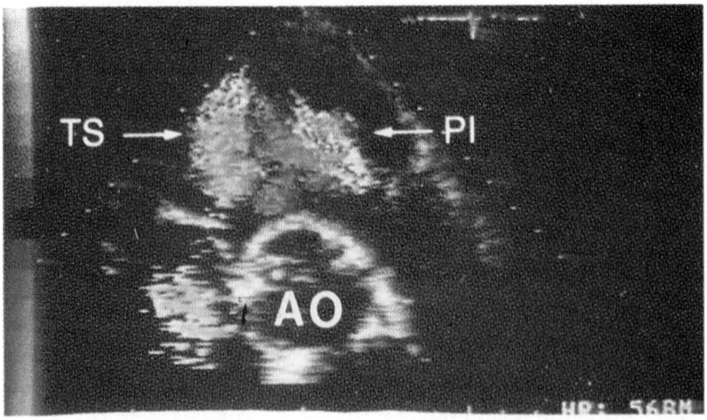

Figure 5–13. Short axis parasternal view at the aortic level. Color flow imaging demonstrates tricuspid stenosis (TS) as a red jet toward the transducer, and pulmonic insufficiency (PI) as a mosaic pattern, also toward the transducer. Both of these lesions occur at the same time in the cardiac cycle. AO = aorta.

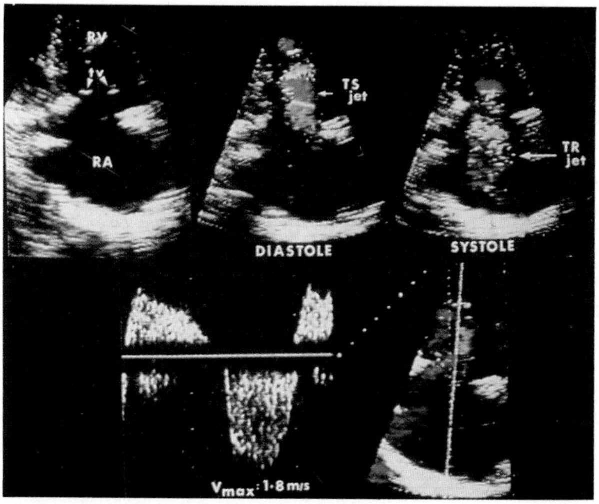

Figure 5–14. Color flow imaging in tricuspid stenosis. *Upper left*: Diastolic frame of 2D echocardiogram in apical view showing thick, retracted tricuspid valve leaflets (tv) with doming. RA = right atrium, RV = right ventricle. *Upper*: Diastolic frame in color flow mode showing the jet of tricuspid stenosis (TS). Note the color reversal in the center of the jet due to aliasing (arrow). The peripheral zone of normal flow velocities is orange-red. *Upper*: Systolic frame showing the jet of tricuspid regurgitation (TR). The jet is mosaic and blue in color, since flow is away from the transducer. Mosaic pattern of the jet indicates turbulent flow. *Lower*: Flow-guided CW Doppler interrogation of the tricuspid valve. The spectral display shows maximum antegrade velocity to be 1.8 m/s. The calculated mean gradient is 13 mmHg. The pressure half-time is 150 ms. Also note the systolic Doppler signal of tricuspid regurgitation with peak velocity of 3 m/s.

REFERENCES

1. Thuillez C, Theroux P, Bourassa M, et al: Pulsed Doppler echocardiographic study of mitral stenosis. *Circulation* 61:381, 1980.
2. Richards K, Cannon S, Crawford M, et al: Noninvasive diagnosis of aortic and mitral valve disease with pulsed Doppler spectrum analysis. *Am J Cardiol* 51:1122, 1983.
3. Hatle L, Angelsen B: *Doppler Ultrasound in Cardiology*, ed 2. Philadelphia, Lea & Febiger, 1985.
4. Holen J, Aaslid R, Landmark K, et al: Determination of pressure gradient in mitral stenosis with a noninvasive ultrasound Doppler technique. *Acta Med Scand* 199:455, 1976.

5. Hatle L, Brubakk A, Tromsdal A, et al: Noninvasive assessment of pressure drop in mitral stenosis by Doppler ultrasound. *Br Heart J* 40:131, 1978.
6. Stamm R, Martin R: Quantification of pressure gradients across stenotic valves by Doppler ultrasound. *J Am Coll Cardiol* 2:707, 1983.
7. Holen J, Simonsen S: Determination of pressure gradient in mitral stenosis with Doppler echocardiography. *Br Heart J* 41:529, 1979.
8. Holen J, Hoie J, Froysaker T: Determination of pre- and postoperative flow obstruction in patients undergoing closed mitral commissurotomy from noninvasive ultrasound Doppler data and cardiac output. *Am Heart J* 97:499, 1979.
9. Knutsen K, Bae E, Sivertssen E, et al: Doppler ultrasound in mitral stenosis. *Acta Med Scand* 211:433, 1982.
10. Libanoff A, Rodbard S: Atrioventricular pressure half-time, measure of mitral valve orifice area. *Circulation* 38:144, 1968.
11. Libanoff A, Rodbard S: Evaluation of the severity of mitral stenosis and regurgitation. *Circulation* 33:218, 1966.
12. Hatle L, Angelsen B, Tromsdal A: Noninvasive assessment of atrioventricular pressure half-time by Doppler ultrasound. *Circulation* 60:1096, 1979.
13. Smith M, Handshoe R, Handshoe S, et al: Comparative accuracy of two-dimensional echocardiography and Doppler pressure half-time methods in assessing severity of mitral stenosis in patients with and without prior commissurotomy. *Circulation* 73:100, 1986.
14. Thomas J, Weyman A: Doppler mitral pressure half-time: A clincial tool in search of theoretical justification. *J Am Coll Cardiol* 10:923, 1987.
15. Theirstein P, Yock P, Popp R: The accuracy of Doppler ultrasound measurement of pressure gradients across irregular, dual, and tunnel-like obstructions to flow. *Circulation* 72:577, 1985.
16. Khandheria B, Tajik J, Reeder G, et al: Doppler color flow imaging: A new technique for visualization and characterizaion of the blood flow jet of mitral stenosis. *Mayo Clin Proc* 61:623, 1986.
17. Kan M, Goyal R, Helmcke F: Color Doppler assessment of severity of mitral stenosis (abstr). *Circulation* 74 (suppl II):145, 1986.
18. Nakamura K, Satomi G, Ogasawata S, et al: Noninvasive evaluation of tricuspid stenosis with Doppler echocardiography. *Circulation* 70:394, 1984.

CHAPTER 6

Pulmonary Stenosis

Obstructive lesions involving the right ventricle and pulmonary arterial tree occur in 25 to 30 percent of all individuals with congenital heart disease.[1] Pulmonary stenosis can occur either as an isolated abnormality or in association with other congenital cardiac defects (see Chap. 17). The clinical course in patients with pulmonary stenosis is determined by several factors: (1) the site or sites of obstruction to flow, (2) the severity of obstruction to flow, and (3) the complexity and severity of associated abnormalities.

The diagnosis of pulmonary stenosis is frequently made by the clinician at the bedside. Characteristic physical findings coupled with electrocardiographic evidence of right ventricular hypertrophy have been used to estimate the severity of isolated valvular pulmonary stenosis.[2] With the advent of echocardiography, first M-mode and then 2D imaging, characteristics of pulmonary stenosis were recognized and reported. M-mode findings of an exaggerated A wave were reported for isolated pulmonary valve stenosis,[3] and systolic fluttering of the pulmonary valve was noted in cases of infundibular pulmonary stenosis.[4] The sensitivity and specificity of these signs are limited,[5] however, and attention turned to the pulmonary valve images obtained with 2D echocardiography. Direct visualization of the valve leaflets suggested that they domed during systole in isolated valvular stenosis.[6] High-resolution 2D imaging allowed visualization of pulmonary obstruction at other levels including subvalvular, supravalvular, and pulmonary branch stenosis.[7,8] As experience increased, new imaging windows and planes were used to display the right ventricular outflow tract in its entirety.[8,9] Despite these improvements in imaging technique and capability, diagnostic accuracy remained suboptimal. In a large study, Gutgesell et al[10] found that 2D echocardiography was 97 percent specific but only 77 percent sensitive for pulmonary valve stenosis. Echocardiography was more sensitive and specific for each of the other major congenital cardiac defects tested in the study.

Concurrent with the rapid advances in noninvasive diagnosis, changes occurred in the management of patients with pulmonary stenosis. Early reports of successful percutaneous balloon dilatation of pulmonary valve stenosis[11,12] were followed by rapid confirmation of the safety and efficacy of the procedure and its acceptance as the standard treatment of choice for this lesion.[13–20] In addition, the availability of prostaglandin E_1 for temporary palliation of pulmonary obstruction in the cyanotic newborn[21] created a demand for accurate, rapid noninvasive diagnosis. In many of these patients, noninvasive diagnostic advances have allowed surgical intervention without cardiac catheterization and its attendant risks.[22,23]

Availability of Doppler techniques for the noninvasive evaluation of pulmonary stenosis has allowed major advances in the management of patients with obstruction to pulmonary blood flow. This chapter will focus on the patterns of blood flow present in pulmonary stenosis. In addition, the method of examination is described, and techniques for quantification of severity of pulmonary stenosis are discussed. The current applications and limitations of Doppler echocardiography for management of patients with pulmonary stenosis complete the discussion.

BLOOD FLOW PATTERNS IN PULMONARY STENOSIS

Isolated pulmonary valve stenosis produces flow patterns that are similar to those seen in other discrete obstructions[24] (see Chap. 4, Fig. 4–1). Blood accelerates proximal to the valve and then flows in a laminar jet through the restricted orifice. Flow at this point accelerates to a velocity that is proportional to the square root of the developed pressure gradient. The central laminar jet is surrounded by an area of flow disturbance in which eddy currents develop. The flow disturbance is transmitted downstream to a point where eventual relaminarization of moving blood cells occurs. The specific characteristics of the jet as well as the extent of the flow disturbance downstream depend on many factors, including the severity of stenosis and the volume of flow through the valve. The pulmonary artery bifurcates asymmetrically, and a central stenotic orifice produces a jet that is directed toward the posterior and lateral wall of the pulmonary artery and into the left pulmonary artery.[25]

Nonvalvular stenosis or the presence of multiple areas of obstruction result in increasingly complicated flow patterns. Most of these flow patterns have not been described in detail. In some instances, the anatomy consists of a series of discrete stenoses. In tetralogy of Fallot the infundibular stenosis represents a long segment narrowing with additional valvular and, frequently, supravalvular sites of obstruction. The flow patterns of infundibular obstruction are further complicated because the obstruction is not static but increases in severity during systole. The flow patterns, therefore, change throughout the course of the cardiac cycle. Despite this apparent hemodynamic complexity, the most important feature of obstruction is the flow disturbance itself, which is invariably present and is the cornerstone on which the Doppler diagnosis of pulmonary stenosis is based.

DOPPLER EXAMINATION IN PULMONARY STENOSIS

The parasternal short axis view at the level of the aortic valve generally allows optimal placement of the Doppler cursor parallel to flow in the right ventricular outflow tract and main pulmonary artery. The normal pattern has a narrow spectral band with a rapid ascending and descending slope, and a peak velocity near midejection (rather than in the first third, as with aortic outflow). The normal mean ejection velocity in children is 0.9 m/s and in adults, 0.75 m/s. Obstructive lesions at any point along the outflow tract induce a high velocity jet and marked systolic turbulence.

An alternative location for Doppler interrogation of the outflow tract and pulmonary artery is from the subcostal or subxiphoid window. This is the preferred location in infants and small children and may yield the highest velocities even in adults.[24] Although suprasternal notch scanning is used for anatomical examination of the pulmonary arteries, Doppler interrogation is at a nearly perpendicular angle to flow, limiting its use from this position.

The Doppler examination follows a careful, complete 2D examination. This should reveal findings suggestive of obstruction to right ventricular outflow, such as prominent muscle in the infundibular region, doming of the pulmonary valve, or hypoplasia of the pulmonary anulus. In addition, dilation of the main pulmonary artery suggests valvular pulmonary stenosis while hypoplasia of the pulmonary artery branches should be apparent and suggests a diffuse stenotic process. The PD sample volume is then placed in the right ventricular outflow tract proximal to the pulmonary valve. At this point, flow should occur primarily in systole away from the transducer and with a relatively low velocity. As the sample volume is moved through the pulmonary valve, valve "clicks" are detected, and there is normally a slight increase in velocity but no disturbance of the laminar pattern, and with a clean audio signal. As the sample volume is placed farther downstream in the main pulmonary artery, velocity should remain constant with no increase in spectral broadening. Finally, further advancement of the sample volume into the left pulmonary artery frequently results in the detection of higher velocity signals, without disturbed flow.

Using this approach, infundibular stenosis is suggested by the presence of turbulent flow and an increase in velocity. However, subpulmonic stenosis usually occurs in association with valvar pulmonic stenosis or with a ventricular septal defect, both of which contribute to the high velocity disturbance in the outflow tract. Therefore, when diagnosing a subpulmonic obstruction, pulmonary valvar stenosis should also be excluded and the perimembranous septum should be carefully evaluated for a defect. Also, rarely, an obstruction of the right ventricular outflow tract may be caused by an aneurysm of the interventricular outflow tract may be caused by an aneurysm of the interventricular septum arising from the region of a closed ventricular septal defect which encroaches on the outflow tract.[26]

In isolated valvar pulmonic stenosis, a much more common congenital lesion, flow proximal to the valve is undisturbed and of normal velocity. As the sample volume is moved across the valve, velocities increase dramatically. Aliasing frequently develops and the peak velocity is unobtainable (Fig. 6–1). In addition to the increase in velocity, movement of the sample volume away from the central jet results in the detection of flow disturbance as an obviously abnormal flow pattern.

If no flow disturbance is detected during the PD examination, there is no need for routine CW Doppler interrogation. If a flow disturbance is detected, however, CW Doppler should be used to obtain the peak instan-

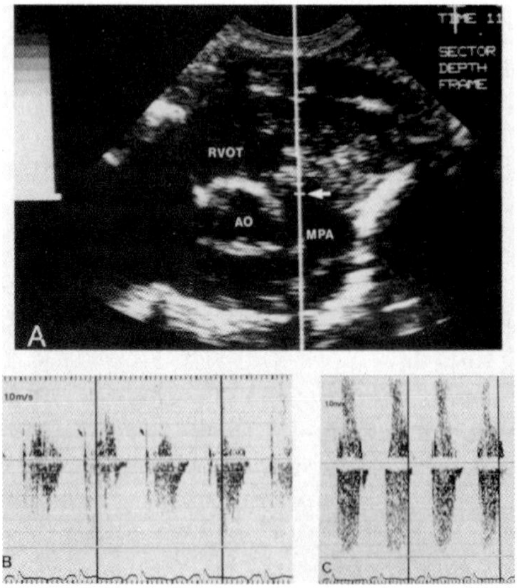

Figure 6–1. Pulsed Doppler interrogation of the pulmonary artery in a patient with valvar pulmonary stenosis. As the sample volume (arrow) is moved through the pulmonary valve (A), Doppler tracing (B) reveals valve artifacts (arrows), increased velocity, and loss of the spectral envelope. A Doppler tracing from the center of the pulmonary artery (C) shows spectral broadening and aliasing indicating a high velocity jet. AO = aorta, MPA = main pulmonary artery, RVOT = right ventricular outflow tract.

taneous velocity in the jet (Figs. 6–2 and 6–3). Continuous wave Doppler can be used in conjunction with 2D imaging or with a separate nonimaging transducer. Quantitation of the severity of pulmonary stenosis by CW Doppler is possible by using the modified Bernoulli equation ($\Delta P = 4V^2$) when a peak velocity has been obtained; the results have been shown to be highly accurate when compared with cardiac catheterization.[27,28] There have been no reports of use of the continuity equation for valve area calculation in pulmonary stenosis, but it should be as useful as it is in aortic stenosis.[29]

COLOR FLOW IMAGING

Normal pulmonary flow is seen as a homogeneous blue color in the main pulmonary artery, streaming into the left and right pulmonary arteries. Aliasing in the center of the pulmonary artery distal to the pulmonary valve is a normal finding. In the absence of increased variance, aliasing does not necessarily suggest a flow disturbance. Stenosis of the valve causes an increase in flow velocity and turbulence. Consequently, the systolic flow jet has a multicolored mosaic appearance; the mosaic pattern or aliased pattern with orange-yellow color, however, may be surrounded by blue coloration (Figs. 6–4 and 6–5). The jet across a stenotic pulmonic valve is often directed toward the left pulmonary artery as seen in Fig. 6–4,

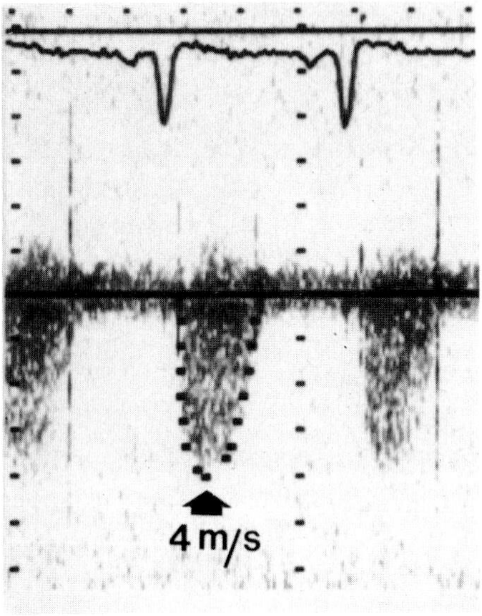

Figure 6 – 2. Continuous wave Doppler tracings of valvar pulmonary stenosis. From the left parasternal position, the peak velocity is 4 m/s and a Doppler estimated gradient ($\Delta P = 4V^2$) of 64 mmHg.

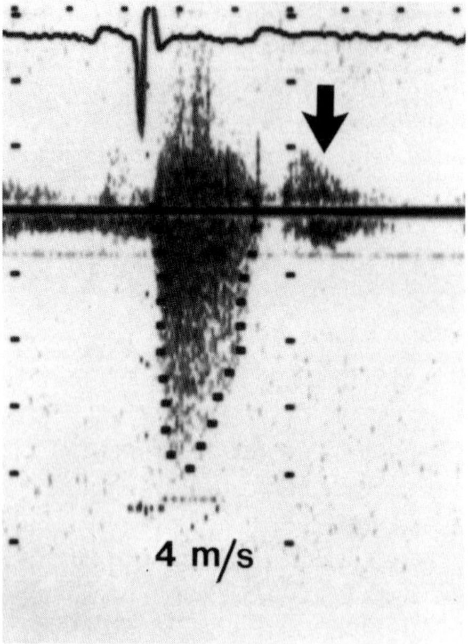

Figure 6 – 3. Continuous wave recording of valvar pulmonary stenosis (4 m/s) and mild pulmonary insufficiency (arrow).

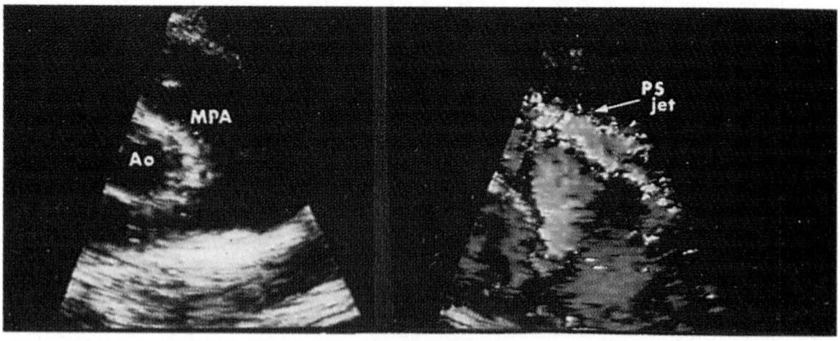

Figure 6 – 4. Color flow imaging in pulmonary stenosis. *Left*: Still-frame of short axis view showing aorta (AO) and main pulmonary artery (MPA). Note the dilated pulmonary artery. *Right*: Systolic frame in color flow mode showing the jet of pulmonary stenosis (PS). Note the mosaic appearance and the discrete jet tracking along the lateral wall of the pulmonary artery (arrow) toward the left pulmonary artery.

or it may be central as displayed in Fig. 6–5. Using color Doppler image guidance, the CW Doppler beam can be aligned with the jet to obtain peak velocity (Fig. 6–5). In infundibular pulmonary stenosis, the flow turbulence, color reversal, and mosaic pattern can be seen proximal to the pulmonary valve.

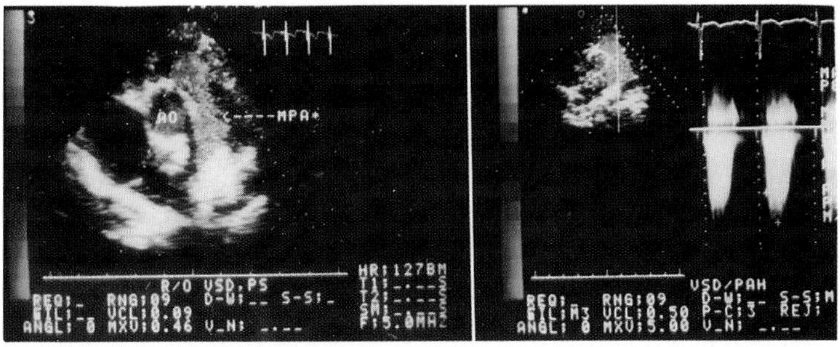

Figure 6–5. Color flow imaging in pulmonary stenosis. *Left*: Systolic frame obtained from parasternal short axis view depicts a central mosaic patterned jet in the main pulmonary artery (MPA) of pulmonary stenosis. AO = aorta. *Right*: Continuous wave Doppler beam aligned parallel to the jet. The maximum velocity obtained was 3.5 m/s. The calculated maximum instantaneous gradient using the modified Bernoulli equation ($\Delta P = 4V^2$) was 49 mmHg.

Pulmonary regurgitation when associated with pulmonary valvular stenosis can also be easily detected by color Doppler imaging. Flow jets due to shunts originating from a patent ductus or surgically created communication may cause abnormal flow jets in the pulmonary artery. These jets are often continuous and will have different directionality and thus can be easily sorted out from pulmonary valve flow.

PATIENT MANAGEMENT BASED ON THE DOPPLER EXAMINATION

For isolated pulmonary valve stenosis, there has been a major change in patient management in the past six years. Percutaneous balloon valvuloplasty has become the standard method of treatment for this defect.[11–19] As information becomes available on the safety and long-term efficacy of this procedure, it is becoming clear that balloon valvuloplasty will be performed routinely for even moderate degrees of pulmonary valvular stenosis. Doppler echocardiography plays a crucial role in the management of these patients. The diagnosis of valvular pulmonary stenosis is made clinically and confirmed echocardiographically. Two-dimensional and Doppler echocardiography are used to exclude associated defects, and Doppler evaluation serves to quantify the severity of the stenosis. Precise estimation of pulmonary pressure gradient is essential in order to avoid unnecessary cardiac catheterization in patients with minimal gradients and to refer patients with moderate or severe obstruction for balloon valvuloplasty. Using Doppler ultrasound, Mullins et al[30] studied 21 patients in the cardiac catheterization laboratory prior to and immediately following balloon pulmonary valvuloplasty, and found an excellent correlation between Doppler estimated gradients and the simultaneous catheter measured gradients. Pressure gradients prior to balloon dilatation also correlated well with similar measurements made in the echocardiography laboratory days or weeks before catheterization. Following balloon valvuloplasty, the patient is assessed serially for the presence of pulmonary regurgitation or for the development of restenosis.[19,30]

REFERENCES

1. Emmanouilides G, Baylen B: Pulmonary stenosis, in Adams F, Emmanouilides G (eds): *Heart Disease in Infants, Children, and Adolescents*. Baltimore, Williams & Wilkins, 1983.
2. Ellison R, Freedom R, Keane J, et al: Indirect assessment of severity in pulmonary stenosis. *Circulation* 56:I-14, 1977.
3. Weyman A, Dillon J, Feigenbaum H, et al: Echocardiographic patterns of pulmonary valve motion in valvular pulmonary stenosis. *Am J Cardiol* 34:644, 1974.
4. Weyman A, Dillon J, Feigenbaum H, et al: Echocardiographic differentiation of infundibular from valvular pulmonary stenosis. *Am J Cardiol* 36:21, 1975.
5. Leblanc M, Paquet M: Echocardiographic assessment of valvular pulmonary stenosis in children. *Br Heart J* 46:363, 1981.
6. Weyman A, Hurwitz R, Girod D, et al: Cross-sectional echocardiographic visualization of the stenotic pulmonary valve. *Circulation* 56:769, 1977.
7. Tinker D, Nanda N, Harris J, et al: Two-dimensional echocardiographic identification of pulmonary artery branch stenosis. *Am J Cardiol* 50:814, 1982.
8. Silove E, DeGiovanni J, Shiu M, et al: Diagnosis of right ventricular outflow obstruction in infants by cross sectional echocardiography. *Br Heart J* 50:416, 1983.
9. Marino B, Ballerini L, Marcelletti C, et al: Right oblique subxiphoid view for two-dimensional echocardiographic visualization of the right ventricle in congenital heart disease. *Am J Cardiol* 54:1064, 1984.
10. Gutgesell H, Huhta J, Latson L, et al: Accuracy of two-dimensional echocardiography in the diagnosis of congenital heart disease. *Am J Cardiol* 55:514, 1985.
11. Kan J, White R, Mitchell S, et al: Percutaneous balloon valvuloplasty: A new method for treating congenital pulmonary valve stenosis. *N Engl J Med* 307:540, 1982.
12. Lababidi Z, Wu J: Percutaneous balloon pulmonary valvuloplasty. *Am J Cardiol* 52:560, 1983.
13. Kan J, White R, Mitchell S, et al: Percutaneous transluminal balloon valvuloplasty for pulmonary valve stenosis. *Circulation* 69:554, 1984.

14. Rocchini A, Kveselis D, Crowley D, et al: Percutaneous balloon valvuloplasty for treatment of congenital pulmonary valvular stenosis in children. *J Am Coll Cardiol* 3:1005, 1984.
15. Shuck J, McCormick D, Cohen I, et al: Percutaneous balloon valvuloplasty of the pulmonary valve: Role of right to left shunting through a patent foramen ovale. *J Am Coll Cardiol* 4:132, 1984.
16. Tynan M, Baker E, Rohmer J, et al: Percutaneous balloon pulmonary valvuloplasty. *Br Heart J* 53:520, 1985.
17. Sullivan I, Robinson P, Macartney F, et al: Percutaneous balloon valvuloplasty for pulmonary valve stenosis in infants and children. *Br Heart J* 54:435, 1985.
18. Ben-Shachar G, Cohen M, Sivakoff M, et al: Development of infundibular obstruction after percutaneous pulmonary balloon valvuloplasty. *J Am Coll Cardiol* 55:754, 1985.
19. Kveselis D, Rocchini A, Snider A, et al: Results of balloon valvuloplasty in the treatment of congenital valvar pulmonary stenosis in children. *J Am Coll Cardiol* 56:527, 1985.
20. Radtke W, Keane J, Fellows K, et al: Percutaneous balloon valvotomy of congenital pulmonary stenosis using oversized balloons. *J Am Coll Cardiol* 8:909, 1986.
21. Leoni F, Huhta J, Douglas J, et al: Effect of prostaglandin on early surgical mortality in obstructive lesions of the systemic circulation. *Br Heart J* 52: 654, 1984.
22. Hagler D, Tajik A, Seward J, et al: Noninvasive assessment of pulmonary valve stenosis, aortic valve stenosis and coarctation of the aorta in critically ill neonates. *Am J Cardiol* 57:369, 1986.
23. Huhta J, Glasow P, Murphy D Jr, et al: Surgery without catheterization for congenital heart defects: Management of 100 patients. *J Am Coll Cardiol* 9:823, 1987.
24. Hatle L, Angelsen B: *Doppler Ultrasound in Cardiology*, ed 2. Philadelphia, Lea & Febiger, 1985.
25. Yoganathan A, Ball J, Woo Y-R, et al: Steady flow velocity measurements in a pulmonary artery model with varying degrees of pulmonic stenosis. *J Biomech* 19:129, 1986.
26. Johnson G, Kwan O, Coltrill C, et al: Detection and quantitation of right ventricular outlet obstruction secondary to aneurysm of the membranous ventricular septum by combined two-dimensional echocardiography: Continuous-wave Doppler ultrasound. *Am J Cardiol* 53:1476, 1984.
27. Lima C, Sahn D, Valdes-Cruz L, et al: Noninvasive prediction of transvalvular pressure gradient in patients with pulmonary stenosis by quantitative two-dimensional echocardiographic Doppler studies. *Circulation* 67:866, 1983.
28. Johnson G, Kwan O, Handshoe, S, et al: Accuracy of combined two-dimensional echocardiography and continuous wave Doppler recordings in the estimation of pressure gradient in right ventricular outlet obstruction. *J Am Coll Cardiol* 3:1013, 1984.

29. Skjaerpe T, Hegrenaes L, Hatle L: Noninvasive estimation of valve area in patients with aortic stenosis by Doppler ultrasound and two-dimensional echocardiography. *Circulation* 72:810, 1985.
30. Mullins C, Ludomirsky A, O'Laughlin M, et al: Balloon valvuloplasty for pulmonic valve stenosis—two-year follow-up: Hemodynamic and Doppler evaluation. *Cathet Cardiovasc Diagn* 11:156, 1985.

CHAPTER 7

Aortic Regurgitation

Doppler echocardiographic techniques provide the optimal noninvasive method by which to diagnose and quantify aortic regurgitation (AR).[1–4] For this application, Doppler echocardiography provides information that complements 2D echocardiographic imaging for assessing AR. In a patient with suspected or known AR, 2D echo generally indicates the etiology of regurgitation, but it provides only indirect clues about its existence and severity. In contrast, Doppler echocardiography allows direct demonstration of retrograde flow across the regurgitant aortic valve and provides a number of methods for assessing the severity of regurgitation. This chapter will summarize the M-mode and 2D echocardiographic findings of AR and review the Doppler echocardiographic techniques that currently can be used to detect and quantify the severity of AR.

SUMMARY OF M-MODE AND TWO-DIMENSIONAL ECHOCARDIOGRAPHIC FINDINGS

Using echocardiography, the diagnosis of AR is suggested on the basis of indirect findings. These M-mode and 2D features may be related to an abnormality of the aortic valve or the aorta, the regurgitant jet direction, or the anatomical and hemodynamic state of the left ventricle. A practical approach to categorize these features is shown in Table 7–1.

Persistent aortic cusp separation during diastole is neither sensitive nor specific in diagnosing AR.[5] This may be due in part to the observation that the aortic valve moves in and out of the imaging plane. When calcific changes are present, dropout of echoes behind the calcium can give the mistaken impression of persistent cusp separation. Fine diastolic fluttering of the aortic cusp is an uncommon M-mode finding; however, when present, it strongly suggests aortic cusp fenestration, which results in AR.[6] Erratic diastolic echoes in the left ventricular outflow tract may be seen in infective aortic valve endocarditis, which leads to the suspicion of a flail

TABLE 7-1. M-Mode and Two-Dimensional Echocardiographic Features of Aortic Regurgitation

Abnormality of aortic valve or aorta

1. Diastolic aortic cusp separation
2. Fine diastolic fluttering of aortic valve
3. Flail aortic cusp with or without vegetations
4. Aortic valve prolapse
5. Aortic root dilatation or dissection

Regurgitant jet direction

1. Fine diastolic fluttering on the anterior mitral leaflet or on the high interventricular septum
2. Partial or complete "diastolic damping" of the anterior mitral leaflet
3. "Diastolic indentation" and "reverse doming" of the anterior mitral leaflet

Anatomical and hemodynamic states of the left ventricle (LV)

1. Dilated LV with hyperdynamic septal motion
2. Early closure of the mitral valve
3. Premature opening of the aortic valve

aortic cusp, with or without vegetations.[7,8] Prolapse of the aortic cusps, frequently associated with AR,[9] can be seen by 2D echocardiography as an isolated entity,[10] or associated with mitral or tricuspid valve prolapse.[9] Two-dimensional echocardiography provides an accurate means for detecting, localizing, and measuring aneurysms of the ascending aorta. Angiographic correlation of size has been reported to be very high ($r = 0.91$).[11] In patients suspected of having aortic root dissection, an intimal flap can be detected in as high as 80 percent of the cases.[12]

The left ventricular outflow tract structure on which the characteristic diastolic fluttering appears depends on the direction of the regurgitant jet and not on the severity of the AR.[13,14] Fine diastolic vibrations of the high interventricular septum may be seen on M-mode in 37 to 58 percent of the cases[13,15]; this indicates that the regurgitant jet is directed anteriorly. Distortion of diastolic mitral valve motion can be detected as a fine fluttering or even as a complete damping of the anterior mitral leaflet excursion in 13 to 95 percent of AR patients.[12,16–18] Unlike the diastolic fluttering of the interventricular septum, fluttering of the anterior mitral leaflet may be seen with any jet direction.[13,14] In mitral stenosis, calcification and fibrosis of the mitral leaflets frequently prevent the development of high-frequency oscillations. With the 2D technique, disturbed motion of the anterior mitral leaflet also can be detected. However, unlike for M-mode, a larger regurgitant volume is required to be detected by 2D methods.[19] The anatomic distortion is seen as "diastolic indentation" in the short axis view or as "reverse doming" (leaflet bowing away from the septum) in the parasternal long axis and apical views.[19]

In acute AR, echocardiography can be particularly useful because the classic bedside findings, i.e., a wide pulse pressure, cardiomegaly, bounding pulses, etc, are usually absent, and the diagnosis of severe AR can be missed. The early hemodynamic response to the sudden increased volume in a nondilated left ventricle is marked elevation of left ventricular end-diastolic pressure (LVEDP), which may approach or even equal aortic diastolic pressure.[20] Because LVEDP may exceed left atrial pressure, premature closure of the mitral valve occurs.[21,22] Also, premature opening of the aortic valve has been reported in patients with acute severe AR in whom LVEDP equals aortic diastolic pressure.[23,24]

DOPPLER TECHNIQUES APPLIED TO AORTIC REGURGITATION

Doppler echocardiography is at present the most important noninvasive modality for the detection and quantification of regurgitant flow into the left ventricle from incompetent aortic valves. Many Doppler approaches to AR can be used to detect and quantify AR (Table 7–2).

Pulsed-Wave Doppler Flow Mapping

Pulsed-wave Doppler techniques were the first to enjoy widespread application. The advent of duplex systems, combining single range-gated PD with 2D echocardiographic imaging,[25,26] made it easier to use a variety of

TABLE 7–2. Doppler Methods for Evaluating Aortic Regurgitation Severity

Pulsed wave flow mapping
Color flow imaging
Continuous wave determination of deceleration rate of aortic regurgitant velocity
Regurgitant velocity waveform intensity
Diastolic flow pattern in the abdominal aorta
Estimations of regurgitant fraction

imaging planes to position the PD sample volume in order to map regurgitant flow disturbances. Thus, apical as well as parasternal windows were used to evaluate the spatial distribution of AR. Although aortic regurgitant flow generally moves approximately perpendicular to a Doppler ultrasound beam directed from a high precordial window, the fact that individual blood cells appear to swirl in vortices as they pass into the left ventricle means that regurgitant flow disturbances are multidirectional. Thus, they can be detected from multiple echocardiographic windows.

Aortic regurgitation is diagnosed by PD by placing the sample volume in the high left ventricular outflow tract and systematically searching beneath the aortic valve for the regurgitant jet. Since velocities of AR flows are uniformly high (greater than 3.0 to 3.5 m/s), they exceed the Nyquist limit and show aliasing (Fig. 7–1). This pandiastolic signal, with its characteristic appearance and sound, provides an accurate, highly sensitive means of detecting AR.

Detection of a flow disturbance using range-gated PD is a reliable indicator of AR, while the absence of such a flow disturbance denotes the absence of AR.[18,25,27–31] It is reassuring to note that despite the fact that these studies used a number of different types of Doppler instrumenta-

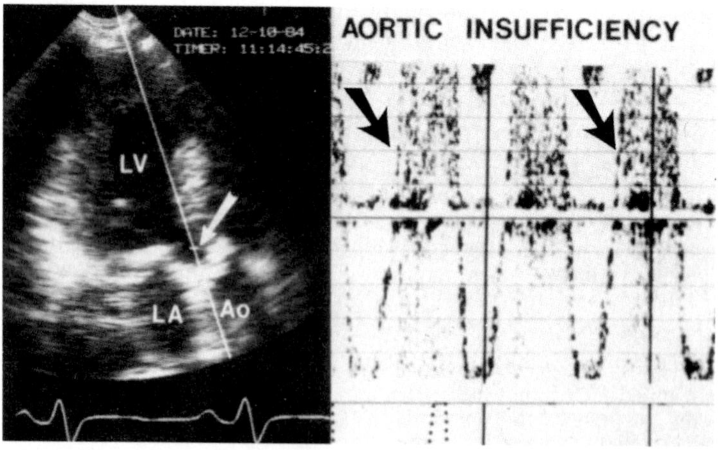

Figure 7–1. Aortic regurgitant flow disturbance recorded from the cardiac apex using pulsed Doppler. *Left*: Diastolic two-dimensional echo image showing the Doppler sample volume (arrow) positioned in the left ventricular (LV) outflow tract just below the thickened aortic leaflets. *Right*: Velocity tracing showing pandiastolic turbulent flow (spectral broadening) which is diagnostic of aortic regurgitation (arrow). The systolic flow, recorded below the baseline, remains laminar. AO = aorta, LA = left atrium.

tion, the sensitivity, specificity, positive and negative predictive values of Doppler findings for AR are fairly consistent from laboratory to laboratory (Table 7–3). When patients from these different series are grouped, forming a composite of 388 patients, PD demonstrates an overall sensitivity of 95 percent; specificity, 96 percent; positive predictive value, 99 percent; and negative predictive value, 99 percent for detecting the presence or absence of AR, using selective aortic root angiography as a standard of reference.

The spatial distribution of the regurgitant flow disturbance in the left ventricle just proximal to the aortic valve is widely used to judge whether AR is mild, moderate, or severe (Fig. 7–2). Investigators using image-guided PD suggested that the severity of AR could be established by determining the length of the regurgitant jet, expressed as the distance from the plane of the aortic valve over which a regurgitant flow disturbance could be detected. Mapping is performed by using the apical position. Two-dimensional images are obtained from apical five chamber or long axis views; the PD sample volume is positioned at the level of the aortic valve and moved progressively through the left ventricular outflow space and body of the left ventricle to the apex. Comparisons of severity grades by Doppler and angiography have generally demonstrated a good correlation[1,18,25,27–33]; deviations are within one grade of severity.

Clinical experience, more recently corroborated by CFI,[34–35] indicates that aortic regurgitant flow disturbances are not uncommonly oblique; moreover, some flow disturbances are narrow while others are broad. Hence, the simple length of an AR jet is an oversimplification of its spatial

TABLE 7–3. Detection of Aortic Regurgitation by Pulsed Doppler Echocardiography vs. Aortic Root Angiography

No. of Patients	Sensitivity, %	Specificity, %	Predictive Value, %		Reference
			Positive	Negative	
45	97	90	97	90	18
25	100	100	100	100	25
65	86	94	98	68	27
35	96	100	100	89	28
46	100	100	100	100	29
26	100	93	92	100	30
52	95	100	100	86	31
94	97	95	99	91	32
Total 388	95	96	99	89	

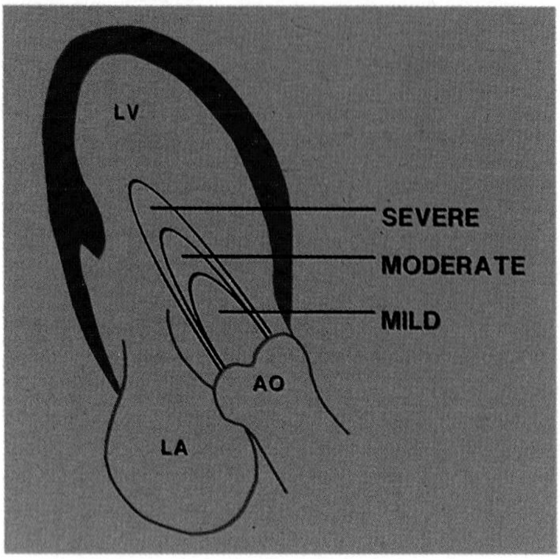

Figure 7 – 2. Schematic diagram showing the grading of severity of aortic regurgitation. LV = left ventricle, LA = left atrium, AO = aorta.

distribution within the left ventricular cavity. For these reasons, our laboratory routinely examine AR jets using parasternal long axis, parasternal short axis, apical four chamber, and apical long axis views, in order to establish whether the jet is localized, generalized, or intermediate in distribution (corresponding respectively to mild, severe, and moderate degrees of regurgitation).

Unfortunately, conventional PD mapping of AR has a number of shortcomings. This technique requires interrogating different portions of the left ventricle from a variety of transducer positions and orientations. The Doppler sample volume needs to be moved back and forth along a given examining line, over a sequence of beats, to define the distribution of disturbed diastolic flow along the scan line. The examining beam must be redirected across another portion of the left ventricle and the process of mapping repeated. Since this same examining sequence is repeated using several transducer positions and orientations, detailed mapping of the left ventricular outflow tract and cavity can be tedious and time consuming. Finally, although the use of a larger sample volume may increase sensitivity, this also may lead to overestimation of the area of the regurgitant flow disturbance. Considering these problems, PD mapping of AR is a semi-quantitative technique. While it usually can distinguish between mild, moderate, and severe degrees of regurgitation, regurgitant flow mapping does not provide a precise numerical descriptor of regurgitant severity.

Color Flow Imaging

Color flow imaging represents a significant advance in the echocardiographic detection and evaluation of AR. A sector of the left ventricular cavity can be interrogated in real time, so CFI should be able to rapidly define the spatial distribution of an AR jet within a given tomographic plane.

The jet of aortic regurgitation generally is well visualized from the parasternal long axis (Figs. 7–3, 7–4, and 7–5A) and the parasternal short axis windows (Fig. 7–5B) as well as low parasternal, right parasternal, and apical windows (Fig. 7–6), despite the fact that the parasternal long and short axis windows are nearly perpendicular to the major direction of flow. This probably is due to the rapid and turbulent nature of the flow, which results in significant velocity vectors pointed in directions other than that of the major axis of the jet.

Color flow imaging can diagnose AR with a sensitivity ranging from 88 to 100 percent in two published series.[36,37] Asaka et al[37] studied 68 consecutive patients with both conventional PD and CFI. They found the sensitivity of the two techniques to be comparable (88 percent for CFI vs 92 percent for conventional PD), but in their series, CFI was more specific (100 percent for CFI vs 83 percent for conventional Doppler). Color Doppler can readily distinguish the jet of AR from that of mitral stenosis[38,39] (Fig. 7–7). Color Doppler may be particularly useful in patients with a mitral prosthesis, because these devices frequently cause turbulence in the left ventricular outflow tract that may confound the diagnosis of AR by conventional PD. Using CFI, Yoshikawa et al[40] were able to diagnose AR with a

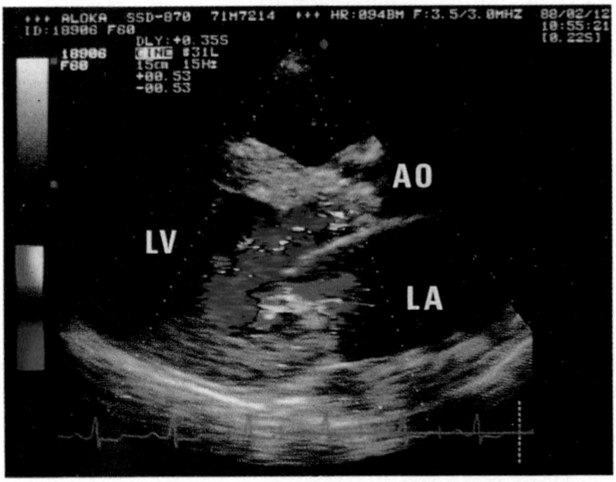

Figure 7–3. Color Doppler flow imaging in a patient with severe aortic regurgitation, parasternal long axis view. The regurgitant jet at its origin occupies two-thirds of the thickness of the left ventricular outflow tract. LV = left ventricle, AO = aorta, LA = left atrium.

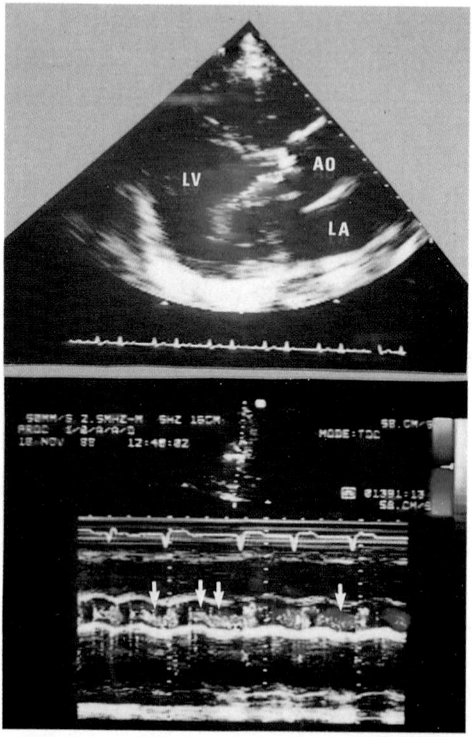

F i g u r e 7 – 4. Mild aortic regurgitation, parasternal long axis view. *Top*: The aortic regurgitant jet is directed toward the anterior mitral valve leaflet. The narrow origin of the jet in the left ventricular outflow tract indicates mild aortic regurgitation. LV = left ventricle, AO = aorta, LA = left atrium. *Bottom*: Color M-mode at aortic valve level demonstrating holodiastolic aortic regurgitation (arrows).

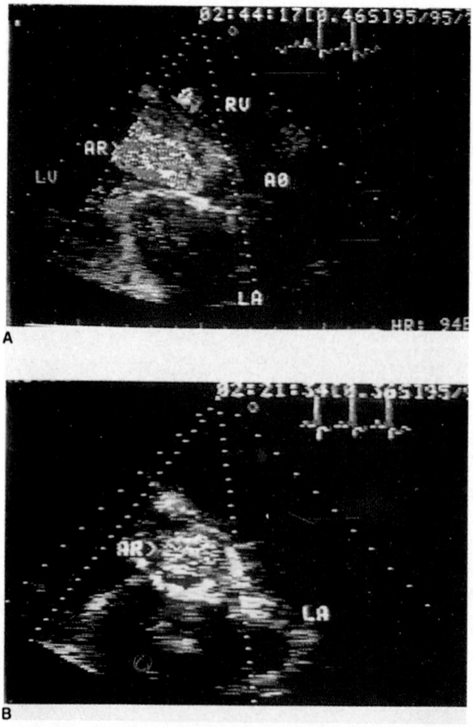

F i g u r e 7 – 5. (A) Parasternal long axis view of a patient with severe aortic regurgitation. The jet occupies nearly the entire area of the left ventricular outflow tract at aortic valve level. AR = aortic regurgitant jet. (B) Aortic regurgitant jet (AR) visualized from the parasternal short axis view at the level of the aortic valve. The jet occupies 100% of the outflow tract, indicating severe aortic regurgitation. LV = left ventricle, RV = right ventricle, AO = aorta, LA = left atrium.

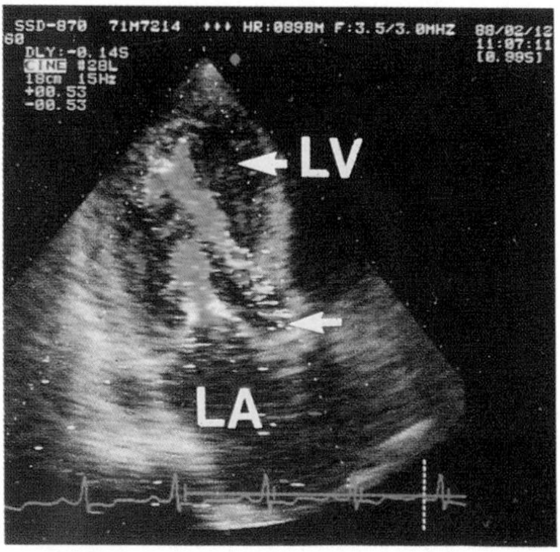

Figure 7–6. Mild aortic regurgitation, apical long axis view. The narrow origin of the jet in the left ventricular outflow tract indicates mild aortic regurgitation (arrow). Mild aortic regurgitation may produce long, thin jets that extend deeply into the left ventricle (LV). The regurgitant jet is readily distinguished from normal mitral inflow in the example, despite a similar direction of flow, due to the higher velocity and turbulence of the regurgitant jet. LA = left atrium.

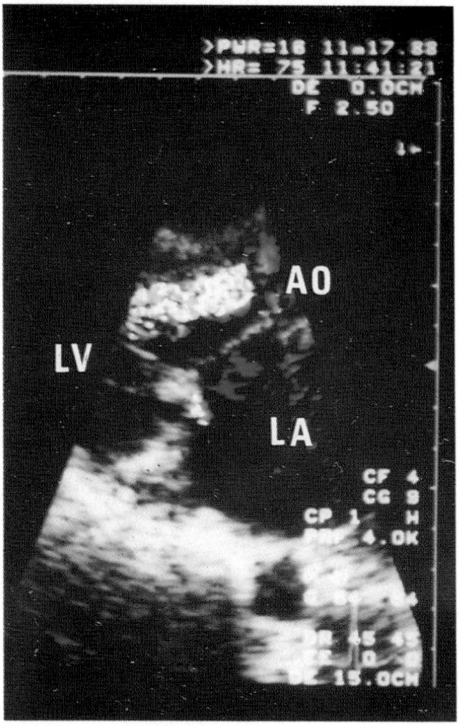

Figure 7–7. Color flow imaging in combined mitral stenosis and aortic regurgitation, parasternal long axis view. The aortic regurgitant jet is clearly imaged in a mosaic pattern. There is minimal flow across the stenotic mitral valve. LV = left ventricle, AO = aorta, LA = left atrium.

sensitivity of 88 percent and a specificity of 100 percent in 42 patients with a coexisting mitral prosthesis.

Several investigators have measured the extent of flow disturbance by CFI as a semiquantitative estimate of the severity of AR. Omoto et al[36] found a moderate association between angiographic and color Doppler estimates of the severity of AR using the maximal distance to which the regurgitant jet extended in the left ventricle in the long axis view as their criterion for severity. Miyatake et al[41] reported on 26 patients in whom AR was visualized by CFI; AR was confirmed at angiography in 23 of 26. No precise attempt at grading was reported, but it was noted that by angiography the extent of the regurgitant flow was more extensive in patients with more severe AR, and the regurgitant jet reached the apical cavity in patients with severe AR.

A recent study by Perry et al[42] has shown that the width of the regurgitant jet relative to the size of the left ventricular outflow tract was more accurate to the area of the regurgitant jet or length to which the jet extends in the left ventricle. A jet width that occupies 50 percent or more of the outflow space represents moderately severe to severe AR (see Fig. 7–3). There is both in vivo and in vitro evidence that supports the concept that the thickness of the AR stream at its origin is predictive of the severity of AR. Jet width in the high left ventricular outflow tract relative to left ventricular outflow tract width measured angiographically from the cranial left anterior oblique projection during the first diastole after aortic root injection correlates with angiographic AR grade.[43] In vitro modeling of AR using a porcine heterograft demonstrates that the width of the regurgitant jet at its origin may reflect the size of the valvular defect.[42] Finally, earlier studies using a conventional PD technique to map the short axis area of the regurgitant jet at the aortic valve level[44] or reconstruct the three-dimensional area of the regurgitant jet in the left ventricular outflow tract[45] have correlated reasonably well with angiographic grading of AR. Some investigators have cautioned that the size of AR jets demonstrated by CFI does vary with instrument gain setting, regurgitant orifice size and shape, driving pressure, and the size and compliance of the left ventricle.[46]

Continuous Wave Doppler Determination of Deceleration Rate of Aortic Regurgitant Velocity

Continuous wave Doppler echocardiography may also be helpful in semiquantitation of the severity of AR. Because the instantaneous maximal velocity should be proportional to the instantaneous gradient between the aortic and left ventricular diastolic pressures, the slope of the Doppler velocity during diastole should indicate how rapidly the left ventricular diastolic pressure is increasing. In severe AR, the left ventricular diastolic pressure increases rapidly; thus, the gradient between the aorta and the left ventricle will decrease rapidly. Consequently, a rapid decline in the slope of the diastolic AR Doppler signal will be evident (Fig. 7–8). If the AR is mild, there will be minimal increase in left ventricular pressure and minimal change in the gradient between the aorta and left ventricle. Therefore, the decline in the slope of the diastolic signal will be slower (Fig. 7–9).

Several groups have shown that the rate of deceleration of AR velocity is directly proportional to the severity of regurgitation.[47–49] Typically, patients with aortic regurgitant deceleration rates of 3.0 m/s^2 or greater have significant regurgitation, while those with less rapid rates of deceleration have mild or moderate regurgitant lesions (Figs. 7–8 and 7–9). This approach is conceptually straightforward, practical, and not too tedious.

Teague el al[50] has suggested a method for estimating the severity of AR that is analogous to the Doppler assessment of mitral stenosis. The CW profile has been quantitated as the Doppler half-time, or the time required for the Doppler velocity profile to decay by 29 percent. The Doppler half-time is intimately related to the pressure half-time across the

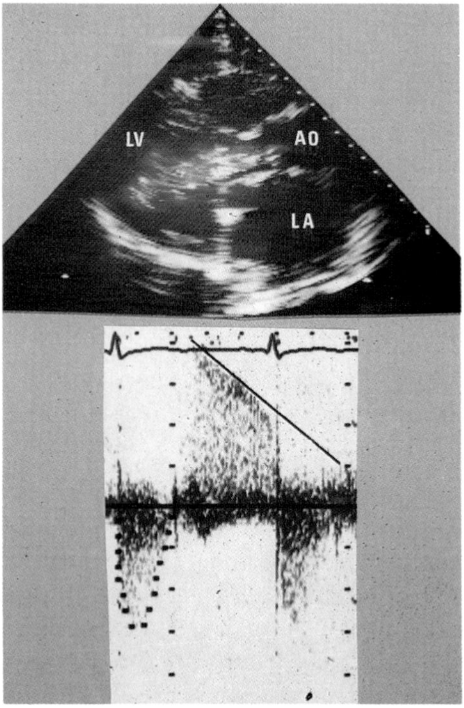

Figure 7–8. Severe aortic regurgitation. *Top*: Parasternal long axis view. The regurgitant jet at its origin occupies two-thirds of the thickness of the left ventricular outflow tract, indicating severe aortic regurgitation. LV = left ventricle, AO = aorta, LA = left atrium. *Bottom*: Continuous wave Doppler recording from an apical view. The high slope is associated with elevated left ventricular end-diastolic pressure and severe regurgitation as demonstrated by angiography. (Scale marks = 1 m/s.)

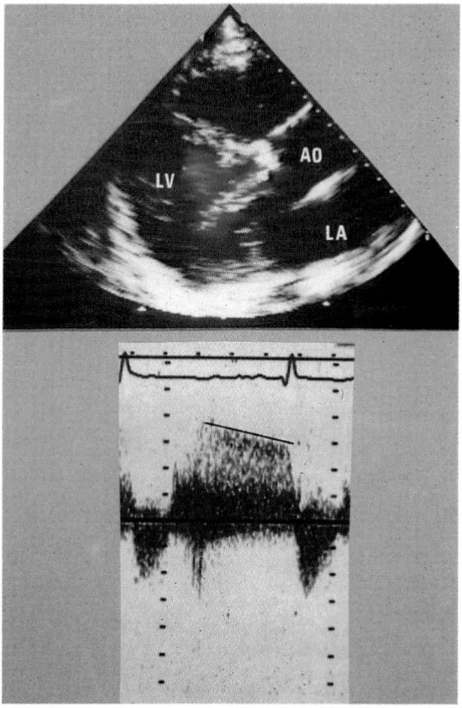

Figure 7–9. Mild aortic regurgitation. *Top*: Parasternal long axis view demonstrating the narrow origin of the aortic regurgitant jet in the left ventricular outflow tract. LV = left ventricle, AO = aorta, LA = left atrium. *Bottom*: Continuous wave Doppler profile of the regurgitant aortic jet recorded from the apex. The low slope is associated with normal left ventricular end-diastolic pressure and mild regurgitation as demonstrated by angiography. (Scale marks = 1 m/s.)

valve, and inversely related to regurgitation severity. Half-times greater than 0.45 s are caused by mild AR, while half-times from 0.45 to 0.30 s are associated with moderate regurgitation. Half-times of 0.25 s or less are almost always associated with severe regurgitation. However, substantial overlap among groups was present. Moreover, extreme elevation of left ventricular end-diastolic pressure, aortic root pressure, and compliance of both the aorta and the ventricle may influence the Doppler half-time independent of the size of the regurgitant orifice.

Regurgitant Velocity Waveform Intensity

The intensity of AR signals, which is most easily appreciated using CW Doppler, does reflect the relative volume of regurgitant as compared to forward transaortic flow. Thus, patients with mild AR typically manifest relatively faint diastolic regurgitant jets (using the intensity of anterograde flow in order to calibrate for differences in ultrasound signal strength in individual patients). In contrast, if the intensity of the regurgitant signal is strong and nearly equal to that of anterograde systolic flow, this suggests that the degree of AR is significant.[51] Assessment of the intensity of the regurgitant waveform only provides a general sense of regurgitant severity, but this is a relatively simple and straightforward approach.

Diastolic Flow Pattern in the Abdominal Aorta

Another method for determining if AR is severe or not has been proposed by Takenaka and coworkers.[52] This approach involves interrogating the abdominal aorta just below the diaphragm, using PD from a subcostal approach. In normal subjects, systolic flow in the abdominal aorta is oriented toward the transducer, causing an upright systolic Doppler waveform. In patients with mild AR, systolic upright flow may be accompanied by brief retrograde diastolic flow. Holodiastolic flow reversal is not recorded unless AR is significant, in which case evidence for holodiastolic retrograde flow is typically recorded in the abdominal aorta. Although this is a simple and rapid method for determining the severity of AR, it is not a quantitative method, and it does not distinguish between mild or absent AR.

Estimations of Regurgitant Fraction

Estimations of regurgitant fraction have also been attempted according to the continuity principle. In theory, it should be possible to estimate the regurgitant fraction by Doppler examination of forward flows from two different sites, one representing forward output and one representing the total left ventricular output (discussed in Chap. 11). The forward output can be assessed by interrogating PD in the pulmonary artery and deriving the cross-sectional area from the 2D echo image. This approach, although practical in children, is not feasible in most adults because of the inability to visualize the walls of the pulmonary artery. Alternate sites to assess forward flow are at the mitral and tricuspid valves, but the accuracy of these approaches is currently not sufficient to be of routine use. Similarly, the accuracy of total left ventricular outflow measures depends on accurate evaluation of the cross-sectional area of the left ventricular outflow space, using the echo image in the parasternal long axis view. Institution of this approach in a given laboratory requires systematic correlative confirmation of its accuracy.

REFERENCES

1. Grayburn P, Smith M, Handshoe R, et al: Detection of aortic insufficiency by standard echocardiography, pulsed Doppler echocardiography, and auscultation: A comparison of accuracies. *Ann Intern Med* 104:599, 1986.

2. Esper R: Detection of mild aortic regurgitation by range-gated pulsed Doppler echocardiography. *Am J Cardiol* 50:1037, 1982.

3. Boughner D: Assessment of aortic insufficiency by transcutaneous Doppler ultrasound. *Circulation* 52:874, 1975.

4. Wautrecht J, Vandenbossche J, Englert M: Sensitivity and specificity of pulsed Doppler echocardiography in detection of aortic and mitral regurgitation. *Eur Heart J* 5:404, 1984.

5. Feigenbaum H: *Echocardiography*, ed 4. Philadelphia, Lea & Febiger, 1986.

6. Estevez C, Dillon J, Walker P, et al: Echocardiographic manifestations of aortic cusp rupture in a case of myxomatous degeneration of the aortic valve. *Chest* 69:544, 1976.

7. Ramirez J, Guardiola J, Flowers N: Echocardiographic diagnosis of ruptured aortic valve leaflet in bacterial endocarditis. *Circulation* 57:634, 1978.

8. Das G, Lee C, Weissler A: Echocardiographic manifestations of ruptured aortic valvular leaflets in the absence of valvular vegetations. *Chest* 72:464, 1977.

9. Ogawa S, Hayashi J, Sasaki H, et al: Evaluation of combined valvular prolapse syndrome by two-dimensional echocardiography. *Circulation* 65:174, 1982.

10. Wolddow A, Parameswaran R, Hartman J, et al: Aortic regurgitation due to aortic valve prolapse. *Am J Cardiol* 55:1435, 1985.

11. DeMaria A, Bommer W, Newmann A, et al: Identification and localization of aneurysms of the ascending aorta by cross-sectional echocardiography. *Circulation* 59:755, 1979.

12. Victor M, Mintz G, Kotler M, et al: Two-dimensional echocardiographic diagnosis of aortic dissection. *Am J Cardiol* 48:1155, 1981.

13. D'Cruz I, Cohen H, Prabhu R, et al: Flutter of left ventricular structures in patients with aortic regurgitation, with special reference to patients with associated mitral stenosis. *Am Heart J* 92:684, 1976.

14. Nakao S, Tanaka H, Tahara M, et al: An experimental study on the mechanisms of echocardiographic findings in aortic regurgitation: With special reference to the direction of regurgitant jet (abstr). *Circulation* 60(II):798, 1979.

15. Cope G, Kisslo J, Johnson M, et al: Diastolic vibration of the interventricular septum in aortic insufficiency. *Circulation* 51:589, 1975.

16. Pridie R, Benham R, Oakley C: Diastolic vibration of the interventricular septum in aortic insufficiency. *Br Heart J* 33:291, 1971.

17. Winsberg F, Gabor E, Hernberg J: Fluttering of the mitral valve in aortic insufficiency. *Circulation* 41:225, 1970.

18. Saal A, Gross B, Franklin D, et al: Noninvasive detection of aortic insufficiency in patients with mitral stenosis by pulsed Doppler echocardiography. *J Am Coll Cardiol* 5:176, 1985.

19. Robertson W, Stewart J, Armstrong W, et al: Reverse doming of the anterior mitral leaflet with severe aortic regurgitation. *J Am Coll Cardiol* 3:431, 1984.

20. Wigle E, Labrosse C: Sudden, severe aortic insufficiency. *Circulation* 32:708, 1965.

21. Mann T, McLaurin L, Grossman W, et al: Assessing the hemodynamic severity of acute aortic regurgitation due to infective endocarditis. *N Engl J Med* 293:108, 1975.

22. Morganroth J, Perloff J, Zeldis S, et al: Acute severe aortic regurgitation: Pathophysiology, clinical recognition and management. *Ann Intern Med* 82:223, 1977.

23. Pietro D, Parisi A, Harrington J, et al: Premature opening of the aortic valve: An index of highly advanced aortic regurgitation. *J Clin Ultrasound* 6:170, 1978.

24. Weaver W, Wilson C, Rourke T, et al: Mid-diastolic aortic valve opening in severe acute aortic regurgitation. *Circulation* 55:145, 1977.

25. Bommer W, Mapes R, Miller L, et al: Quantitation of aortic insufficiency with two-dimensional Doppler echocardiography (abstr). *Am J Cardiol* 47:412, 1981.

26. Pearlman A, Dooley T, Franklin D, et al: Detection of regurgitant flow using Duplex (two-dimensional/Doppler) echocardiography (abstr). *Circulation* 60(II):154, 1979.

27. Ward J, Baker D, Rubenstein S, et al: Detection of aortic insufficiency by pulse Doppler echocardiography. *J Clin Ultrasound* 5:5, 1977.

28. Ciobanu M, Abbasi A, Allen M, et al: Pulsed Doppler echocardiography in the diagnosis and estimation of severity of aortic insufficiency. *Am J Cardiol* 49:339, 1982.

29. Esper R: Detection of mild aortic regurgitation by range-gated pulsed Doppler echocardiography. *Am J Cardiol* 50:1037, 1982.

30. Richards K, Cannon S, Crawford M, et al: Noninvasive diagnosis of aortic and mitral valve disease with pulsed-Doppler spectral analysis. *Am J Cardiol* 51:1122, 1983.

31. Veyrat C, Cholot N, Abitbol G, et al: Noninvasive diagnosis and assessment of aortic valve disease and evaluation of aortic prosthesis function using echo pulsed Doppler velocimetry. *Br Heart J* 43:393, 1983.

32. Saal A, Pearlman A, Hossack K, et al: Detection of aortic insufficiency: Relative strengths and limitations of auscultation, M-mode echocardiography, and pulsed Doppler echocardiography in 94 catheterized patients, in *Fifth Symposium on Echocardiography*. Rotterdam, Ultrasonoor Bull, 1983.

33. Meyers D, Olson T, Hansen D: Auscultation, M-mode echocardiography and pulsed Doppler echocardiography compared with angiography for the diagnosis of chronic aortic regurgitation. *Am J Cardiol* 56:811, 1985.

34. Perry G, Nanda N: Diagnosis and quantitation of valvular regurgitation by color Doppler flow mapping. *Echocardiography* 3:493, 1986.

35. Pearlman A, Otto C, Janko C, et al: Direction and width of aortic regurgitation jets: Assessment by Doppler color flow mapping (abstr). *J Am Coll Cardiol* 7:100A, 1986.

36. Omoto R, Yokote Y, Takamoto S, et al: The development of real-time two-dimensional Doppler echocardiography and its clinical significance in acquired valvular disease. *Jpn Heart J* 25:325, 1984.

37. Asaka T, Yoshikawa J, Yoshida K, et al: Sensitivity and specificity of real-time two-dimensional Doppler flow imaging system in the detection of valvular regurgitation (abstr). *Circulation* 70(II): 38, 1984.

38. Byard C, Perry G, Roitman D, et al: Quantitative assessment of aortic regurgitation by color Doppler (abstr). *Circulation* 72(III):146, 1985.

39. Kitabatake A, Ito H, Tanouchi J, et al: A new approach to quantitate aortic regurgitation by real-time two-dimensional Doppler echocardiography (abstr). *Circulation* 72(III): 306A, 1985.

40. Yoshikawa J, Kato H, Yoshida K, et al: Real-time two-dimensional Doppler echocardiographic diagnosis of aortic regurgitation in the presence of a mitral prosthesis (abstr). *Circulation* 70(II):39, 1984.

41. Miyatake K, Okamoto M, Kinoshita N, et al: Clinical applications of a new type of real-time two-dimensional Doppler flow imaging system. *Am J Cardiol* 54:857, 1984.

42. Perry G, Helmcke F, Nanda N, et al: Evaluation of aortic insufficiency by Doppler color flow mapping. *J Am Coll Cardiol* 9:952, 1987.

43. Helmcke F, Perry G, Soto B, et al: Correlation of angiographic and color Doppler parameters of aortic insufficiency (abstr). *Clin Res* 34:307A, 1986.

44. Veyrat C, Lessana A, Abitbol G, et al: New indexes for assessing aortic regurgitation with two-dimensional Doppler echocardiographic measurements of the regurgitant aortic valvular area. *Circulation* 68:998, 1983.

45. Veyrat C, Ameur A, Gourtchiglouian C, et al: Calculation of pulsed Doppler left ventricular outflow tract regurgitant index for grading the severity of aortic regurgitation. *Am Heart J* 108:507, 1984.

46. Bolger A, Eigler N, Pfaff J, et al: Relationship of color Doppler jet area to flow volume: Reliability and limitations (abstr). *Circulation* 74(II):216, 1986.

47. Grayburn P, Handshoe R, Smith M, et al: Quantitative assessment of the hemodynamic consequences of aortic regurgitation by means of continuous wave Doppler recordings. *J Am Coll Cardiol* 10:135, 1987.

48. Beyer R, Ramirez M, Josephson M, et al: Correlation of continuous-wave Doppler assessment of chronic aortic regurgitation with hemodynamics and angiography. *Am J Cardiol* 60:852, 1987.

49. Labovitz A, Ferrara R, Kern M, et al: Quantitative evaluation of aortic insufficiency by continuous wave Doppler echocardiography. *J Am Coll Cardiol* 8:1341, 1986.

50. Teague S, Heinsimer J, Anderson J, et al: Quantification of aortic regurgitation utilizing continuous wave Doppler ultrasound. *J Am Coll Cardiol* 8:592, 1986.

51. Hatle L, Angelsen B: *Doppler Ultrasound in Cardiology*, ed 2. Philadelphia, Lea & Febiger, 1985.

52. Takenaka K, Dabestani A, Gardin J, et al: A simple Doppler echocardiographic method for estimating severity of aortic regurgitation. *Am J Cardiol* 57:1340, 1986.

CHAPTER 8

Mitral Regurgitation

Mitral regurgitation (MR) may be caused by dysfunction of any part of the mitral valve apparatus, including the leaflets, anulus, chordae tendineae, and papillary muscles.[1] M-mode echocardiographic findings of MR are usually nonspecific. Although 2D echocardiography can image the valve and its apparatus in real time and identify the cause of MR, only Doppler echocardiography can accurately detect and quantify the severity of MR.

Mitral regurgitation results in a high velocity, turbulent flow disturbance in the left atrium that is readily distinguished from normal intracardiac flow by Doppler technology. Detection of this high velocity flow disturbance by either pulsed, continuous wave, or color Doppler flow imaging allows accurate diagnosis of the presence of MR.

PULSED WAVE DOPPLER

Detection of Mitral Regurgitation

The PD technique permits detection and semiquantitation of MR. The diagnosis of MR by PD examination consists of detection of a systolic turbulence when the sample volume is placed in the left atrium[2] (Fig. 8–1). Normally, no systolic signal is detected at the mitral valve coaptation point except for the high-pitched "clicks" produced by the opening and closing of the valve. The turbulent sound of MR should be sought by imaging from both the parasternal and the apical transducer positions[3,4] because the regurgitant jet may not be noted if it is directed out of the plane of any single 2D view. In many instances, mild MR will be detected from only one or the other position. Frequently, a pansystolic signal is observed below the baseline, designating flow away from the transducer or into the left atrium. Signal aliasing is commonly noted, especially closer to the valve.

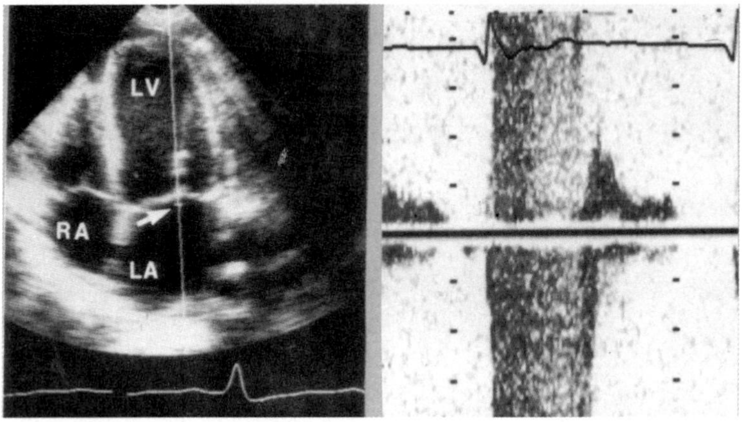

Figure 8–1. Mitral regurgitant flow disturbance recorded from the apex using pulsed-Doppler. *Left*: Systolic 2D echo image showing the Doppler sample volume (arrow) positioned in the left atrium (LA) just behind the plane of the closed mitral leaflets. LV = left ventricle, RA = right atrium. *Right*: Doppler velocity tracing showing pansystolic turbulent flow (spectral broadening) diagnostic of mitral regurgitation. Signal aliasing is noted.

Many investigators have evaluated the ability of PD to determine the presence of MR (Table 8–1). When patients from these different series are grouped, forming a composite of 389 patients in whom selective left ventricular cineangiographic data were available for comparison, the overall sensitivity and specificity of PD was 90 and 93 percent, respectively. As

TABLE 8–1. Detection of Mitral Regurgitation by Pulsed Doppler Echocardiography

No. of Patients	Sensitivity, %	Specificity, %	Predictive Value, % Positive	Predictive Value, % Negative	Reference
92	95	90	89	96	5
45	100	100	100	100	6
47	91	95	95	92	7
31	91	95	95	82	8
48	93	100	100	91	9
34	72	100	100	56	10
27	100	100	100	100	11
65	83	85	68	93	12
Total 389	90	93	92	91	

would be expected, the sensitivity of the technique in detecting MR increases with the increasing severity of the MR because the area of systolic turbulence into the left atrium becomes larger.[13]

The cause of MR is also a factor in the accuracy of the Doppler detection of MR. Rheumatic MR tends to produce a wide regurgitant jet[14,15]; the sensitivity of the Doppler examination approaches 100 percent[7,16] In contrast, the regurgitant jet produced by mitral valve prolapse, dysfunction of the papillary muscle, or a cleft mitral valve leaflet may be more difficult to detect.[7,8,16] In mitral valve prolapse, a small localized jet is usually located directly behind the opposite valve leaflet. In prolapse of the anterior leaflet, the jet is directly behind the posterior leaflet, whereas in prolapse of the posterior leaflet, the jet is directly behind the anterior leaflet.[15]

Quantitation of Mitral Regurgitation

Quantitation of MR by PD mapping relies on the depth and width to which the regurgitant velocity can be detected (Fig. 8–2). Abasi et al[7] estimated the degree of MR on the basis of the location and distribution of the regurgitant jet within the left atrium. Mild MR was detected only immediately beneath the mitral valve in the left atrium. As MR increased in severity, the distribution of abnormal flow within the left atrium became more widespread. Comparing this semiquantitative approach to the angiographic assessment of MR, there was a high correlation ($r = 0.88$).[7] However, in another study, 4 of 11 patients with moderate to severe MR by angiography had no detectable systolic turbulence in the left atrium.[10]

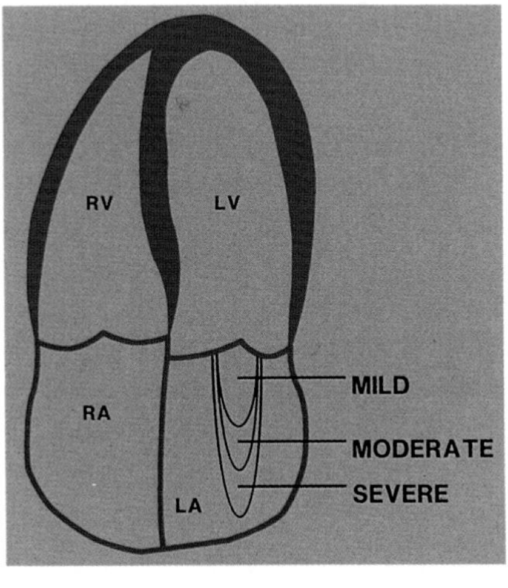

Figure 8–2. Schematic diagram showing the grading of severity of mitral regurgitation. LA = left atrium, LV = left ventricle, RA = right atrium, RV = right ventricle.

Mapping the spatial distribution of MR flow requires examination from a variety of transducer positions and orientations in order to define properly the 3D spatial distribution of the systolic regurgitant flow disturbance within the left atrium. As in the case with aortic regurgitation, it is important to distinguish between broad and narrow regurgitant jets. Moreover, MR may be oblique in orientation, and CFI shows that many MR jets hug the walls of the left atrium, leading to complex systolic flow patterns within the left atrium. For all of these reasons, examination from apical and parasternal echo windows is important. Although the apical views are theoretically better suited for mapping MR jets, a practical limitation in adults with substantial enlargement of the left ventricle and atrium is the inability to interrogate the sample volume at desired depths. Hence, failure to detect MR flow in distant regions of the left atrium may be due to inadequate signal strength rather than absence of MR flow. In these patients, the precordial echo window usually places the sample volume closer to the transducer than does the apical window; moreover, as the sample volume is moved away from the plane of the mitral valve, its depth changes little. Thus, standard and low parasternal windows have been particularly helpful in mapping MR flow disturbances. This is true using either conventional PD or CFI techniques.

CONTINUOUS WAVE DOPPLER

Continuous wave Doppler echocardiography has been as accurate as the PD mode in detection of MR. Examination of the mitral valve is usually done from the apical position with the transducer angulated until the typical M-shaped diastolic flow pattern of the mitral valve is found; then the angulation is altered slightly until a characteristic holosystolic high-velocity signal, directed away from the transducer, is detected (Fig. 8–3).

An indirect quantitative evaluation of MR severity may be provided by the strength of the CW Doppler signal (by comparison to mitral diastolic forward flow). Because it is related to the volume of flow, a weak signal indicates a mild or trivial lesion; a strong high-velocity signal indicates moderate to severe regurgitation[17] (Fig. 8–2 and 8–3). Thus, CW Doppler provides a clue to distinguishing mild from more severe regurgitant lesions. The peak MR velocity is nearly always in excess of 4 m/s and does not provide a clue to severity.

The hemodynamic profile of acute severe MR makes it sufficiently unique to result in an altered profile of MR velocity waveform. The characteristic high V wave in mid-late systole noted in the left atrial pressure

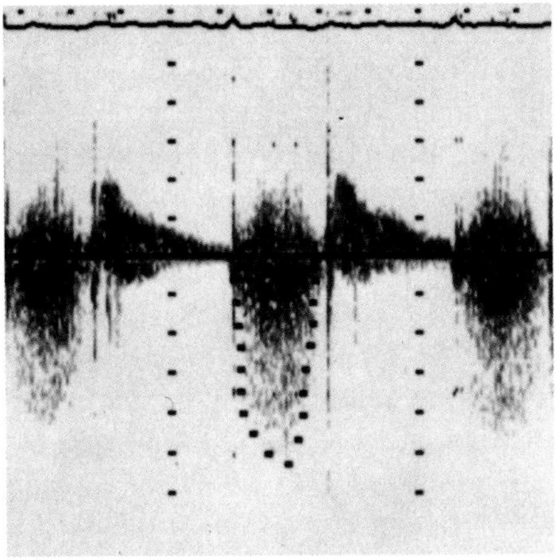

Figure 8–3. Mitral regurgitation recorded from the cardiac apex using continuous wave Doppler. Mitral regurgitation causes a pansystolic jet that accelerates rapidly and has a symmetric, rounded peak (dashed lines) resembling an inverted left ventricular pressure trace. The systolic waveform is relatively dense indicating moderate regurgitation. (Scale marks = 1 m/s.)

pulse alters the profile of the left ventricular-left atrial pressure gradient. The pressure drop is high in early systole and rapidly decreases as the left atrial V wave rises to approach left ventricular systolic pressure. The MR velocity profile in such cases mirrors this altered pressure gradient profile. Thus, the velocity waveform reaches its peak in early systole and then decreases rapidly toward baseline (Fig. 8–4). This shape resembles that of normal aortic outflow velocity with an early systolic peak. The velocity waveform shape may change following acute interventions such as administration of vasodilators, which result in a decrease in the height of the V wave.

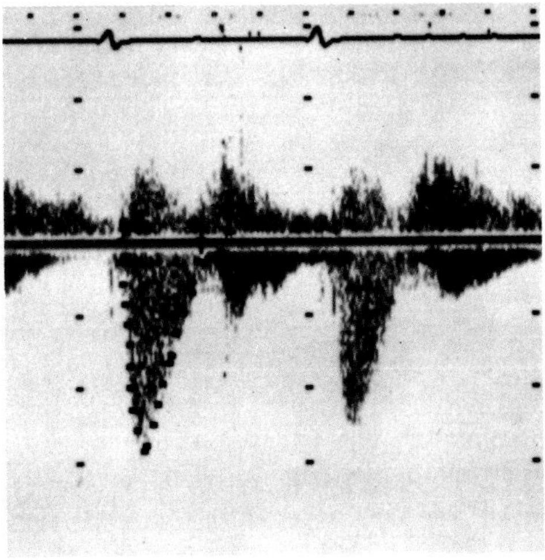

Figure 8–4. Acute severe mitral regurgitation recorded from the cardiac apex using continuous wave Doppler. The velocity waveform reaches its peak in early systole and decreases rapidly toward baseline resulting from a prominent left atrial V wave (see Fig. 8–3 for comparison). (Scale marks = 1 m/s.)

COLOR FLOW IMAGING

Mitral regurgitation is diagnosed by CFI by demonstrating turbulent or abnormally directed systolic flow in the left atrium originating from the mitral valve (Fig. 8–5). Color Doppler, like conventional Doppler, is less sensitive in the diagnosis of MR compared to aortic regurgitation due to the depth of the left atrium. Color Doppler does allow more rapid examination for the regurgitant jet, however, and should diminish the likelihood of missing an eccentric jet provided multiple planes are interrogated.

Color Doppler may be slightly more sensitive in the diagnosis of MR than is PD, perhaps because the former is less likely to miss small eccentric jets. In three series published to date, the sensitivity of CFI in 189 patients with angiographically documented MR was 94 percent (range 86 to 100 percent),[18–20] while the specificity in 97 patients with angiographically competent mitral valves was 100 percent.[18,20] However, caution is necessary when comparing sensitivities of PD and CFI series, due to the operator dependency of the techniques and the multiple patient population factors that will influence sensitivity of either Doppler technique.

Color flow quantification of MR has been validated by angiography. In a system of grading MR on a scale of 0 to 4 on the length of the jet from the mitral orifice (see Fig. 8–2), Miyatake et al[21] found a moderate correlation

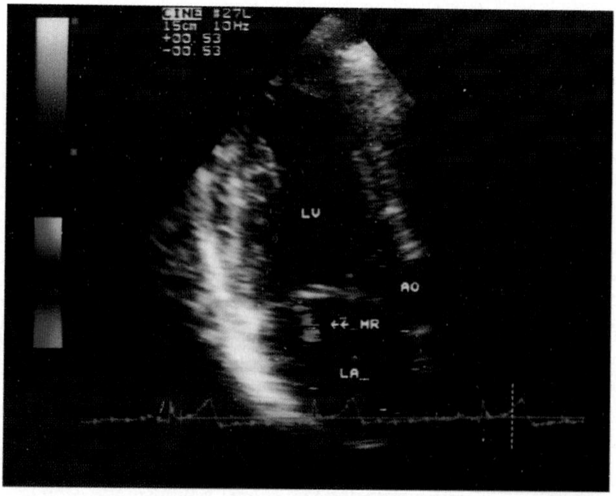

Figure 8–5. Color Doppler flow imaging from the apical long axis view in a patient with mild mitral regurgitation. The eccentric blue jet of mitral regurgitation (MR) can be clearly appreciated. AO = aorta, LA = left atrium, LV = left ventricle.

between angiographic grading and both the maximal depth of the regurgitant jet ($r = 0.87$) and the maximal 2D area ($r = 0.83$). Helmcke et al[20] found a poor correlation between the regurgitant jet area in any one plane and the angiographic grade of MR in 147 patients. Averaging jet area from several orthogonal planes improved the relationship. The best correlation with angiography was observed when the ratio of the 2D area of the MR jet to the planimetered area of the left atrium was obtained in two or more orthogonal views and these ratios were then averaged. If the average ratio was less than 20 percent, it represented mild MR (Fig. 8–6); moderate MR was diagnosed if the ratio was 20 to 40 percent (Fig. 8–7 and 8–8); and severe MR was indicated if the ratio exceeded 40 percent (Fig. 8–9).

When grading the severity of an MR jet with CFI, the examiner needs to consider the dynamic nature of the jet and its dependence on multiple hemodynamic factors. For example, with atrial fibrillation, beat-to-beat variation in the regurgitant area will vary significantly (occasionally greater than 100 percent),[22] and an average of at least 10 beats should be used for grading. Acute afterload alteration will also dramatically change the severity of the MR jet. For example, during sustained hand grip, the size of the jet may increase to the next higher degree of severity.[22] Additionally, the gold standard for quantification of MR is cardiac catheterization, which may be performed under different afterload and preload conditions, heart

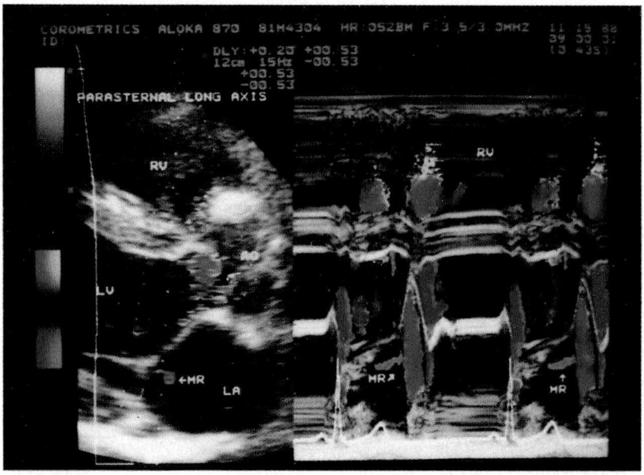

Figure 8–6. Simultaneous Doppler flow imaging and color M-mode demonstrating mild mitral regurgitation (MR). Color M-mode is valuable in determining the timing of the onset and cessation of flow. AO = aorta, LA = left atrium, LV = left ventricle, RV = right ventricle.

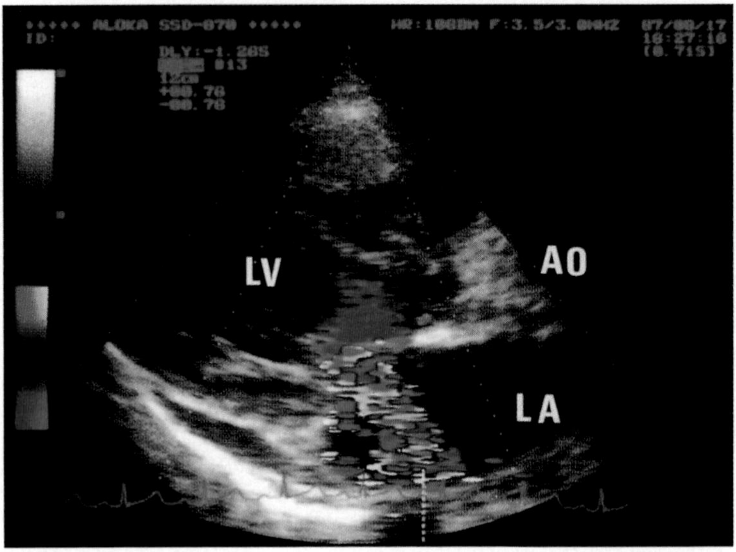

Figure 8–7. Mitral regurgitation from parasternal long axis view. Mitral regurgitant jet occupies 20% to 40% of the left atrium indicating severe mitral regurgitation. Note the high velocity, turbulent flow (mosaic) at the center of the jet, and the lower velocity flow (blue) at the periphery of the jet. AO = aorta, LA = left atrium, LV = left ventricle.

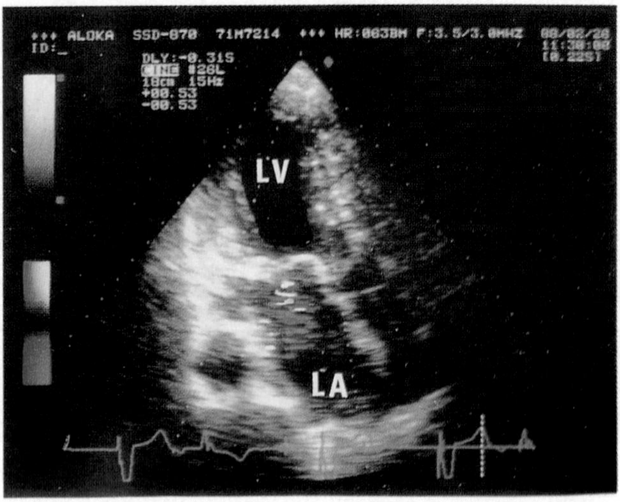

Figure 8–8. Moderate mitral regurgitation, apical long axis view. LA = left atrium, LV = left ventricle.

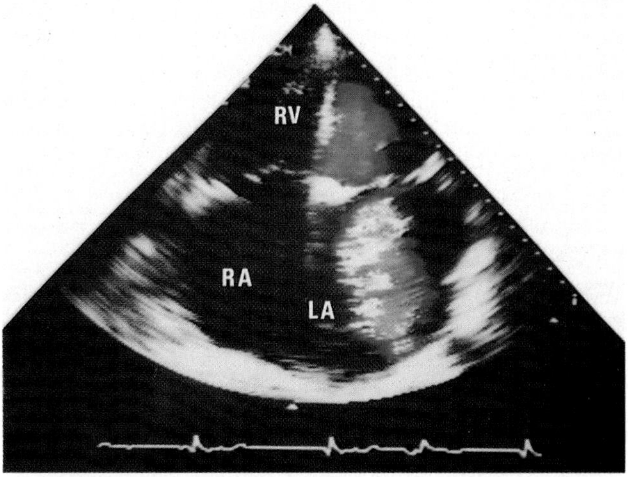

Figure 8 – 9. Mitral regurgitation, from apical four chamber view. The mitral regurgitant jet occupies almost the entire left atrium in this view, indicating severe mitral regurgitation. LA = left atrium, RA = right atrium, RV = right ventricle.

rate, and pharmacologic circumstances than would a routine Doppler examination in a quiet office. Thus, absolute quantification via any technique may be difficult to achieve.

The clinical estimation of the severity of MR should incorporate not only the regurgitant jet area, left atrial size, and the ratio of the two, but should also consider left ventricular function and dimension. Since clinical management of patients is guided by left ventricular adaptation to volume overload, 2D echocardiographic evaluation of left ventricular dimension and contractility is essential.

REFERENCES

1. Roberts W: Morphologic features of the normal and abnormal mitral valve. *Am J Cardiol* 51:1005, 1983.
2. Miyatake K, Kinoshita N, Nagata S, et al: Intracardiac flow pattern in mitral regurgitation studied with combined use of the ultrasonic pulsed Doppler technique and cross-sectional echocardiography. *Am J Cardiol* 45:155, 1980.
3. Kalmanson D, Veyrat C, Bouchareine F, et al: Noninvasive recording of mitral valve flow velocity patterns using pulsed Doppler echocardiography: Application to diagnosis and evaluation of mitral valve disease. *Br Heart J* 39:517, 1977.
4. Diebold B, Theroux P, Bourassa M, et al: Non-invasive pulsed Doppler study of mitral stenosis and mitral regurgitation: Preliminary study. *Br Heart J* 42:168, 1979.

5. Dooley T, Rubenstein S, Stevenson J: Pulsed Doppler echocardiography: The detection of mitral regurgitation, in Lyons WD (ed): *Ultrasound in Medicine*, ed 4. New York, Plenum Press, 1978.
6. Pearlman A, Gentile R, Rubenstein S, et al: Echocardiographic detection of mitral regurgitation (MR) in mitral valve prolapse (MVP), in Lancee CT (ed): *Echocardiology*. The Hague, Martinus Nijhoff, 1979.
7. Abbasi A, Allen M, De Cristofaro D, et al: Detection and estimation of the degree of mitral regurgitation by range-gated pulsed Doppler echocardiography. *Circulation* 61:143, 1980.
8. Shah A, Waggoner A, Young J, et al: Mitral regurgitation in mitral valve prolapse: Detection by pulsed Doppler echocardiography versus angiography and cardiac auscultation (abstr). *Am J Cardiol* 45:442, 1980.
9. Kalmanson D, Veyrat C, Abitbol G, et al: Doppler echocardiography and valvular regurgitation, with special emphasis on mitral insufficiency: Advantages of two-dimensional echocardiography with real-time spectral analysis, in Rijsterborgh H (ed): *Echocardiology*. The Hague, Martinus Nijhoff, 1981.
10. Patel A, Rowe G, Thomsen J, et al: Detection and estimation of rheumatic mitral regurgitation in the presence of mitral stenosis by pulsed Doppler echocardiography. *Am J Cardiol* 51:986, 1983.
11. Richards K, Cannon S, Crawford M, et al: Noninvasive diagnosis of aortic and mitral valve disease with pulsed-Doppler spectral analysis. *Am J Cardiol* 51:1122, 1983.
12. Kwan O, Handshoe R, Handshoe S, et al: Sensitivity and specificity of Doppler ultrasound in the detection of valvular regurgitation: Comparison of continuous and pulsed wave techniques (abstr). *Circulation* 68(III):229, 1983.
13. Blanchard D, Diebold B, Peronneau P, et al: Non-invasive diagnosis of mitral regurgitation by Doppler echocardiography. *Br Heart J* 45:589, 1981.
14. Veyrat C, Ameur C, Bas S, et al: Pulsed Doppler echocardiographic indices for assessing mitral regurgitation. *Br Heart J* 51:130, 1984.
15. Miyatake K, Nimura Y, Sakakibara H, et al: Localization and direction of mitral regurgitant flow in mitral orifice studied with the combined use of ultrasonic pulsed Doppler technique and two dimensional echocardiography. *Br Heart J* 48:449, 1982.
16. Areias J, Goldberg S, de Villeneuve U: Use and limitations of time interval histogram output from echo Doppler to detect mitral regurgitation. *Am Heart J* 101:805, 1981.
17. Hatle L, Angelsen B: *Doppler Ultrasound in Cardiology*, ed 2. Philadelphia, Lea & Febiger, 1985.
18. Miyatake K, Okamoto M, Kinoshita N, et al: Clinical applications of a new type of real-time two-dimensional Doppler flow imaging system. *Am J Cardiol* 54:857, 1984.
19. Omoto R, Yokote Y, Takamoto S, et al: The development of real-time two-dimensional Doppler echocardiography and its clinical significance in acquired valvular diseases. *Jpn Heart J* 25:325, 1984.

20. Helmcke F, Nanda N, Hsiung M, et al: Color Doppler assessment of mitral regurgitation using orthogonal planes. *Circulation* 75:175, 1987.

21. Miyatake K, Izumi S, Okamoto M, et al: Semiquantitative grading of severity of mitral regurgitation by real-time two-dimensional Doppler flow imaging technique. J *Am Coll Cardiol* 7:82, 1986.

22. Saenz C, Deumite N, Roitman D, et al: Limitations of color Doppler in quantitative assessment of mitral regurgitation (abstr). *Circulation* 72(III):99, 1985.

CHAPTER 9

Tricuspid and Pulmonic Regurgitation

The clinical detection of right-sided cardiac valve regurgitation of either tricuspid or pulmonary origin may often be difficult. Tricuspid regurgitation (TR) may occur as a functional result of right ventricular pressure or volume overload or may be caused by rheumatic heart disease, infective endocarditis, congenital malformations, trauma, and, infrequently, carcinoid disease.[1–3] Pulmonic regurgitation (PR), as an isolated lesion, has been shown to be well tolerated and seldom leads to right ventricular failure. When symptoms occur, pulmonary hypertension or additional disease must be suspected.[4,5] Thus, detection of right-sided valve regurgitation may assume clinical importance as a marker of a more serious underlying disease process, particularly in patients with coexistent left-sided heart disease.

Invasive procedures such as angiography have certain limitations in the identification of right-sided heart valve regurgitation but are probably reliable in establishing the absence of valve regurgitation.[6–8] Although noninvasive techniques such as echocardiography and phonocardiography are relatively insensitive indicators of right-sided heart valve regurgitation, echocardiography can provide useful information on right ventricular size, abnormalities of ventricular septal motion due to right ventricular volume overload, abnormalities of pulmonary valve motion that may suggest the presence of pulmonary hypertension, and for assessing the integrity of the tricuspid valve and estimating the tricuspid anular area.[9] In contrast, Doppler echocardiography allows direct demonstration of right-sided heart valve regurgitation and provides a number of methods for assessing the severity of the regurgitation.

TRICUSPID REGURGITATION

Conventional Doppler Techniques

The diagnosis of TR is made by PD echocardiology by searching the right atrium for a turbulent flow disturbance (Fig. 9–1), using the apical four chamber or the parasternal short axis views, or by CW Doppler from an apical window (Fig. 9–2). The subcostal view also may be useful, particularly to demonstrate reverse flow in the hepatic veins which is often present in severe TR.[10] In some patients with normal tricuspid valves a short systolic signal is recorded due to closure of the tricuspid valve.[11] Thus, to diagnose TR, the flow disturbance must occupy more than half of the period of systole.

Validation of the diagnosis of TR with Doppler techniques has been clearly demonstrated by many clinical studies.[5,11–13] These studies have shown 85 to 100 percent sensitivity and specificity for the diagnosis of TR by PD. In our experience TR detected by Doppler examination is frequently unsuspected clinically.[4] Although the presence of TR can also be demonstrated by contrast echo and M-mode recordings from the inferior vena cava,[14,15] Doppler echo is a more sensitive method when the regurgitation is mild or moderate.[16,17] Mild regurgitation is recorded only a short distance behind the tricuspid valve plane, making detection of contrast in the vena cava highly unlikely. The combined use of contrast echo and

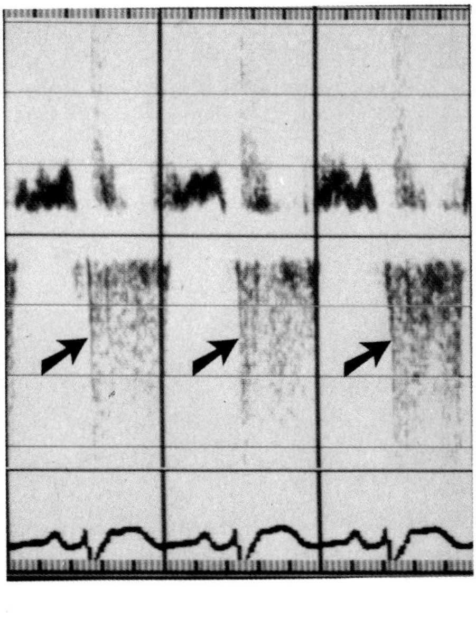

Figure 9–1. Pulsed wave recording of tricuspid regurgitation. Note the holosystolic turbulence displayed below the baseline (arrows). Forward diastolic flow is decreased because of sampling deep in the right atrium. (Scale marks = 20 cm/s.)

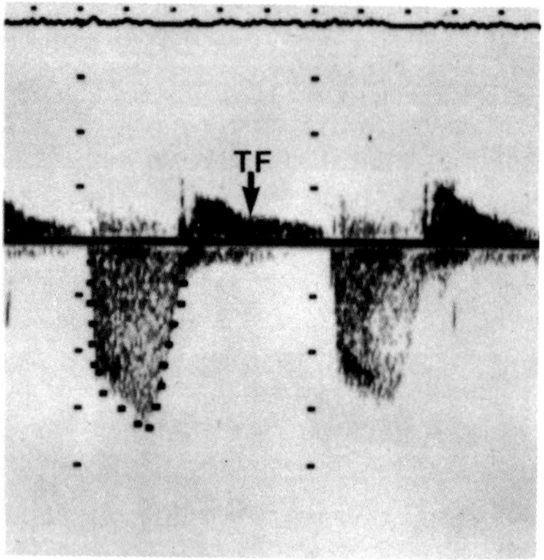

Figure 9–2. Continuous wave recording of tricuspid regurgitation from an apical window. Tricuspid inflow (TF) is displayed above the baseline. (Scale marks = 1 m/s.)

Doppler echo, however, might improve the sensitivity for the diagnosis of TR,[18] because microbubbles are easily detected with Doppler methods.

Doppler echocardiographic assessment of the severity of TR uses methods similar to those used in mitral regurgitation, although there is less validation for TR due to the lack of a suitable gold standard for comparison. The severity of TR can be graded by mapping the area of turbulence into the right atrium,[11] similar to the approach used to quantify mitral regurgitation (see Fig. 8–2). Quantification of TR is also possible by dividing the retrograde flow by the total flow in the inferior vena cava.[10,19] Color flow imaging (discussed below) appears to be the most accurate technique because it shows the extension and direction of reverse flow in the right atrium.[20]

Color Flow Imaging

With CFI, the apical four chamber and parasternal short axis views are usually the best windows. The subcostal and right parasternal approaches are also often helpful in many patients and can be used to differentiate the extent of TR from superior and inferior vena caval inflows. Similar to the jets seen in mitral regurgitation, TR is usually visualized as a systolic blue jet originating from the incompetent area of the tricuspid valve and projecting for a variable distance into the right atrium (Figs. 9–3, 9–4, and 9–5).

In the presence of moderate or severe TR there will be systolic flow reversal in the dilated hepatic veins; this is often appreciated from a subcostal examination[21] (Fig. 9–6). Normally, only blue flow is seen in the

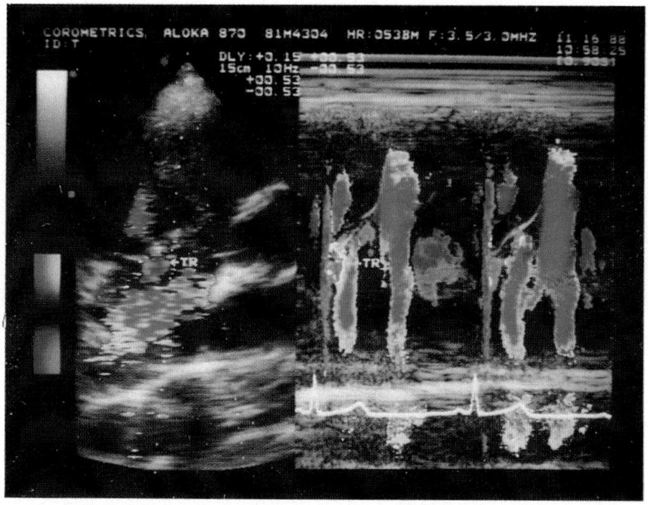

Figure 9–3. Color Doppler study of mild tricuspid regurgitation. *Left*: From a parasternal short axis view, tricuspid regurgitation (TR) is seen as a discrete blue systolic jet. *Right*: Color Doppler signals superimposed on an M-mode through the tricuspid valve shows regurgitant flow reversal (blue) during systole and normal red-colored flow with diastole (corresponding to right ventricular inflow). AO = aorta, RV = right ventricle.

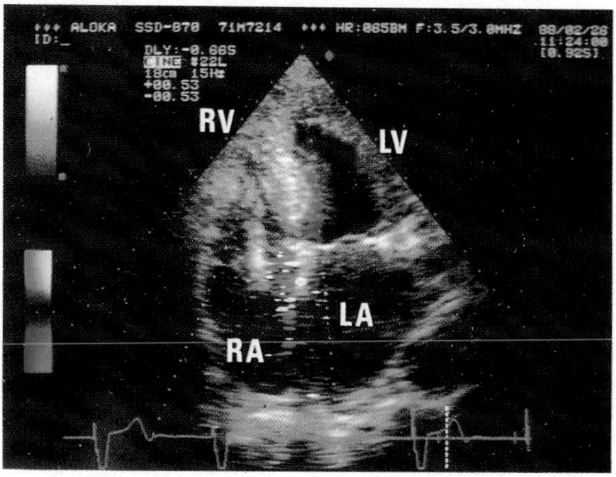

Figure 9–4. Color Doppler study of mild-moderate tricuspid regurgitation, apical four chamber view. An eccentric jet of tricuspid regurgitation is seen as a blue systolic jet that originates from the tricuspid valve and is directed along the intraatrial septum. RV = right ventricle, LV = left ventricle, RA = right atrium, LA = left atrium.

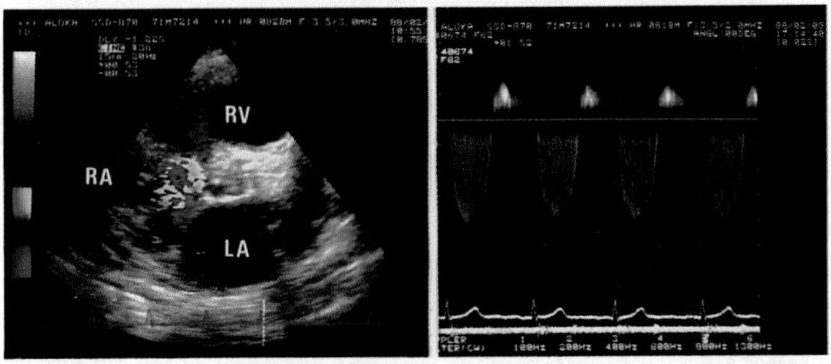

Figure 9–5. Tricuspid regurgitation. *Left*: From the parasternal short axis view, the regurgitant jet occupies more than 40% of the right atrium, indicating severe tricuspid regurgitation. Note the mosaic of colors indicating turbulence. RV = right ventricle, RA = right atrium, LA = left atrium. *Right*: Using color flow guided continuous wave Doppler, the velocity of the regurgitant jet was 4.2 m/s. This corresponds to a peak systolic pressure gradient of 71 mmHg between the right ventricle and right atrium (by using the Bernoulli equation $\Delta P = 4V^2$). Adding the clinically estimated mean right atrium pressure provided an estimated right ventricle systolic pressure of 81 mmHg. (Scale marks = 1 m/s.)

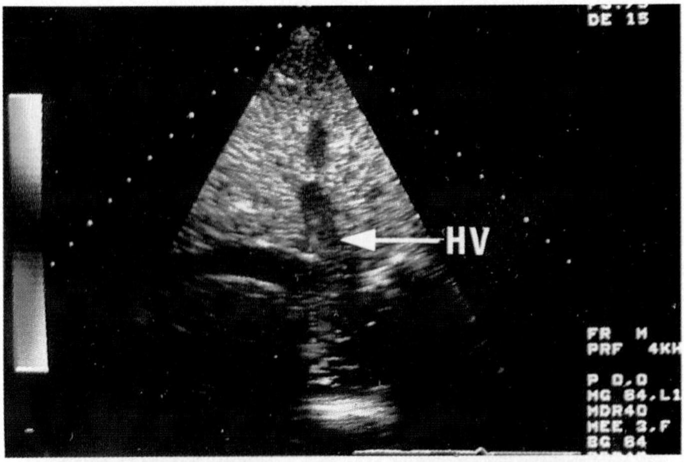

Figure 9–6. Color Doppler study of severe tricuspid regurgitation. From a subcostal approach, prominent systolic flow reversal was seen in the vertical hepatic veins (HV) indicating severe tricuspid regurgitation. This is shown by the prominent red color within the hepatic vein during each systole.

vertical hepatic veins, predominantly during diastole. Occasionally, a small retrograde (red) component is noted during atrial systole in the normal subject, but with significant TR, a prominent red-colored systolic flow is seen in these veins, corresponding to the pulsatile flow reversal due to the TR. Less commonly, a similar pattern can also be found within the superior vena cava from the right suprasternal approach when the TR is severe.

Trivial TR is often observed by conventional PD and CFI in normal subjects and should not be considered a pathologic finding[22–24] (Fig. 9–7). However, significant TR in the adult often reflects right ventricular dysfunction, either as a result of left ventricular dysfunction or as a result of elevated pulmonary pressures. The right ventricular systolic pressure and, thereby, the pulmonary systolic pressure may be estimated by measuring the peak velocity of the TR jet by CW Doppler and adding the clinically estimated right atrial pressure [25] (discussed in Chap. 13). Color Doppler imaging may improve this technique by facilitating optimal alignment of the CW Doppler beam with the regurgitant jet (Fig. 9–5).

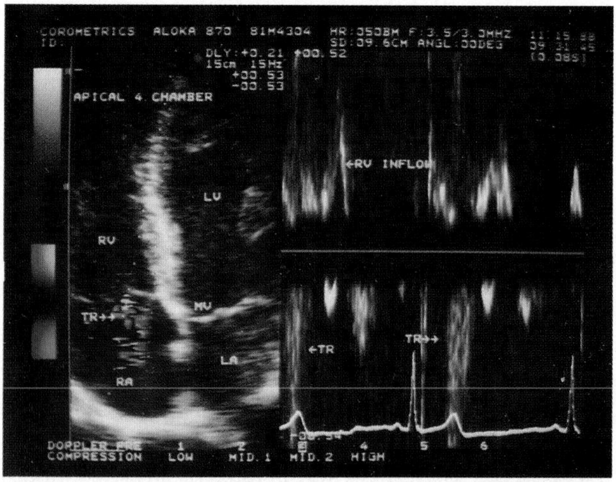

Figure 9–7. Tricuspid regurgitation (TR) in a normal subject. *Left*: The apical four chamber view shows minimal regurgitation (blue systolic jet). RV = right ventricle, LV = left ventricle, RA = right atrium, LA = left atrium, MV = mitral valve. *Right*: Pulsed wave Doppler recorded at the level of the tricuspid valve demonstrating TR below the baseline and the normal right ventricular diastolic inflow above the baseline.

PULMONIC REGURGITATION

The Doppler examination for PR is performed primarily from a parasternal short axis view or mitral-pulmonic plane to visualize the right ventricular outflow tract and plane of the pulmonic valve. Pulmonic regurgitation frequently is noted in normal patients,[22–24] in whom the distribution of pulmonic regurgitant signals typically is localized, either by conventional PD or by CFI (Figs. 9–8 and 9–9). On color Doppler imaging PR appears as an orange-red jet originating from the plane of the pulmonic valve, and projecting into the right ventricular outflow tract (Figs. 9–8 and 9–9).

The severity of PR should be graded in a manner similar to that reviewed for aortic regurgitation (discussed in Chap. 7). Attention should be given to the maximum depth of the jet into the right ventricular outflow tract and also to the maximum width of the jet. Also, the evolution of the jet during the diastolic interval should be evaluated since a small jet seen primarily in early diastole has less physiologic relevance than a pandiastolic jet.

Pulmonary regurgitation is a sensitive marker for pulmonary hypertension.[26] In a group of 50 healthy individuals, holodiastolic PR originating from the valve's coaptation site could be detected in 39 by CFI and was always found when 2D image of the pulmonic valve was visualized clearly.[27] In these normal subjects, the depth of the regurgitant jet was

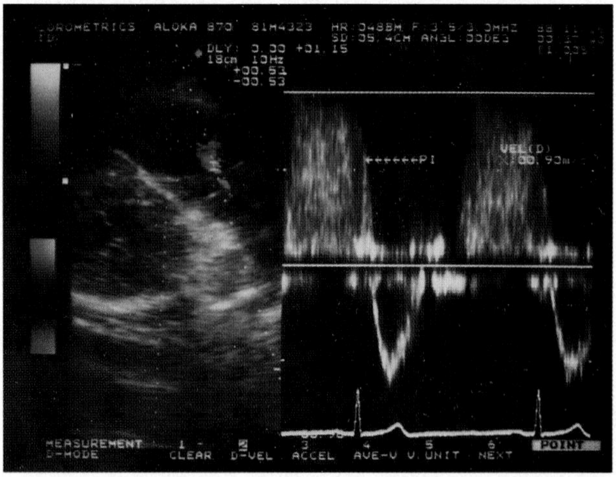

Figure 9–8. Mild pulmonic regurgitation in a normal subject. *Left*: Parasternal short axis view demonstrating a red jet of pandiastolic flow emerging from the center of the pulmonic valve. AO = aorta, RV = right ventricle. *Right*: Pulsed wave Doppler view of pulmonic insufficiency (PI). Holodiastolic spectral broadening is recorded above the baseline.

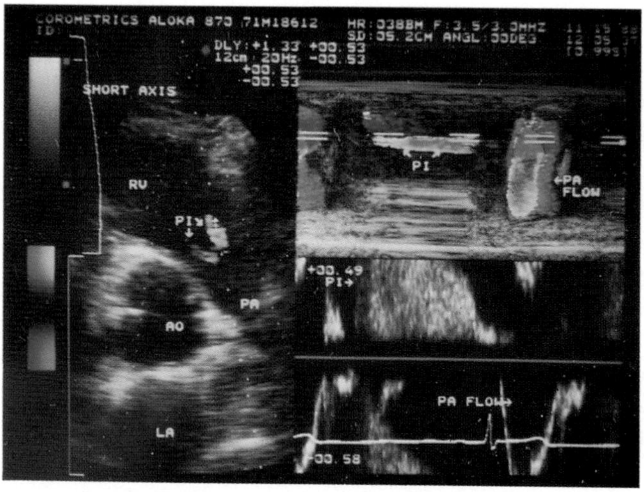

Figure 9–9. Color Doppler study of mild pulmonic insufficiency (PI). *Left*: In this patient without pulmonary hypertension, two jets of mild PI were imaged within the same plane. RV = right ventricle, AO = aorta, LA = left atrium, PA = pulmonary artery. *Upper right*: Color Doppler signals superimposed on an M-mode showing both diastolic regurgitant signals (PI) and normal pulmonary systolic flow. The center of the jet is orange-red due to aliasing. *Lower right*: Pulsed wave tracing demonstrating holodiastolic spectral broadening of PI.

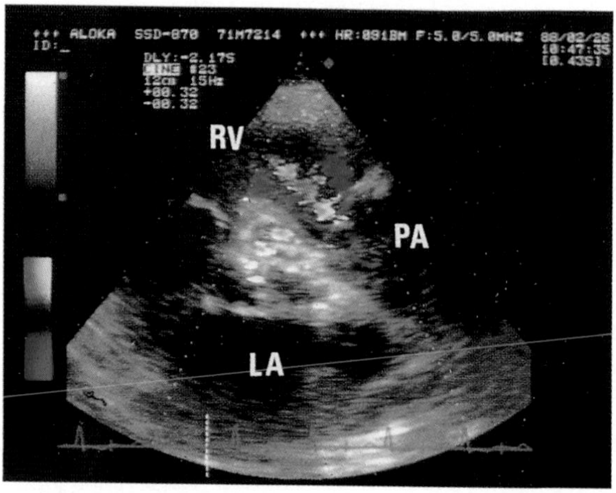

Figure 9–10. Color Doppler study of pulmonic regurgitation in a patient with pulmonary hypertension. A red jet of pandiastolic flow is seen emerging from the pulmonic valve. Note that the jet extends further than 2 cm into the right ventricular (RV) outflow tract, indicating significant pulmonic regurgitation. LA = left atrium, PA = pulmonary artery.

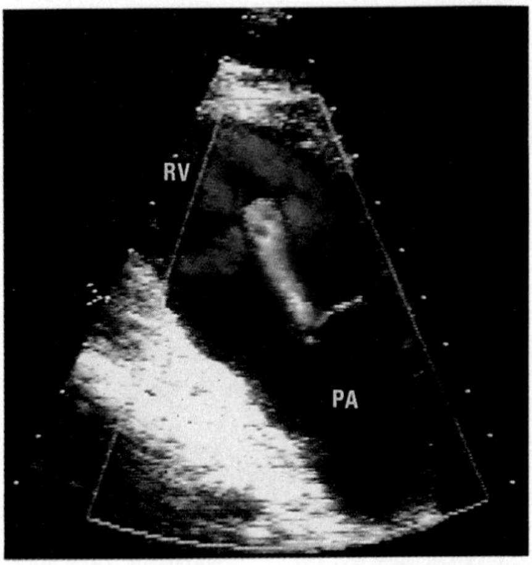

Figure 9–11. Severe pulmonic regurgitation in a patient with pulmonary hypertension. The regurgitant red jet extends beyond 2 cm into a dilated right ventricle (RV). PA = pulmonary artery.

less than 1 cm in 38 of 39 subjects. However, in patients with pulmonary hypertension and a PR murmur, the length of the jet was always greater than 2 cm. Thus, PR should be considered pathologic when the jet is pandiastolic, wide, and extends deeper than 2 cm into the right ventricular outflow tract (Figs. 9–10 and 9–11).

REFERENCES

1. Hauck A, Freeman D, Ackerman D, et al: Surgical pathology of the tricuspid valve: A study of 363 cases spanning 25 years. *Mayo Clin Proc* 63:851, 1988.
2. Ahn A, Segal B: Isolated tricuspid insufficiency, clinical features, diagnosis and management. *Prog Cardiovasc Dis* 9:166, 1967.
3. Grahame-Smith D: The carcinoid syndrome. *Am J Cardiol* 21:376, 1968.
4. Missri J, Agnarsson U, Sverrisson J: The clinical spectrum of tricuspid regurgitation detected by pulsed Doppler echocardiography. *Angiology* 36:746, 1985.
5. Waggoner A, Quinones M, Young J, et al: Pulsed Doppler echocardiographic detection of right-sided valve regurgitation. *Am J Cardiol* 47:279, 1981.
6. Collins N, Braunwald E, Morrow A: Isolated congenital pulmonic valvular regurgitation. *Am J Med* 28:159, 1960.
7. Cairns K, Kloster F, Bristow J, et al: Problems in the hemodynamic diagnosis of tricuspid insufficiency. *Am Heart J* 75:173, 1968.
8. Runco V, Levin H, Vahabzadeh H, et al: Basal diastolic murmurs in rheumatic heart disease: intracardiac phonocardiography and cineangiography. *Am Heart J* 75:153, 1968.

9. Mikami T, Kudo T, Sakurai N, et al: Mechanisms for development of functional tricuspid regurgitation determined by pulsed Doppler and two-dimensional echocardiography. *Am J Cardiol* 53:160, 1984.

10. Pennestri F, Loperfido F, Salvatori M, et al: Assessment of tricuspid regurgitation by pulsed Doppler ultrasonography of the hepatic veins. *Am J Cardiol* 54:383, 1984.

11. Miyatake K, Okamoto M, Kinoshita N, et al: Evaluation of tricuspid regurgitation by pulsed Doppler and two-dimensional echocardiography. *Circulation* 66:777, 1982.

12. Veyrat C, Kalmanson D, Farjon M, et al: Non-invasive diagnosis and assessment of tricuspid regurgitation and stenosis using one and two-dimensional echo-pulsed Doppler. *Br Heart J* 47:596, 1982.

13. Stevenson J, Kawabori I, Guntheroth W: Validation of Doppler diagnosis of tricuspid regurgitation (abstr). *Circulation* 64(IV):255, 1981.

14. Lieppe W, Behar U, Scallion R, et al: Detection of tricuspid regurgitation with two-dimensional echocardiography and peripheral vein injection. *Circulation* 57:128, 1978.

15. Meltzer R, van Hoogenhuyze D, Serruys P, et al: Diagnosis of tricuspid regurgitation by contrast echocardiography. *Circulation* 63:1093, 1981.

16. Hatle L, Angelsen B: *Doppler Ultrasound in Cardiology*, ed 2. Philadelphia, Lea & Febiger, 1985.

17. Wranne B: Evaluation of tricuspid regurgitation: A comparison between pulsed Doppler, contrast echocardiography, jugular vein and liver pulse recordings and angiography, in Spencer M (ed): *Cardiac Doppler Diagnosis*. The Hague, Martinus Nijhoff, 1983.

18. Goldberg S, Valdes-Cruz L, Feldman L, et al: Range-gated Doppler ultrasound detection of contrast echocardiographic microbubbles for cardiac and great vessel blood flow patterns. *Am Heart J* 101:793, 1981.

19. Dabestani A, French J, Gardin J, et al: Doppler hepatic vein blood flow in patients with tricuspid regurgitation (abstr). *J Am Coll Cardiol* 1:658, 1983.

20. Stevenson J, Kawabori I, Brandestini M: A twenty-month experience comparing conventional pulsed Doppler echocardiography and color-coded digital multigate Doppler for detection of atrioventricular valve regurgitation and its severity, in Rijsterborgh H (ed): *Echocardiology*. The Hague, Martinus Nijhoff, 1981.

21. Omoto R: Acquired valvular diseases, in Omoto R (ed): *Color Atlas Of Real-Time Two-Dimensional Doppler Echocardiography*. Philadelphia, Lea & Febiger, 1984.

22. Yoshida K, Yoshikawa J, Shakudo M, et al: Color Doppler evaluation of valvular regurgitation in normal subjects. *Circulation* 78:840, 1988.

23. Pollak S, McMillan S, Knopff W, et al: Cardiac evaluation of women distance runners by echocardiographic color Doppler flow mapping. *J Am Coll Cardiol* 11:89, 1988.

24. Kostucki W, Vandenbossche J-L, Friart A, et al: Pulsed Doppler regurgitant flow patterns of normal valves. *Am J Cardiol* 58:309, 1986.

25. Yock P, Popp R: Noninvasive estimation of right ventricular systolic pressure by Doppler ultrasound in patients with tricuspid regurgitation. *Circulation* 70:657, 1984.

26. Miyatake K, Okamoto M, Kinoshita N, et al: Pulmonary regurgitation studied with the ultrasonic pulsed Doppler technique. *Circulation* 65:969, 1982.

27. Takao S, Miyatake K, Izumi S, et al: Physiological pulmonary regurgitation detected by the Doppler technique and its differential diagnosis. *J Am Coll Cardiol* 5:499, 1985.

CHAPTER 10

Evaluation of Prosthetic Heart Valves

The first successful prosthetic valve replacements were reported by Harken et al.[1] and Starr and Edwards[2] over 28 years ago. Since then the design of prosthetic valves has steadily improved, leading to increased durability and a lesser incidence of prosthetic valve dysfunction. Just the same, serial evaluation of the patient following valve replacement is essential to monitor both prosthetic valve function and ventricular performance. Often a combination of cardiac imaging tools is necessary, since persistent or recurrent symptoms in these patients may be related to prosthetic valve dysfunction, left ventricular dysfunction, other cardiac disease, or a combination of these.

The assessment of prosthetic valve dysfunction by cardiac imaging techniques was initially performed using combined M-mode echocardiography and phonocardiography.[3] In assessing the mitral prosthesis function, for example, the A_2–mitral valve opening interval was measured. However, a prolonged A_2–mitral valve opening interval was found to be nonspecific and could indicate high left atrial pressure from valve obstruction, perivalvular leak, or left ventricular dysfunction; these various etiologies could not always be separated. There were other problems with this approach: the A_2 was not clearly recorded in some patients, and arrhythmias could further confuse the interpretation of these time intervals. For these studies it was essential to use the patient as his or her own control. In these original M-mode echocardiographic studies, emphasis was also placed on measuring ball excursion and opening and closing velocities. However, a variety of factors including heart rate and hemodynamic status could affect these variables, and these velocities did not prove to be a good method for measuring prosthetic valve dysfunction. Several other reasons have led to relatively poor sensitivities and specificities in detecting prosthetic valve dysfunction using echophonocardiographic approaches in a variety of mechanical cardiac valve prostheses in various valve positions.[4]

More recently, 2D echocardiography has been used to assess for abnormalities of prosthetic valve function. In general, 2D echocardiography has been disappointing in its ability to evaluate mechanical valve dysfunction because of excessive reverberations and beam width artifacts limiting the clarity of the studies. Thus, detailed visualization of disc or ball motion is often difficult. However, evaluation of the bioprosthetic valve has been somewhat easier.[5,6] Increased cusp thickness, a focal mass or masses of echoes attached to the valve leaflets, excessive rocking or erratic motion of the valves, and systolic displacement of the cusp leaflets into the left atrium may all suggest valve dysfunction. Since the incidence of dysfunction of porcine bioprosthetic valves is as great as 20 percent at 10 years for patients older than 35 years,[7] careful serial 2D echocardiographic follow-up of these patients is indicated.

Doppler echocardiography holds great promise as a tool that provides accurate and noninvasive assessment of prosthetic valve function. Recent advances in Doppler echocardiographic technology allow both qualitative and quantitative evaluation of stenotic and regurgitant lesions of prosthetic heart valves.[8–13] In addition, color flow imaging (CFI) can provide important spatial orientation to stenotic and regurgitant flow across prosthetic valves and allow rational angle correction of Doppler velocities for pressure gradient calculations. Determination of quantitative flow parameters such as peak velocities, however, still requires PD or CW Doppler echocardiography.

TYPES OF PROSTHESES

Prosthetic heart valves may be mechanical or made from tissue (Table 10–1). Mechanical prostheses consist of three separate components: a moving part (occluder) that can occlude an orifice or allow flow to occur, a seat for the occluder to seal against, and a cloth sewing ring. Three major types of mechanical prostheses are presently in widespread use. The prototype mechanical prosthesis is the central ball occluder (Starr-Edwards) prosthesis. It consists of a circular seat attached to a wire cage. Inside the cage is a ball that alternately falls into the cage or seals against the metal ring. Because of its high profile and central occluder, this valve, although durable, has not proved ideal for all uses. The second type of mechanical prosthesis also has a circular metal seat, but with a disc occluder. Various forms of this valve are available, utilizing different methods of fixing the disc to the ring. These valves appear more efficient since the narrow disc

TABLE 10–1. Types of Prosthetic Heart Valves

A. Mechanical
   1. Ball Occluder
      a. Starr-Edwards
   2. Disc Occluder
      a. Beall-Surgitool
      b. Lillehei-Kaster
      c. Hall-Kaster
      d. Björk-Shiley
   3. Bileaflet
      a. St. Jude Medical

B. Bioprosthetic
   1. Porcine heterograft
      a. Carpentier-Edwards
      b. Hancock
   2. Pericardial xenograft
      a. Ionescu-Shiley
   3. Muscle fascia
   4. Aortic Homograft

should offer less obstruction to blood flow than do central occluder valves. The third type of mechanical prosthesis is the split disc, consisting of two halves of the disc, each individually hinged (St. Jude).

Bioprosthetic or tissue valves are also of two major types. Most common in the United States are fixed porcine aortic valves, which are supported by cloth-covered wire stents and surrounded by a cushioned sewing ring. Other types of tissue prosthesis have been constructed from pericardium (Ionescu-Shiley) or muscle fascia.

COMPLICATIONS IN MECHANICAL AND TISSUE PROSTHESES

The most common complication of mechanical prostheses is thrombosis.[14,15] This can occur as a sudden catastrophic event or can be more gradual. Thrombosis and fibrosis on the atrial side of a disc-type prosthesis in the mitral position can be an insidious complication. Thrombosis can produce varying degrees both of stenosis (by obstructing the valve orifice) and of regurgitation (by preventing complete valve closure). Infective endocarditis is a less common complication of mechanical prostheses, and can be associated with perivalvular abscesses and valvular dehiscence with perivalvular regurgitation. Problems due to changes in ball or disc size (variance) are a relatively uncommon cause of mechanical valve dysfunction.

The two major complications of bioprosthetic valves are infective endocarditis and valvular degeneration. Endocarditis can affect both the valve sewing area and the tissue leaflets, which results in disruption of valve tissue.[16] Degeneration of bioprostheses is a common complication, and can be associated with valve disruption and regurgitation or with calcification and progressive valvular stenosis. Valvular dehiscence can occur in the presence of endocarditis or as an isolated complication.

DOPPLER ECHOCARDIOGRAPHIC TECHNIQUE

Evaluating prosthetic valves by Doppler echocardiography is similar to evaluating native valves. The mitral valve is interrogated from the apex of the left ventricle and left parasternal window, and the aortic valve from the apex, right parasternal area, and suprasternal notch.

Each type of valve should be interrogated with its specific characteristics in mind.

Mechanical Prostheses

Flow around the ball occluder of the Starr-Edwards valve is mostly laminar as blood is passing between the ring and the ball, and then breaks down into disturbed flow distally. To properly sample flow around a Starr-Edwards prosthesis, the CW beam or PD sample volume must be placed close to the base of the valve in an area where nondisturbed flow occurs. The Björk-Shiley type of disc valve does not open a full 90°. The majority of flow across these valves occurs through the major (larger) orifice and is oriented in the direction of the disc opening. Flow is most easily recognized at the major orifice or at the level of the disc tip. One variation of the disc valve is the Medtronic prosthesis. The disc of this prosthesis does not have a fixed opening angle, but in the open position rests on a hook-shaped stent out of the orifice. As a result, the flow velocities can be recorded across the entire valve orifice. Flow through a St. Jude valve occurs in a similar fashion. Flow is relatively laminar across the entire valve orifice,[17] and can be recorded well at almost any point in the opening. With both valves, an attempt should be made to record centrally so as to avoid problems with contamination by lower velocities at the sides of the jet. Proper alignment of the CW beam and placement of the PD sample volume is facilitated by the use of CFI.

Bioprostheses

Bioprostheses are designed to perform like native valves. Flow occurs centrally and is relatively undisturbed. Because of the physical size of the stent and sewing ring, the orifice of the bioprosthetic valve is smaller than the anulus diameter, and the resultant blood flow acts like the jet through a stenotic lesion.[17] Blood flow is of relatively high velocity and more discrete, but breaks down to disturbed flow several centimeters below the valve plane. For this reason, recordings are made as close to the orifice of the valve as possible.

PITFALLS IN THE DOPPLER EVALUATION OF PROSTHETIC VALVE REGURGITATION

Understanding the role of Doppler echocardiography for detection of abnormal flows through prosthetic valves begins with appreciation of the problems of acoustic shadowing.[18] Once emitted from the transducer into the tissues, ultrasound either is reflected, is attenuated (absorbed), or continues on to another tissue interface where the process is repeated. All prosthetic valves contain some degree of nonbiologic material which can be plastic, metal or cloth. Each of these materials may have highly reflective or attenuative properties that may not allow the ultrasound to penetrate and pass through the nonbiologic portion of the valve.

The nonbiologic material can interfere with the transmission of sound waves to such a degree that it may be impossible to detect some valvular regurgitation. All of the cardiac prosthetic valves cast characteristic shadows on the chamber behind them that obscure proper flow detection by Doppler echocardiography. Figure 10–1 shows a diagrammatic representation of acoustic shadowing from three valves. The largest shadow emanates from behind the Starr-Edwards Silastic ball and St. Jude valves, and the smallest from the porcine heterograft (Carpentier-Edwards), whose acoustic shadowing is limited to the sewing ring of the prosthesis.

This concept has important implications for the clinical detection of prosthetic valvular regurgitation using conventional Doppler echocardiography or CFI. These physical properties of prosthetic valves may significantly alter the ability of Doppler systems to detect abnormal flow even when present. Considerable clinical caution must, therefore, be exercised when one encounters patients with prosthetic valves. It may be impossible to detect any flow on the opposite side of a prosthetic valve when the valve is interposed between the interrogating transducer and the area being examined.

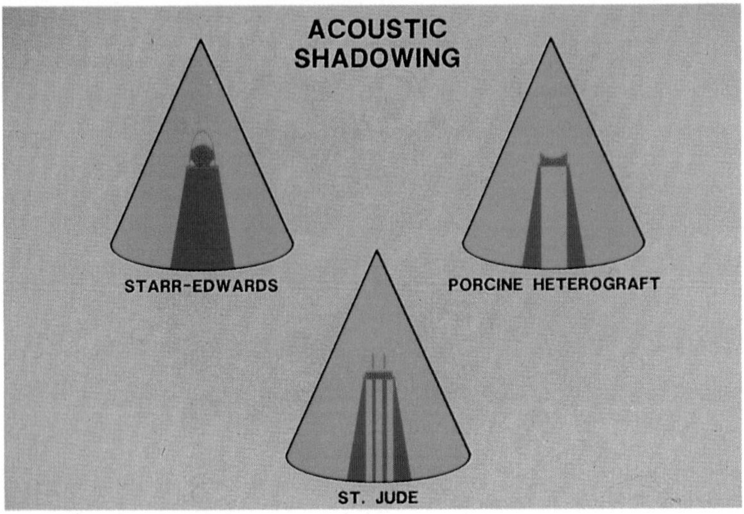

Figure 10–1. Various degrees of acoustic shadowing are seen behind ball occluder, disc occluder, and bioprosthetic valves.

An example of this problem occurs in the evaluation of prosthetic mitral regurgitation from the apical view. From this approach almost the whole of the left atrium may be masked by a mechanical prosthesis, and one might incorrectly conclude that no mitral regurgitation existed. The problem can usually be minimized when the body of the left atrium is interrogated using parasternal long and short axis views and subcostal views. Furthermore, CFI should theoretically improve on both CW Doppler echocardiography, in recognizing mitral regurgitation, and PD echocardiography, in determining the spatial extent of mitral regurgitation.

MITRAL VALVE PROSTHESES

All prosthetic mitral valves offer some obstruction to flow, which resembles mild mitral stenosis on a Doppler tracing. There are three methods of expressing the severity of obstruction (Table 10–2): the mean transprosthetic diastolic gradient, the mitral prosthetic pressure half-time, and the effective prosthetic mitral valve area. Normal values for mechanical prostheses are listed in Table 10–3, and for tissue prostheses in Table 10–4.

The pressure gradient across a prosthetic mitral valve can be calculated by Doppler echocardiography using the simplified Bernoulli equation: Pressure gradient (ΔP) = $4\ V^2$ (discussed in Chap. 2). The reliability of Doppler measurements of the pressure gradient across native and pros-

TABLE 10–2. Doppler Echocardiographic Evaluation of Mitral Valve Prosthesis Function

A. Obstruction of flow
   1. Mean diastolic gradient
   2. Pressure half-time
   3. Effective valve area

B. Regurgitation
   1. Detection of regurgitation
   2. Quantification of regurgitation

thetic valves has been validated by angiographic methods.[21,29] The gradient, however, is a function of the volume of transvalvular flow and will therefore give a false impression of more severe obstruction in the presence of prosthetic regurgitation, in the same manner as in combined stenosis and regurgitation of the native valve.

A method identical to that employed for native mitral stenosis may be used to calculate the pressure half-time for mitral valve prostheses[30] (method illustrated in Fig. 5–5). Normal values are listed in Tables 10–3 and 10–4. Measurements of pressure half-time appear more useful than peak flow velocities in distinguishing between prosthetic mitral valve stenosis and mitral regurgitation.[11,30] Although peak inflow velocities are elevated in both mitral stenosis and mitral regurgitation, pressure half-time is prolonged only in prosthetic mitral valve stenosis. A pressure half-time exceeding 160 ms identifies patients with prosthetic mitral valve stenosis. Pressure half-time measurements therefore provide very good separation between stenotic prostheses and normally functioning or purely regurgitant prosthetic valves. It is particularly useful when a postoperative baseline value has been established, and the patient may serve as his or her own control on subsequent examinations.

The pressure half-time method can then be used to calculate the effective orifice area (method illustrated in Fig. 5–5). Comparing the calculated orifice areas with the manufacturers' specified orifice areas yielded relatively good correlation for mechanical and bioprosthetic valves;[31] correlations were better for tissue valves than for mechanical valves. However, the calculated orifice areas were generally lower than the manufacturers' specified areas by about 10 percent. This difference may arise because the viscosity of blood in the human heart is higher than the viscosity of the fluid medium used in the manufacturers' laboratory measurements.

TABLE 10–3. Normal Doppler Values for Mechanical Prostheses in the Mitral Position

Prosthesis	Peak Velocity (m/s)	Peak Gradient (mmHg)	Mean Velocity (m/s)	Mean Gradient (mmHg)	Pressure Half-Time (ms)	Valve Area Mean (cm^2)	Valve Area Range (cm^2)	Mild Regurgitation (%)	Reference
Starr-Edwards	1.8 ± 0.4	15 ± 6	1.1 ± 0.3	4.6 ± 2.4	110 ± 27	2.1	1.2–2.5	36	9,19,20
Björk-Shiley	1.6 ± 0.3	11 ± 3	0.8 ± 0.2	2.9 ± 1.6	90 ± 22	2.4	1.6–3.7	25	9,12,19,21–23
Beall	1.8 ± 0.2	13 ± 4	1.2 ± 0.2	6.0 ± 2.0	129 ± 15	1.7	1.3–2.0	NI[a]	19
St. Jude Medical	1.6 ± 0.3	10 ± 4	0.9 ± 0.2	3.5 ± 1.3	77 ± 17	2.8	1.8–5.0	30	19,24–26

[a]NI = no information

TABLE 10–4. Normal Doppler Values for Tissue Prostheses in the Mitral Position

Prosthesis	Peak Velocity (m/s)	Peak Gradient (mmHg)	Mean Velocity (m/s)	Mean Gradient (mmHg)	Pressure Half-Time (ms)	Valve Area Mean (cm^2)	Valve Area Range (cm^2)	Mild Regurgitation (%)	Reference
Ionescu-Shiley	1.5 ± 0.3	9 ± 3	0.9 ± 0.2	3.3 ± 1.2	93 ± 25	2.4	1.2–4.0	NI[a]	27
Hancock	1.5 ± 0.3	10 ± 3	1.1 ± 0.3	4.3 ± 2.1	129 ± 31	1.7	1.1–2.7	20	8,11–13,20,22
Carpentier-Edwards	1.8 ± 0.2	12 ± 4	1.3 ± 0.2	6.5 ± 2.1	90 ± 25	2.5	1.1–4.0	30	24,27,28

[a]NI = no information

Minimal or mild degrees of mitral regurgitation have been found by both angiography and Doppler echocardiography in patients with normally functioning mechanical and tissue valves (Tables 10–3 and 10–4). Because it may be difficult to distinguish paravalvular from transvalvular leaks, and "physiologic" from pathologic regurgitation, by PD studies, the use of CFI to map the regurgitant jet may be helpful. Detection of the regurgitant jet more than 2 cm into the left atrium is often suggestive of significant mitral regurgitation.[9] Another useful sign suggesting the presence of significant regurgitation is the recording of a high forward peak velocity across the prosthesis, provided that the patient has preserved cardiac output. However, the mere presence of increased antegrade transprosthetic velocity is probably not helpful unless a postoperative baseline study is available for comparison.

Continuous wave Doppler recordings from the apexes of normal prostheses show characteristic patterns (Figs. 10–2, 10–3, and 10–4). Flow through the prosthesis starts simultaneously with the opening of the disc or leaflet and reaches its maximum velocity at the time of complete valve opening, with subsequent linear deceleration to near zero at closure of the valve.

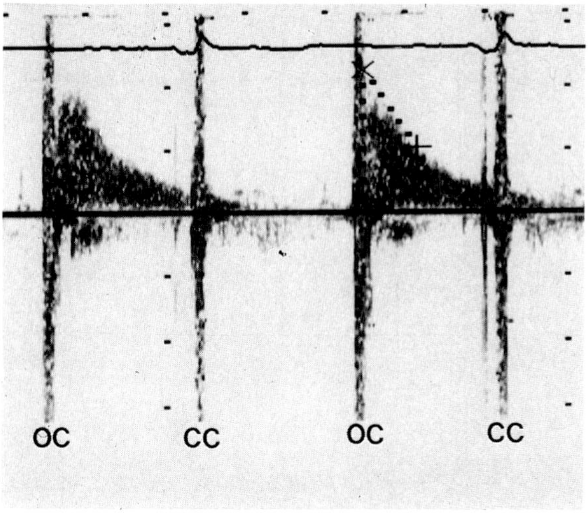

Figure 10–2. Apical continuous wave Doppler tracing of a normally functioning Björk-Shiley mitral valve. The peak velocity is 2 m/s, the pressure half-time 73 ms, and the valve area 3.0 cm^2. Note the sharp opening (oc) and closing (cc) clicks. It is important not to include the opening click as part of the flow velocities when calculating pressure half-times. (Scale marks = 1 m/s)

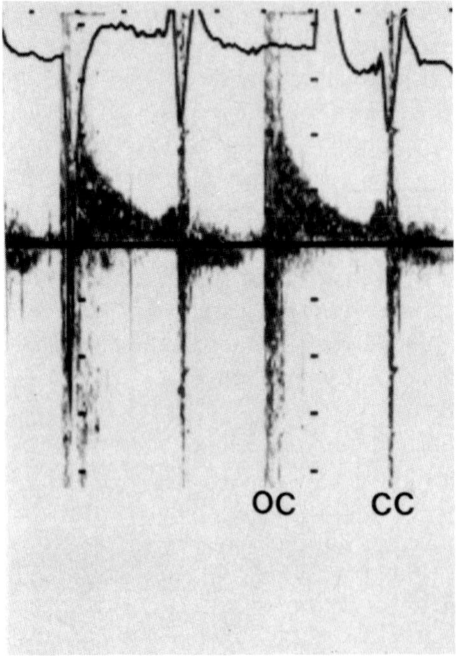

Figure 10–3. Apical continuous wave tracing of a normally functioning St. Jude Medical mitral prosthesis. The flow pattern resembles that of a normal native mitral valve. The pressure half-time is 74 ms and the valve area is calculated at 2.9 cm^2. Note the sharp opening (oc) and closing (cc) clicks. (Scale marks = 1 m/s)

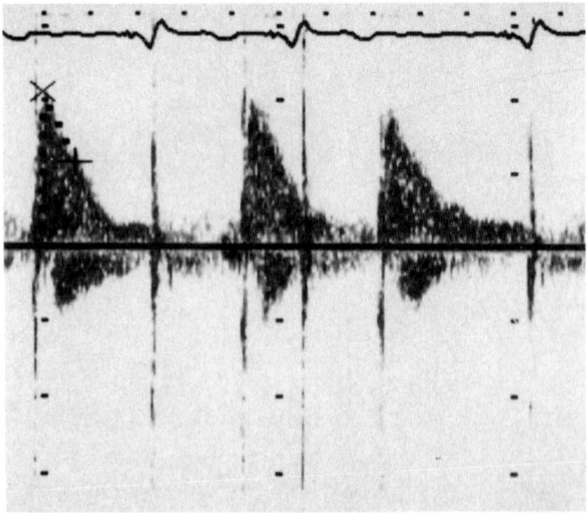

Figure 10–4. Apical continuous wave recording of a normally functioning Carpentier-Edwards bioprosthesis in the mitral position in a patient with atrial fibrillation. The peak velocity across the prosthetic valve is 2 m/s, the pressure half-time 91 ms, and the valve area 2.4 cm^2. All calculations were based on the average of 10 beats. (Scale marks = 1 m/s)

In some patients with atrial fibrillation a nonuniform deceleration rate has been observed, resulting in either concavity or convexity of the curve.[32] In patients with an extreme form of concavity this was associated with prosthetic regurgitation. Convex curves (Fig. 10–5) could be obtained across most values during short cardiac cycles, but in a small number of patients with atrial fibrillation there was a constant finding, unrelated to heart rate. Constant convexity was associated with grossly impaired left ventricular contractility, aortic regurgitation, or mean transprosthetic diastolic gradient >5 mmHg.

Color flow imaging provides a means for spatial identification of flows through mitral prosthetic valves if the proper transducer orientations and limitations are kept in mind.[33] Flow through a Starr-Edwards valve has turbulent, high-velocity peripheral circumferential jets (Fig. 10–6). The areas of the jets adjacent to the left ventricular outflow tract appear larger than the areas adjacent to the left ventricular free wall. There are regions of flow reversal just distal to the cage during mid- and late diastole. Turbulence displayed as a mosaic green/yellow is detected along the edges of the forward flow jets.

Color Doppler flow imaging of tilting disc valves (e.g., Björk-Shiley) characteristically has two high-velocity jets in both the major and minor

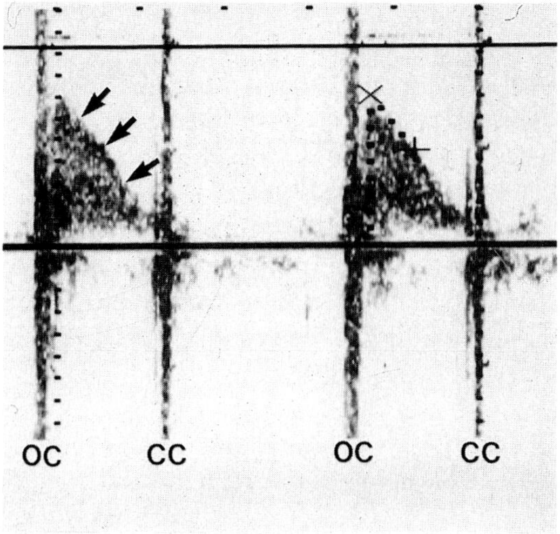

Figure 10–5. Diastolic flow pattern across a St. Jude Medical mitral prosthesis. Nonlinear deceleration (arrows) results in a convex curve. This patient had severe left ventricular dysfunction. The pressure half-time is 84 ms and the valve area 2.6 cm^2. Note the opening (oc) and closing (cc) clicks.

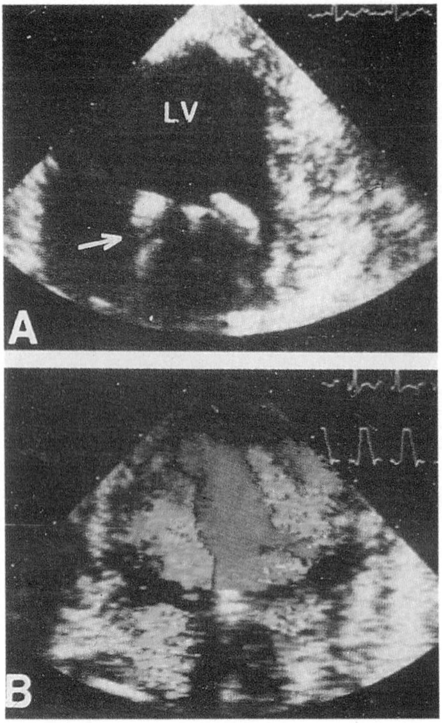

Figure 10–6. (A) Two-dimensional echocardiogram of the left ventricle from an apical window with a Starr-Edwards prosthesis in the mitral position. The arrow points to the valve cage. LV = left ventricle. (B) Color flow imaging of ball-and-cage valve. The portion of the circumferential peripheral flow field, on the left, that is adjacent to the outflow tract is wider than the portion on the right, which is adjacent to the free wall. Flow reversal (blue) occurs distal to the cage.

orifices (Fig. 10–7). The area of flow through the major orifice is two or more times larger than the area of flow through the minor orifice. When the major orifice is oriented toward the septum, greater intraventricular turbulence occurs than with the major orifice oriented toward the left ventricular free wall.[33] This finding indicates that tilting disc valves in the mitral position have better velocity profiles with the major orifice oriented toward the left ventricular free wall than with the same orifice oriented toward the septum. Flow through a normal tilting disc valve should always be imaged through the major and minor orifices. Absence of flow through either orifice is indicative of obstruction.

Color flow imaging of the St. Jude mitral valve is characterized by three jets (Fig. 10–8). The two jets from the lateral orifices are directed toward the septum and free wall. The jet from the central orifice is usually delayed by 20 to 30 ms.[33] Compared to the other mechanical valve designs, the bileaflet valve appears to create lower levels of turbulence, at least during mitral inflow.

The porcine bioprosthetic valve has a high-velocity, turbulent, eccentric jet, usually directed toward the septum during ventricular diastole

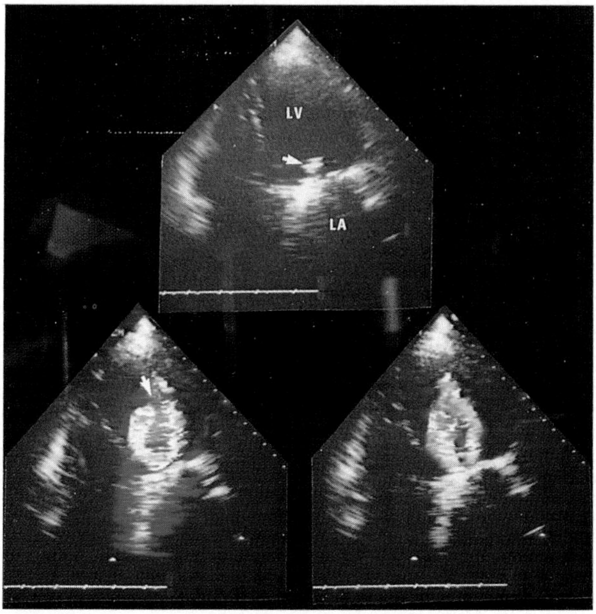

Figure 10–7. *Top*: Two-dimensional echocardiogram from an apical four-chamber view of a Björk-Shiley mitral prosthesis. The major orifice is oriented toward the free wall. The arrow points to the open disc. LV = left ventricle; LA = left atrium. *Bottom Left*: Color flow imaging in mid-diastole. The jet from the major orifice is on the right, and the jet from the minor orifice on the left. There is turbulence and aliasing of both jets. The arrow points to eddies of velocity reversal distal to the disc. *Bottom Right*: In late diastole the turbulence has decayed; a laminar, low-velocity flow field (orange-red) is directed toward the left ventricular apex.

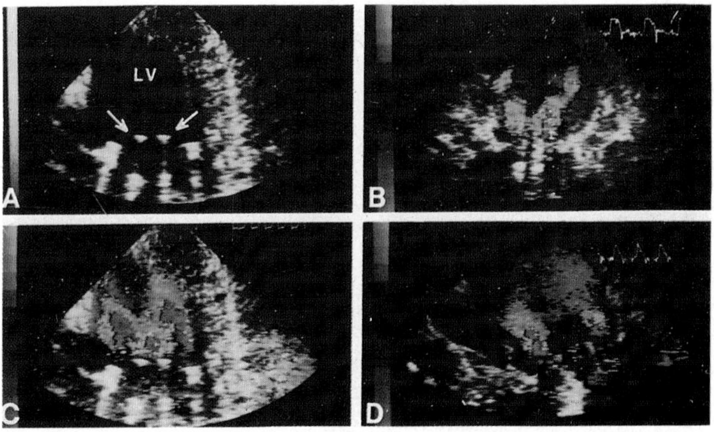

Figure 10–8. (A) Two-dimensional echocardiogram of a St. Jude Medical mitral prosthesis. Arrows point to the two open hemidiscs. LV = left ventricle. (B) In early diastole there are two jets through the lateral orifices, one directed toward the left ventricular outflow tract and the other toward the free wall. The jet through the central orifice is delayed. (C) In mid-diastole there are three jets extending downstream into the left ventricular cavity. (D) In late diastole there is a low-velocity laminar flow field extending toward the left ventricular apex.

(Fig. 10–9). The jet takes on a "candle-flame" appearance similar to that of mitral stenosis, with areas of aliasing and turbulence. In mid- to late diastole the flow profiles become laminar before reaching the left ventricular apex.

AORTIC VALVE PROSTHESES

The criteria for evaluation of aortic prosthetic systolic function, as for native aortic valve stenosis, are the magnitude of the transprosthetic pressure drop, or gradient, and its time course[35] (Table 10–5). Prosthetic aortic valves have hemodynamics similar to those of mild aortic stenosis. Doppler interrogation of prosthetic aortic valves reveals mild systolic pressure gradients that can be calculated with the modified Bernoulli equation: $\Delta P = 4\,V^2$. Normal values for mechanical prostheses are listed in Table 10–6, and for tissue prostheses in Table 10–7.

The increase in velocity across an aortic valve prosthesis can usually be adequately recorded from the apex. However, other approaches should be routinely utilized, including the right parasternal, subcostal, and suprasternal windows. When recording aortic transprosthetic flow velocity from an apical location, the high-velocity jet is on the opposite side of the prosthesis from the incident ultrasound beam. The problems that may occur due to shadowing or reverberations are the same ones encountered in examining for regurgitation of a mechanical mitral prosthesis.

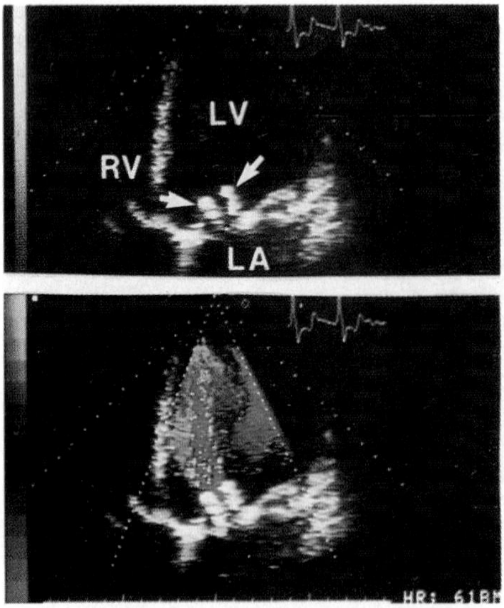

Figure 10–9. *Top*: Two-dimensional echocardiogram of a Carpentier-Edwards bioprosthetic mitral valve. Arrows point to the valve's struts. RV = right ventricle, LV = left ventricle, LA = left atrium. *Bottom*: Color flow image demonstrates a forward flow jet in which the central portion of the flow is high-velocity and therefore aliased (blue), whereas the peripheral aspects of the jet are of slower velocity and normally colored for direction (red). A prominent flow stream that has been reflected from the cardiac apex backward toward the mitral orifice can be seen, in blue, in the lateral aspect of the left ventricle.

TABLE 10-5. Doppler Echocardiographic Evaluation of Aortic Valve Prosthesis Function

A. Obstruction of flow
  1. Peak systolic gradient
  2. Mean systolic gradient
  3. Time course of pressure drop

B. Regurgitation
  1. Detection of regurgitation
  2. Quantification of regurgitation

The increase in velocity across an aortic prosthesis varies with valve size as well as with cardiac output or stroke volume. In general, all but the smallest aortic valves have Doppler peak gradients less than 40 mmHg. A decrease in mean pressure drop with increasing valve size is seen. Individual variability will be seen on Doppler imaging in patients with normally functioning prosthetic valves secondary to valve size and position as well as to left ventricular function. For this reason, a baseline Doppler evaluation is recommended in order to aid in the future diagnosis of valve dysfunction. The maximal velocities recorded across a normal mechanical and tissue valve are shown in Figs. 10–10 and 10–11.

The time course of the pressure drop is also useful as a rough guide to the severity of aortic prosthesis function.[35] As with stenosis of the native aortic valve, the more severe the obstruction, the more prolonged the duration of the systolic gradient. Since the gradient, or pressure drop, is the driving force behind the transprosthetic blood flow velocity measured by Doppler ultrasound, the more severe the obstruction, the longer the duration of high-velocity flow. Therefore, prolongation of high velocities into late systole indicates persistent obstruction. The combination of the mean transprosthetic gradient and the time course of the pressure drop is the best method now available for assessment of the severity of obstruction produced by an aortic prosthetic valve.[35]

Mild aortic prosthetic valve regurgitation is very common (Tables 10–6 and 10–7). The Doppler examination for transprosthetic or paraprosthetic regurgitation is performed in the same manner as that for regurgitation of the native valve (discussed in Chap. 7). The diagnosis of prosthetic aortic valve incompetence can be made by recording from the apex and parasternal long axis view, using CW, PD, or CFI, and the severity of the disorder can be assessed from the extension of the regurgitant flow into the left ventricle. Detection of the regurgitant jet more than 2 cm into the left ventricular cavity is often suggestive of significant aortic regurgitation.

TABLE 10–6. Normal Doppler Values for Mechanical Prostheses in the Aortic Position

Prosthesis	Peak Velocity (m/s)	Peak Gradient (mmHg)	Mean Velocity (m/s)	Mean Gradient (mmHg)	Mild Regurgitation (%)	Reference
Starr-Edwards	3.1 ± 0.5	37 ± 12	2.5 ± 0.2	24 ± 4	52	9,19,20,34
Björk-Shiley	2.6 ± 0.4	24 ± 9	1.8 ± 0.3	14 ± 5	22	9,12,19,34
St. Jude Medical	2.4 ± 0.3	26 ± 5	1.7 ± 0.5	13 ± 6	58	19,24,25

TABLE 10–7. Normal Doppler Values for Tissue Prostheses in the Aortic Position

Prosthesis	Peak Velocity (m/s)	Peak Gradient (mmHg)	Mean Velocity (m/s)	Mean Gradient (mmHg)	Mild Regurgitation (%)	Reference
Ionescu-Shiley	2.5 ± 1.7	25 ± 7	1.9 ± 0.3	14 ± 4	NI[a]	24,27
Hancock	2.4 ± 0.4	23 ± 7	1.7 ± 0.2	11 ± 2	27	9,12,20,34
Carpentier-Edwards	2.4 ± 0.5	23 ± 9	1.9 ± 0.4	14 ± 6	20	24,27,28,34

[a]NI = no information

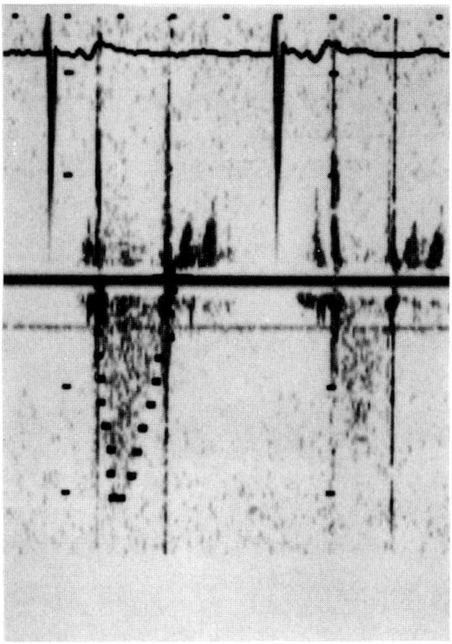

Figure 10–10. Continuous wave recording from the apex of a normally functioning St. Jude Medical aortic prosthesis. The peak flow velocity measures 2 m/s with a calculated peak pressure gradient of 16 mmHg and a mean gradient of 8 mmHg. (Scale marks = 1 m/s)

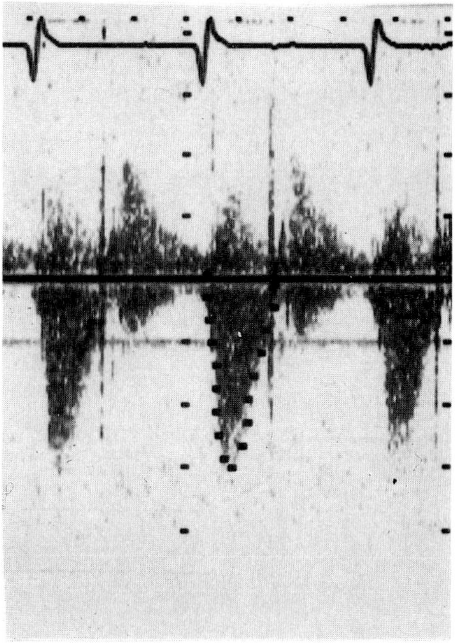

Figure 10–11. Continuous wave recording from the apex of a normally functioning Carpentier-Edwards aortic bioprosthesis. The peak flow velocity measures 3 m/s with a calculated peak pressure gradient of 36 mmHg and a mean gradient of 17 mmHg. Note the diastolic inflow above the baseline. (Scale marks = 1 m/s)

TRICUSPID VALVE PROSTHESES

Evaluation of a tricuspid valve prosthesis is relatively easy with conventional Doppler echocardiography and CFI. Techniques identical to those employed for assessment of obstruction to forward flow and regurgitation in the native tricuspid valve are employed; these, in turn, are analogous to those used for evaluation of mitral prostheses. The tricuspid pressure half-time, however, has not been as thoroughly investigated as its mitral counterpart. It does seem to offer comparable ability to differentiate an abnormally high transtricuspid gradient due to regurgitation from one due to obstruction.[30] Finally, it is extremely important in dealing with tricuspid prostheses that a sufficient number of cycles be averaged to account for respiratory variations.

Tricuspid annuloplasty is a much more common procedure for alleviation of tricuspid regurgitation than is valve replacement. The degree of obstruction to antegrade flow produced by the annuloplasty procedure may be quantified by calculation of the mean transvalvular gradient in the same manner as for a tricuspid or a mitral prosthesis, and the tricuspid pressure half-time may also be useful as noted above.

PROSTHETIC VALVE MALFUNCTION

Markedly elevated aortic transvalvular gradients (Fig. 10–12), reduced mitral valve orifice (Fig. 10–13), and moderate to severe prosthetic regur-

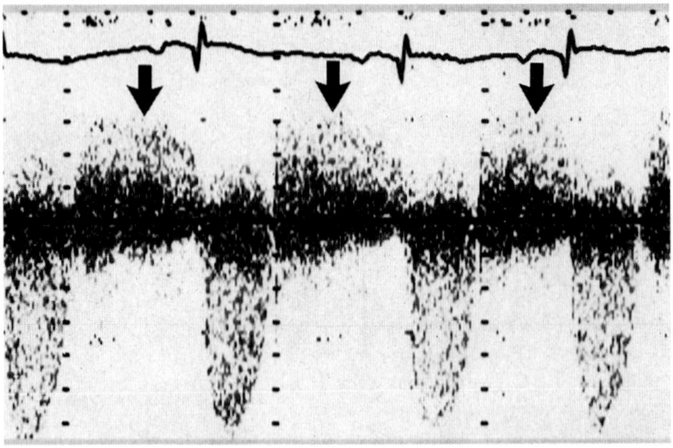

Figure 10–12. Apical continuous wave recording of an obstructed Björk-Shiley aortic prosthesis. Aortic regurgitation is recorded above the baseline (arrows). Peak velocities of 6 m/s are present. (Scale marks = 1 m/s)

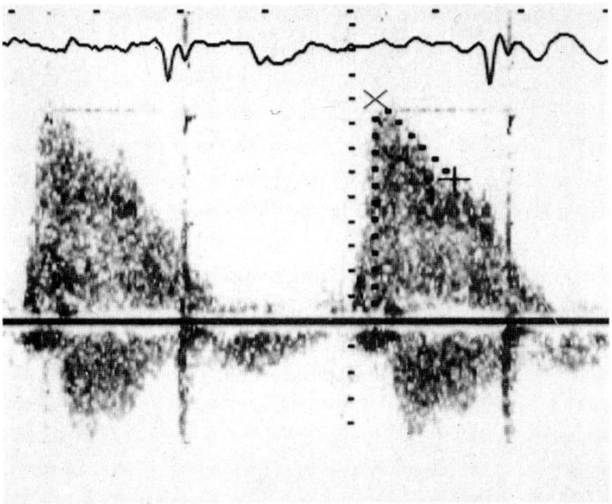

Figure 10–13. Apical continuous wave recording of an obstructed Carpentier-Edwards mitral bioprosthesis. Pressure half-time is prolonged to 220 ms, consistent with a valve area of 1.0 cm^2. (Scale marks = 20 cm/s)

gitation (Figs. 10–12, 10–14) are pathognomonic of severe prosthetic valvular malfunction. Although the sensitivity of Doppler echocardiography has not been assessed in this situation, it has been shown to be highly specific.[9,10,36] In patients with known regurgitation, CFI is useful in localizing regurgitant jets and in distinguishing central valve regurgitation from perivalvular regurgitation. In our laboratory, a peak transvalvular aortic gradient of more than 40 mmHg, a smaller than normal (1 cm^2) mitral orifice, or the presence of moderate to severe regurgitation is an indication that valve dysfunction has occurred.

GUIDELINES FOR PERFORMING DOPPLER ECHOCARDIOGRAPHIC STUDIES IN PATIENTS WITH PROSTHETIC VALVES

Guidelines for performing Doppler echocardiographic studies in patients with prosthetic valves are summarized in Table 10–8. Every patient receiving a prosthetic valve should have a Doppler echocardiographic examination performed while still in the hospital. This provides a baseline against which to compare any later recordings when a patient is suspected of having valve malfunction.

The frequency of serial Doppler echocardiographic examinations must be tailored to each patient. If no mechanical prosthesis abnormality is

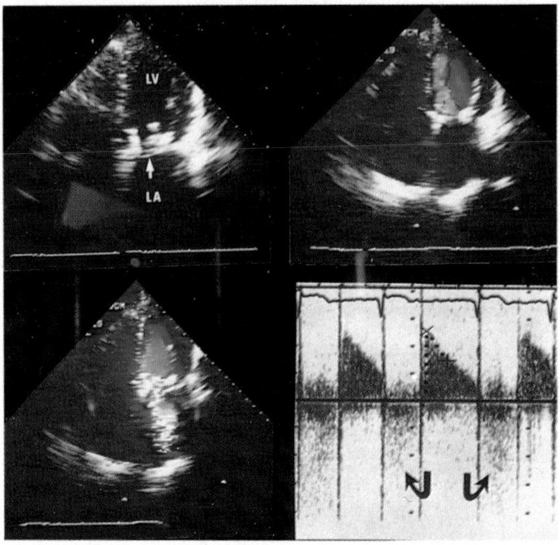

Figure 10–14. *Top Left*: Two-dimensional echocardiographic apical four-chamber view of a Carpentier-Edwards mitral prosthesis. The leaflets appear thickened (arrow). LV = left ventricle, LA = left atrium. *Top Right*: Color flow imaging in diastole. The jet (red) is directed eccentrically toward the left ventricular septum. The blue area on the right represents the velocity of blood that has turned from the apex. *Bottom Left*: Systolic image demonstrating severe prosthetic mitral regurgitation. Note the mosaic pattern, due to turbulence. *Bottom Right*: Apical continuous wave Doppler tracing demonstrating holosystolic regurgitation (arrows). The pressure half-time is 130 ms and the valve area 1.7 cm^2. (Scale marks = 1 m/s)

suspected from history, physical examination, or laboratory studies, there is probably no need for routine serial Doppler examinations. On the other hand, if the gradient is already high at the time of the baseline postoperative study and a diagnosis of patient-prosthesis mismatch is entertained, serial Doppler examinations are of considerable value for detection of any further increase in the gradient due to superimposed intrinsic malfunction of the prosthesis.

Bioprosthetic valve malfunction is increased in certain groups of patients, including the young[37,38] and those with chronic renal disease[39] or certain metabolic abnormalities.[40] In these patients a more rigorous follow-up strategy appears warranted. Doppler echocardiography is well suited to provide this close scrutiny, although the proper interval between serial examinations has not been determined.

Finally, immediate Doppler examination is indicated for anyone with suspected prosthetic valve obstruction or regurgitation. In many patients

TABLE 10–8. Guidelines for Performing Doppler Echocardiographic Studies in Patients with Prosthetic Valves

Patient Category	Indications for Doppler Study
A. Early postoperative	
1. Mechanical and bioprosthetic valves	Baseline in all patients
B. Long-term follow-up	
1. Mechanical valves	Abnormal history, physical examination, laboratory data (serial studies indicated if high gradient present on baseline examination, possibly due to patient-prosthesis mismatch)
2. Bioprosthetic valves	
a. Adults	Abnormal history, physical examination, laboratory data (serial studies indicated if high gradient present on baseline examination)
b. Children	Routine serial studies[a]
c. Chronic renal disease	Routine serial studies[a]
d. Abnormality of calcium metabolism	Routine serial studies[a]
C. Suspected obstruction or regurgitation	Immediate study

[a]Interval not known

the Doppler findings are sufficiently diagnostic that corrective surgery can be performed without preoperative cardiac catheterization.

REFERENCES

1. Harken D, Soroff H, Taylor W, et al: Partial and complete prosthesis in aortic insufficiency. *J Thorac Cardiovasc Surg* 40:744, 1960.
2. Starr A, Edwards M: Mitral replacement: Clinical experience with a ball-valve prosthesis. *Ann Surg* 154:726, 1961.
3. Kotler M, Mintz G, Panidis I, et al: Noninvasive evaluation of normal and abnormal prosthetic valve function. *J Am Coll Cardiol* 2:151, 1983.
4. Mintz G, Carlson E, Kotler M: Comparison of noninvasive techniques in evaluation of the nontissue cardiac valve prosthesis. *Am J Cardiol* 49:39, 1982.
5. Alain M, Madrazo A, Magilligan D, et al: M-mode and two-dimensional echocardiographic features of porcine valve dysfunction. *Am J Cardiol* 43:502, 1979.
6. Shapira J, Martin R, Fowles R, et al: Two-dimensional echocardiographic assessment of patients with bioprosthetic valves. *Am J Cardiol* 43:510, 1979.
7. Magilligan D Jr, Lewis J Jr, Tilley B, et al: The porcine bioprosthetic valve—Twelve years later. *J Thorac Cardiovasc Surg* 89:499, 1985.
8. Hollen J, Simonsen S, Froysaker T: Determination of pressure gradient in the Hancock mitral valve from non-invasive ultrasound Doppler data. *Scand J Clin Invest* 41:177, 1981.
9. Williams G, Labovitz A: Doppler hemodynamic evaluation of prosthetic and bioprosthetic cardiac valves. *Am J Cardiol* 56:325, 1985.
10. Gross C, Wann L: Doppler echocardiographic diagnosis of porcine bioprosthetic cardiac valve malfunction. *Am J Cardiol* 53:1203, 1984.
11. Ryan T, Armstrong W, Dillon J, Feigenbaum H: Doppler echocardiographic evaluation of patients with porcine mitral valves. *Am Heart J* 111:237, 1986.
12. Sagar K, Wann L, Paulsen W, et al: Doppler echocardiographic evaluation of Hancock and Björk-Shiley prosthetic valves. *J Am Coll Cardiol* 7:681, 1986.
13. Fawzy M, Halim M, Ziady G, et al: Hemodynamic evaluation of porcine bioprostheses in the mitral position by Doppler echocardiography. *Am J Cardiol* 59:643, 1987.
14. Murphy E, Kloster F: Late results of valve replacement surgery: II. Complications of prosthetic heart valves. *Mod Concepts Cardiovasc Dis* 18:59, 1979.
15. Copans H, Lakier J, Kinsley R, et al: Thrombosed Björk-Shiley mitral prostheses. *Circulation* 61:169, 1980.
16. Ivert T, Dismukes W, Cobbs C, et al: Prosthetic valve endocarditis. *Circulation* 69:223, 1984.
17. Yoganathan A, Chaux A, Gray R, et al: Tilting disc and porcine aortic valve substitutes: In vitro hydrodynamic characteristics. *J Am Coll Cardiol* 3:313, 1984.

18. Come P: Pitfalls in the diagnosis of periprosthetic valvular regurgitation by pulsed Doppler echocardiography. *J Am Coll Cardiol* 9:1176, 1987.

19. Panidis I, Ross J, Mintz G: Normal and abnormal prosthetic valve function as assessed by Doppler echocardiography. *J Am Coll Cardiol* 8:317, 1986.

20. Rothbard R, Smucker L, Gibson R: Pulsed and continuous Doppler examination of prosthetic valves: Correlation with clinical and cardiac catheterization data (abstr). *Circulation* 72(III):373, 1985.

21. Holen J, Simonsen S, Frøysaker T: An ultrasound Doppler technique for the noninvasive determination of the pressure gradient in the Björk-Shiley mitral valve. *Circulation* 59:436, 1979.

22. Holen J, Høie J, Semb B: Obstructive characteristics of Björk-Shiley, Hancock, and Lillehei-Kaster prosthetic mitral valves in the immediate postoperative period. *Acta Med Scand* 204:5, 1978.

23. Dubach-Reber P, Vargus-Barron J: Velocidad maxima del flujo en la prostesis mitrale de Björk-Shiley normofuncionante. *Arch Inst Cardiol Mex* 56:57, 1986.

24. Cooper D, Stewart W, Schiavone W, et al: Evaluation of normal prosthetic valve function by Doppler echocardiography. *Am Heart J* 114:576, 1987.

25. Weinstein I, Marbager J, Perez J: Ultrasonic assessment of the St. Jude prosthetic valve: M-mode, two-dimensional, and Doppler echocardiography. *Circulation* 68:897, 1983.

26. Burckhardt D, Hoffman A, Vogt S, et al: Clinical evaluation of the St. Jude Medical heart valve prosthesis. *J Thorac Cardiovasc Surg* 88:432, 1984.

27. Lesbre J, Chasset C, Lesperance J, et al: Evaluation des nouvelles bioprosthèses pericardiques par Doppler pulsé et continu. *Arch Mal Coeur* 79:1439, 1986.

28. Gibbs J, Wharton G, Williams G: Doppler echocardiographic characteristics of the Carpentier-Edwards xenograft. *Eur Heart J* 7:353, 1986.

29. Stamm R, Martin R: Quantification of pressure gradients across stenotic valves by Doppler ultrasound. *J Am Coll Cardiol* 2:707, 1983.

30. Hatle L, Angelsen B: *Doppler Ultrasound in Cardiology*, 2d ed. Philadelphia, Lea & Febiger, 1985.

31. Diazumba S, Cornman C, Joyner C: Estimation of mitral prosthetic valve area by Doppler echocardiography (abstr). *J Am Coll Cardiol* 5:526, 1985.

32. Goldrath N, Zimes R, Vered Z: Analysis of Doppler-obtained velocity curves in functional evaluation of mechanical prosthetic valves in the mitral and aortic positions. *J Am Soc Echo* 1:211, 1988.

33. Jones M, McMillan S, Eidbo B, et al: Evaluation of prosthetic heart valves by Doppler flow imaging. *Echocardiography* 3:513, 1986.

34. Ramirez M, Wong M, Sadler N, Shah P: Doppler evaluation of 106 bioprosthetic and mechanical aortic valves (abstr). *J Am Coll Cardiol* 5:527, 1985.

35. Hatle L: Combined 2D-echo and Doppler compared to Doppler without imaging. Assessment of prosthetic valves, in Spencer M (ed): *Cardiac Doppler Diagnosis*. Boston, Nijhoff, 1983.

36. Ferrara R, Labovitz A, Wiens R, et al: Prosthetic mitral regurgitation detected by Doppler echocardiography. *Am J Cardiol* 55:229, 1985.

37. Curcio C, Commerford P, Rose A, et al: Calcification of glutaraldehyde-preserved porcine xenografts in young patients. *J Thorac Cardiovasc Surg* 81:621, 1981.

38. Miller D, Stinson E, Oyer P, et al: The durability of porcine xenograft valves and conduits in children. *Circulation* 66(I):172, 1982.

39. Fishbein M, Gissen S, Collins J Jr, et al: Pathologic findings after cardiac valve replacement with glutaraldehyde-fixed porcine valves. *Am J Cardiol* 40:331, 1977.

40. Lamberti J, Wainer B, Fisher K, et al: Calcific stenosis of the porcine heterograft. *Ann Thorac Surg* 28:28, 1979.

CHAPTER 11

Evaluation of Systolic Cardiac Function

Doppler echocardiography evaluates intracardiac blood flow and provides an estimate of ventricular performance that is independent of ventricular geometry. An accurate determination of forward volume flow does not in itself define whether ventricular function is normal or abnormal. For example, the dilated, hypokinetic left ventricle in a patient with dilated cardiomyopathy may eject a relatively normal forward stroke volume and cardiac output despite marked increases in end-diastolic and end-systolic volumes and marked depression of systolic indexes, such as ejection fraction, rate of increase of left ventricular pressure (dP/dt), and mean velocity of circumferential fiber shortening. However, when combined with M-mode and 2D echocardiography for assessment of regional and global ventricular function, a quantitative measure of stroke volume would add important hemodynamic information in the comprehensive assessment of cardiac function, and in following the response of the failing ventricle to therapeutic interventions.

MEASUREMENT OF STROKE VOLUME AND CARDIAC OUTPUT

Cardiac output is one ejection phase index of function that can be calculated from the Doppler examination. Doppler-derived values for cardiac output have correlated closely with those measured invasively.[1–4] Sampling sites from which cardiac output measurements have been obtained include: ascending and descending aorta from the suprasternal notch, apical mitral and tricuspid valves, left ventricular outflow tract, and main pulmonary artery from the parasternal short axis view.

For any given window, the stroke volume (SV) is calculated as the product of the cross-sectional area (CSA) of the valve or vessel through which the blood is flowing and the flow velocity integral (FVI) (Fig. 11–1):

$$SV = FVI \times CSA$$

The cardiac output (CO) is then obtained by multiplying the stroke volume by the heart rate (HR):

$$CO = SV \times HR$$

Derias et al[5] recently presented a simplified formula to calculate cardiac output based on quantitative Doppler-derived flows. They measured the aortic anulus (D) with electronic calipers in a parasternal long axis view. Peak flow velocity (PFV) and left ventricular ejection time (ET) were measured using PD interrogation of the ascending aorta visualized from an apical view. An equation was derived to correlate these data with stroke volume by conventional techniques:

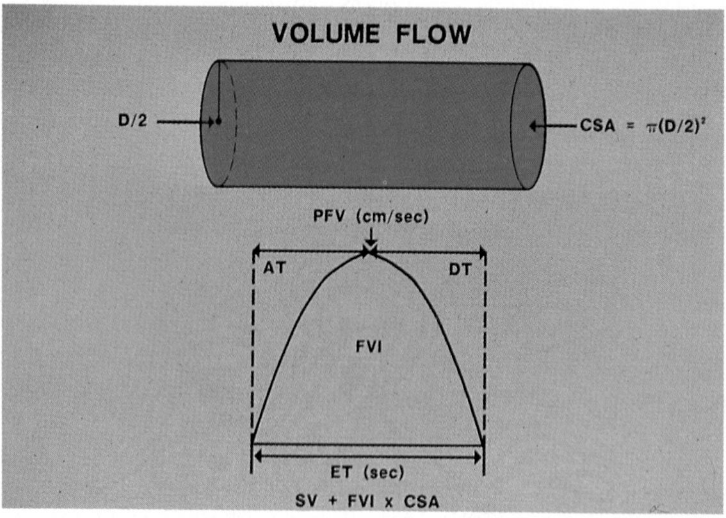

Figure 11–1. Schematic diagram of method for measuring volume flow. Stroke volume (SV) (in milliliters) can be estimated by multiplying the planimetered area under the flow velocity curve [flow velocity integral (FVI) or stroke distance, in centimeters] by the cross-sectional area (CSA) of the vessel through which blood is flowing [$\pi(D/2)^2$, in square centimeters], where D = mean diameter of the vessel (or anulus) through which blood is flowing. The tracing is labeled to show how the peak flow velocity (PFV), ejection time (ET), acceleration time (AT), and deceleration time (DT) are measured.

$$SV = [0.53 (D^2 \times PFV \times ET)] + 0.92$$

Stroke volume determined by this method correlated well ($r = 0.915$) with thermodilution techniques done close in time.

Adding the Doppler-derived stroke volume to the cardiac output equation:

$$CO(l/min) = SV \times HR$$

also showed a close correlation ($r = 0.87$) with thermodilution-derived cardiac output.

The advantage of this very accurate technique is the simplicity of the measurements and the ease of calculation without a need for computer interfacing.

AORTIC FLOW

Flow Velocity Parameters

Measurements of blood flow velocity parameters from the ascending aorta are shown in Fig. 11–1, and the normal data are listed in Table 11–1. Peak flow velocity (in centimeters per second) is measured at the center of the Doppler flow spectrum at the time of maximum blood flow velocity. Acceleration time is calculated as the time in milliseconds from the onset of ejection to peak flow velocity. Similarly, deceleration time is measured in milliseconds as the time from peak flow velocity to the end of deceleration. The average acceleration can be calculated in centimeters per second per second (cm/s^2) by dividing peak flow velocity by the acceleration time. Average deceleration is calculated in centimeters per second per second by dividing peak flow velocity by the deceleration time. Ejection

TABLE 11–1. Normal Flow Velocity Parameters from the Ascending Aorta

	Range	Mean
Peak flow velocity (cm/s)	72–120	92
Acceleration time (ms)	83–118	98
Average acceleration (cm/s^2)	735–1318	955
Deceleration time (ms)	170–230	197
Average deceleration (cm/s^2)	355–630	473
Ejection time (ms)	265–325	294
Flow velocity integral (cm)	12.6–22.5	15.7

time is measured in milliseconds from the onset of ejection to the end of systolic ejection. The area under the systolic flow velocity curve, or the FVI (discussed below), is expressed in centimeters.

Flow Velocity Integral

Measurement of the FVI in the aorta has been shown to be useful in monitoring changes in stroke volume.[6,7] The aortic FVI is generally determined by planimetering the area under the flow velocity curve for one or more beats either manually or using computer software (Fig. 11–2). The FVI is directly proportional to the stroke volume and is expressed in units of distance (centimeters). For this reason, it is sometimes referred to as "stroke distance." This distance represents how far red blood cells would have moved through a tube of a constant cross-sectional area. Alternatively, the FVI may be estimated in centimeters using the following formula:

$$\text{FVI} = \frac{\text{PFV} \times \text{ET}}{2}$$

where PFV = peak flow velocity in centimeters per second, and ET = ejection time in seconds. This equation usually underestimates the true FVI and should be recognized as only an estimate. Measurement of these velocity parameters is depicted in Fig. 11–1.

The technique of measuring the FVI can significantly alter the results of cardiac output calculations. It is important to use the best possible tracings from the area being interrogated—namely, those with the highest velocity and the least spectral broadening. Because some spectral broadening is present during deceleration in all Doppler tracings, it is important to estimate the "modal" velocity of the red cells.[8,9] This can be approximated by outlining the darkest portion of the spectral tracing (Fig. 11–2), which represents the velocities at which the majority of red cells are traveling. Outlining of only the highest portions of the spectral tracing produces overestimation of cardiac output; using only the lowest velocities produces underestimation of stroke volume.

The suprasternal notch can be used to record both ascending and descending aortic velocities (Fig. 11–3). Since there may be variation in velocity throughout the aortic profile,[10,11,12] it is important to record velocities from as close to the center of the aorta as possible. Both PD and CW Doppler systems have been used to interrogate the aortic arch.[2,6,13,14] In this laboratory, CW Doppler echocardiography, using a small nonimaging transducer, is used. This provides the best velocity pattern. When PD is used, the sample volume depth is varied until the best recordings are

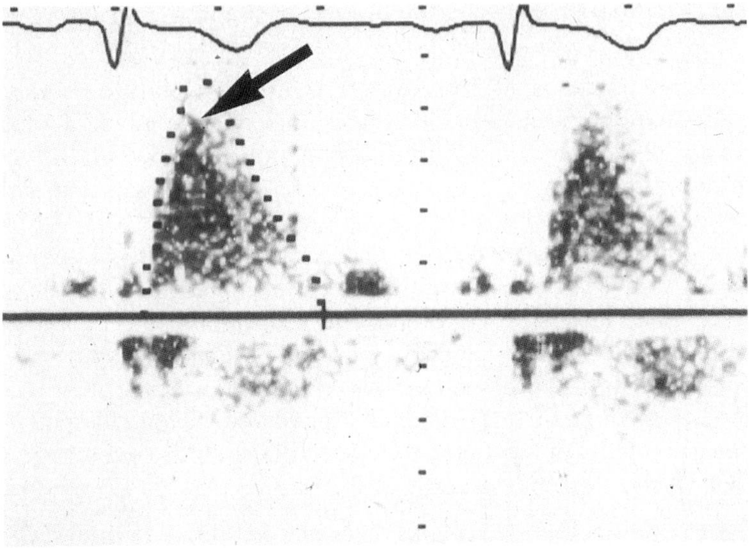

Figure 11–2. Continuous wave aortic flow velocity recording from the suprasternal notch. The systolic velocities are toward the transducer (above the baseline). The velocities are outlined showing peak velocity. Peak velocity is the highest velocity at any given time. Peak modal velocity is identified as the velocity with the darkest spectral recording (arrow). Modal velocity is that which occurs most often or is dominant. The FVI determined from the modal velocity is 19 cm. (Scale marks = 20 cm/s)

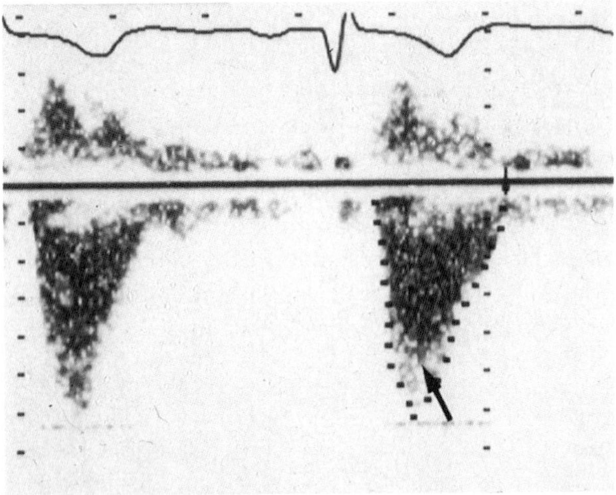

Figure 11–3. Continuous wave flow velocity recording from the descending aorta from the suprasternal notch; recorded from the same patient as in Fig. 11–12. The curve is similar to that from the ascending aorta. The arrow points to the peak modal velocity. The FVI of 22 cm is similar to that of the ascending aorta. (Scale marks = 20 cm/s)

again obtained. Because a "cross section" of the cell velocities is important to adequately sample aortic flow, a sample volume length of 7 to 10 mm is used. The beam can also be carefully oriented and the sample volume depth adjusted by 2D visualization to an area where flow is approximately parallel to the interrogating beam.

Since approximately 25 percent of the cardiac output is lost to the head and neck, a lower velocity would be expected in the distal aortic arch and descending aorta. The distribution of velocities in the descending aorta has been shown to be similar to that in the ascending aorta[15] due to narrowing of the aortic cross section. The time-velocity profiles have been shown to be similar in the experimental preparation[16] and in patients.[17,18] Thus, measurements of the FVI in the aorta can be made from either the ascending or the descending aortic arch.

Cross-Sectional Area

The most difficult part of calculating stroke volume is measuring the CSA of the aorta, which can be obtained using the following formula (Fig. 11–1):

$$\text{CSA}(\text{cm}^2) = \pi(\text{D}/2)^2$$

where π is approximately 3.14 and D = diameter of aorta. Several reasons exist for this difficulty. The calculation of the CSA supposes an aorta of circular cross section, which may not be found in all patients. Also, the cross-sectional area of the aorta varies by as much as 11 to 17 percent during systole.[19] Because of the squaring of the radius, errors in diameter measurements are doubled in area calculations.

The diameter of the aorta has been measured by M-mode[2] and 2D echocardiography.[18,20–22] Two-dimensional measurements appear to be more reliable than those taken by M mode.[21] The diameter is usually measured either at the aortic valve anulus or at a level just above the sinuses of Valsalva (Fig. 11–4). An inner-to-inner-wall measurement is used to provide aortic diameter. For serial studies in one patient, the aortic diameter is measured during the initial study and is assumed to be constant for all following studies.

Cardiac Output

Excellent results have been obtained in Doppler echocardiographic calculation of cardiac output from the aorta, to judge from comparisons of such estimates with those made by thermodilution.[1,4,17,20–24] These calculations, however, are not valid across a stenotic or regurgitant valve, because

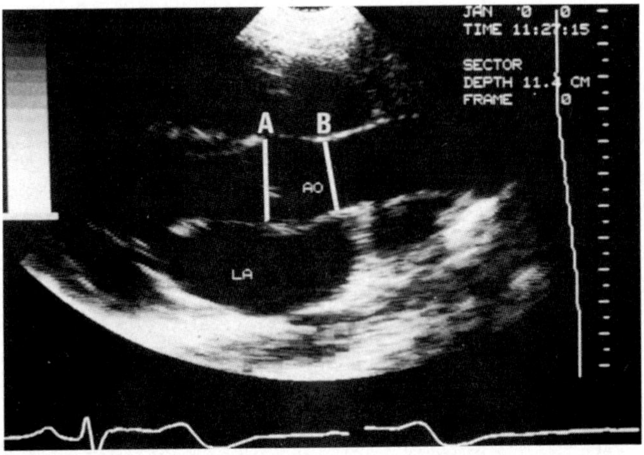

Figure 11–4. Two-dimensional parasternal long axis view illustrating the two commonly used sites for measuring aortic root diameter: (A) at the level of the aortic leaflets, and (B) just distal to the aortic sinuses. An inner-to-inner-wall measurement is used. AO = aorta, LA = left atrium.

increases in velocity in the vicinity of an abnormal valve produce a false increase in the calculated integral.

Although serial determinations of cardiac output can be accurately measured using Doppler echocardiography, potential errors in the determination of the cross-sectional area of flow have limited the application of this technique. One recent study[25] in open-chest dogs and healthy human volunteers used CFI to determine the flow diameter area, and to explore the relationship between the anatomic, echo-derived diameter of a valve or vessel and its corresponding diameter as measured with CFI, so as to assess which of these would most reliably estimate flow area for volume flow calculation. These studies concluded that aortic flows calculated from CFI-derived diameters were more accurate at low cardiac outputs, suggesting that CFI may be particularly valuable in these low flow states. Generally, output determinations made with CFI were not as accurate as those using anatomic diameters. These findings are probably due to low velocity threshold cutoffs, low signal-to-noise ratio, and gain dependence of the area of flow imaging with current Doppler systems.

PULMONARY ARTERY FLOW

In recording volume flow in the pulmonary artery, measurement of pulmonary artery diameter seems to be a more difficult problem than measuring pulmonary flow velocity. The difficulty lies in the fact that although one attempts to record Doppler flow as parallel as possible to the flow stream (Doppler angle ~0°), the best resolution for imaging of structures (e.g., the pulmonary artery walls) is obtained when images are obtained perpendicularly to the structures. It often is difficult to visualize the walls of the pulmonary artery in the parasternal short axis view, though in general this is an excellent view for recording Doppler pulmonary artery flow signals. Solutions that have been suggested include: (1) obtaining images in the steep left lateral decubitus position (in an attempt to find a relatively lung-free window for imaging the pulmonary artery), (2) using images of the right ventricular outflow tract just proximal to the pulmonary valve, and (3) obtaining the pulmonary artery diameter from other views. Investigators have reported a good correlation between Doppler stroke volume obtained from the pulmonary artery and invasively measured stroke volume.[26–28]

MITRAL AND TRICUSPID FLOW

A number of investigators have reported that stroke volume can be reliably measured in the region of the mitral and tricuspid valves.[22,28–30] As in measuring aortic and pulmonary artery volume flow, measurement of the area through which blood is flowing appears to be the major difficulty in estimating mitral or tricuspid volume flow. For the mitral valve, techniques that have been suggested for use in calculating the appropriate volume flow area include using measurements of (1) the maximal mitral orifice area, planimetered from the parasternal short axis 2D image, multiplied by the ratio of the mean-to-maximal mitral leaflet separation on M-mode echocardiography,[29] and (2) the mitral anulus diameter measured from 2D apical two- or four-chamber images.[22,28,30]

Use of 2D measurements of mitral orifice area have not proved reliable in estimating stroke volume in adult patients.[31] Lewis and associates[22] have reported a good correlation between thermodilution and Doppler stroke volume estimates using the Doppler mitral FVI and the mitral anular diameter to estimate mitral flow area (Fig. 11–5). However, these investigators noted a mean interobserver variability of 15 ± 10% in measuring mitral CSA, emphasizing the variability involved in this measurement.[22]

The tricuspid valve is more difficult to assess than the other valves. The velocities are lower and more difficult to record, despite the fact that recordings can be made from either the apex or the left parasternal window. However, this method has been shown to be useful in both animals and children. The maximal tricuspid valve velocities were integrated and

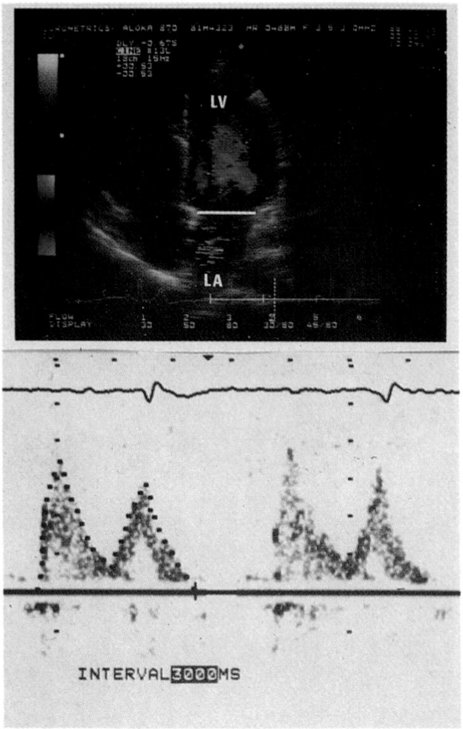

Figure 11–5. Apical four-chamber view with color flow imaging (CFI) demonstrating mitral diastolic inflow (red), anulus diameter measurement (horizontal line), and mitral FVI (dotted line). The mitral anulus is measured as an internal dimension in mid-diastole and treated as a circular structure. LV = left ventricle, LA = left atrium.

multiplied by the area of the tricuspid anulus calculated from the maximal diastolic anulus diameter in the four-chamber view. In 10 patients, a correlation of 0.89 was obtained with thermodilution.[32] When calculated flows were compared in the short axis and four-chamber views, the best results were obtained when velocities were averaged between inspiration and expiration.

ERRORS IN DETERMINING CARDIAC OUTPUT

As noted above, error can be introduced into the flow estimate at several levels. The major sources of error are summarized in Table 11–2. They can be divided into errors of velocity estimate, errors of area measurement, and inappropriate combinations of area and velocity measurements.

Velocity Estimate

Two major sources of error are present in the velocity estimate. The major error is that of position. When the sampling is performed, the Doppler

TABLE 11-2. Errors in Determining Cardiac Output

A. Velocity estimate
1. Technique
   a. Inadequate beam alignment
   b. Failure to outline modal velocity
   c. Measurement of too few beats
2. Inappropriate velocity
   a. Stenotic valve velocity
   b. Regurgitant valve
   c. Arterial stenosis

B. Area measurement
1. Site of area measurement
2. Measurement of area and velocity at different sites

beam must be aligned as well as possible with the blood flow. The adequacy of alignment is reflected in the spectral tracing as a well-defined outline and a narrow spectral bandwidth, especially during deceleration. During measurement, the velocity tracing is outlined at the darkest area, the "modal" velocity. Estimation through only the highest velocity can overestimate cardiac output. In many patients, the systolic profile varies slightly from beat to beat during respiration. As a result, multiple (usually three to five) cycles should be measured.

A second major source of error is that of sampling inappropriate sites. Sampling distal to a stenotic value will yield velocities that are representative of both flow and the pressure gradient across the valve. The elevated velocity represents flow at the narrowed orifice, not in the vessel being sampled. Similarly, the calculated flow across a regurgitant valve represents systemic and regurgitant flow.[33] Prosthetic heart valves are always mildly stenotic, and reliable flow estimates are not obtainable when prosthetic valve velocities are used.

The mitral valve FVI is sensitive not only to sampling site but also to Doppler modality. For accurate results, measurements must be made from the same site; Doppler and 2D echocardiography must be used together at the tips of the valve, or paired at the anular level.

Anatomic Area

To accurately estimate aortic flow, measurements of the anatomic area are made at the aortic valve anulus or in the ascending aorta during systole. As noted, multiple conventions have been used successfully to measure anatomic area. In an individual laboratory, it is important to use one convention consistently in all patients. For serial studies in one patient the same area is applied for all measurements, unless the patient is in the pediatric age group, in which case growth is expected.

Measurement of Area and Velocity at Different Sites

As noted, the aortic velocity profile is similar in the ascending and distal arch areas. The resultant FVIs thus can be interchanged and used with the ascending aortic area. When measuring both inflow and outflow valves, it is important to remember that velocity, and therefore the FVI, rises distal to the valve. For accuracy, subvalvular velocities are paired with areas taken at the same site.

Arterial Obstruction

Congenital abnormalities may cause alterations in the flow profile. Supravalvular aortic stenosis or coarctation of the aorta may elevate velocities similarly to other stenotic lesions, and use of velocities distal to these obstructions may produce artifactual high estimates of cardiac output.

CLINICAL APPLICATIONS OF DOPPLER CARDIAC OUTPUT

The measurements of the components of Doppler cardiac output have been shown to have several important clinical applications (Table 11–3). Doppler echocardiography can be used to provide ongoing evaluation of patients in determining the effects of therapeutic interventions on ventricular performance.[34] To compare changes over time in stroke volume or cardiac output in the same individual, however, the cross-sectional area need not be calculated, since the change in the measured FVI is directly proportional to the change in stroke volume.

TABLE 11–3. Clinical Applications of Doppler Cardiac Output

Evaluation of left ventricular function
Evaluation of therapeutic interventions
Evaluation of pacemaker hemodynamics
Regurgitant fractions
Change in cardiac output with exercise
Shunt calculations

The ability of Doppler echocardiography to objectively assess ventricular performance has been the basis of several investigations of optimal pacemaker hemodynamics (Fig. 11–6). Doppler echocardiography has been shown to help predict which patients will benefit most from dual-chamber as opposed to ventricular-demand pacing modes.[35–38] In addition, the optimal atrioventricular delay may also be assessed by these means.[36]

The volume of valvular regurgitation and regurgitant fraction can also be estimated. This was recently demonstrated to be reliable in the estimation of mitral regurgitation.[33] The aortic valve stroke volume was calculated from the left ventricular outflow tract, and the mitral valve flow was calculated from the mitral integral. The regurgitant fraction is estimated using the formula:

$$\text{Regurgitant fraction} = \frac{\text{Mitral SV} - \text{Aortic SV}}{\text{Mitral SV}}$$

Similar estimation of aortic regurgitant volumes and regurgitant fraction may be useful.

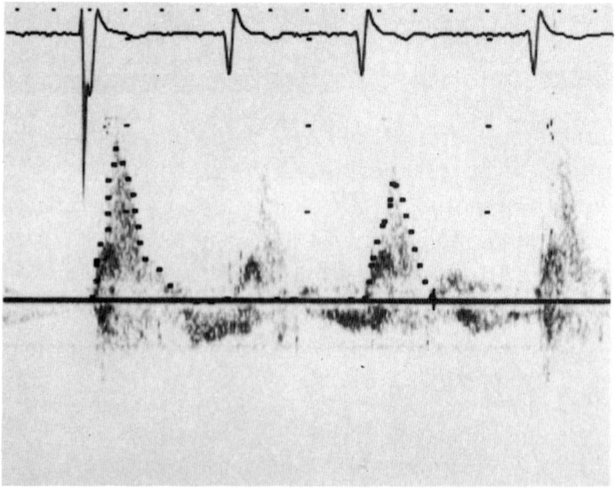

Figure 11–6. Beat-to-beat changes in stroke volume demonstrated with Doppler echocardiography in a patient with atrial fibrillation and ventricular demand pacing. This is a continuous wave tracing from the suprasternal notch. The first beat is a ventricular paced beat that was preceded by a long R–R interval, allowing increased left ventricular diastolic filling and augmentation in stroke volume. The second and third beats follow a short R–R interval and reflect a drop in stroke volume. (Scale marks = 1 m/s)

In a similar way, the ratio of pulmonary to systemic flow (Q_p/Q_s) can be calculated by measuring right and left ventricular stroke volumes at the pulmonic and aortic valves, respectively.[26,27,32] This information can be used for atrial level shunts. In ventricular level shunts, the mitral valve flow can be used to represent pulmonary artery flow (Q_p) and the aortic flow to represent systemic flow (Q_s). In extracardiac shunts (e.g., patent ductus arteriosus), mitral or ascending aortic flow reflects forward flow plus the shunt flow (Q_p), while tricuspid or pulmonary valve flow represents the actual forward (systemic) flow returning to the lungs.

Measurement of Doppler FVIs from the suprasternal notch during both supine and upright exercise shows the potential value of this technique in evaluating left ventricular function with exercise[13,39,40] (discussed in Chap. 14). An important finding is that it appears feasible to measure these changes before and immediately after exercise, thus eliminating the potentially difficult task of acquiring the information during exercise.

REFERENCES

1. Colocousis J, Huntsman L, Curreri P: Estimation of stroke volume changes by ultrasonic Doppler. *Circulation* 56:914, 1977.
2. Huntsman L, Stewart D, Barnes S, et al: Noninvasive Doppler determination of cardiac output in man. Clinical validation. *Circulation* 67:593, 1983.
3. Alverson D, Eldridge M, Dillon T, et al: Noninvasive pulsed Doppler determination of cardiac output in neonates and children. *J Pediatr* 101:46, 1982.
4. Nishimura R, Callahan M, Schaff H, et al: Noninvasive measurement of cardiac output by continuous wave Doppler echocardiography: Initial experience and review of the literature. *Mayo Clin Proc* 59:484, 1984.
5. Derias S, Zoghbi W, Lewis J, et al: Simplified Doppler method for determining stroke volume and cardiac output from the aortic annulus without computer assistance (abstr). *Circulation* 72(III):351, 1985.
6. Buchtal A, Hanson G, Peisach A: Transcutaneous aortovelography: Potential useful technique in management of critically ill patients. *Br Heart J* 38:451, 1976.
7. Elkayam U, Gardin J, Berkley R, et al: Doppler flow velocity measurements in the assessment of hemodynamic response to vasodilators in patients with heart failure. *Circulation* 67:377, 1982.
8. Sagar K, Wann S, Boerboom L, et al: Comparison of peak and modal aortic blood flow velocities with invasive measures of left ventricular performance. *J Am Soc Echo* 1:194, 1988.
9. Goldberg S, Sahn D, Allen H, et al: Evaluation of pulmonary and systemic blood flow by 2-dimensional Doppler echocardiography using fast Fourier transform spectral analysis. *Am J Cardiol* 50:1394, 1982.
10. Seed W, Wood N: Velocity patterns in the aorta. *Cardiovasc Res* 5:319, 1971.

11. Nerem R, Seed W, Wood N: An experimental study of the velocity distribution and transition to turbulence in the aorta. *J Fluid Mechanics* 52:137, 1972.
12. Steingart R, Meller J, Barovick J, et al: Pulsed Doppler echocardiographic measurement of beat-to-beat changes in stroke volume in dogs. *Circulation* 62:542, 1980.
13. Gardin J, Kozlowski J, Dabestani A, et al: Studies of Doppler aortic flow velocity during supine bicycle exercise. *Am J Cardiol* 57:327, 1986.
14. Mehta N, Bennett D: Impaired left ventricular function in acute myocardial infarction assessed by Doppler measurement of ascending aortic blood velocity and maximum acceleration. *Am J Cardiol* 57:1052, 1986.
15. Clark C, Schultz D: Velocity distribution in aortic flow. *Cardiovasc Res* 7:601, 1973.
16. Farthing S, Peronneau P: Flow in the thoracic aorta. *Cardiovasc Res* 11:607, 1979.
17. Goldberg S, Loeber C: Can Doppler velocities measured anywhere in the aortic arch be substituted for ascending aortic velocities? (abstr) *Circulation* 68(III):260, 1983.
18. Labovitz A, Buckingham T, Habermehl K, et al: The effects of sampling site on the two-dimensional echo-Doppler determination of cardiac output. *Am Heart J* 109:327, 1985.
19. Greenfield J, Patel D: Relation between pressure and diameter in the ascending aorta of man. *Circ Res* 10:778, 1962.
20. Magnin P, Stewart J, Myers S, et al: Combined Doppler and phased-array echocardiographic estimation of cardiac output. *Circulation* 63:338, 1981.
21. Gardin J, Tobis J, Dabestani A, et al: Superiority of two-dimensional measurement of aortic vessel diameter in Doppler echocardiographic estimates of left ventricular stroke volume. *J Am Coll Cardiol* 6:66, 1985.
22. Lewis J, Kuo L, Nelson J, et al: Pulsed Doppler echocardiographic determination of stroke volume and cardiac output: Clinical validation of two new methods using the apical window. *Circulation* 70:425, 1984.
23. Chandraratna P, Nanna M, McKay C, et al: Determination of cardiac output by transcutaneous continuous-wave ultrasonic Doppler computer. *Am J Cardiol* 53:234, 1984.
24. Rose J, Nanna M, Rahimtoola S, et al: Accuracy of determination of changes in cardiac output by transcutaneous continuous-wave Doppler computer. *Am J Cardiol* 54:1099, 1984.
25. Hoit B, Valdes-Cruz L, Sahn D: Use of Doppler color flow mapping in the echocardiographic determination of cardiac output. *Echocardiography* 4:535, 1987.
26. Kitabatake A, Inoue M, Asao M, et al: Noninvasive evaluation of the ratio of pulmonary to systemic flow in atrial septal defect by Duplex Doppler echocardiography. *Circulation* 69:73, 1984.
27. Valdes-Cruz L, Horowitz S, Mesel E, et al: A pulsed Doppler echocardiographic method for calculating pulmonary and systemic blood flow in atrial level shunts: Validation studies in animals and initial human experience. *Circulation* 69:80, 1984.

28. Loeber C, Goldberg S, Allen H: Doppler echocardiographic comparison of flows distal to the four cardiac valves. *J Am Coll Cardiol* 4:268, 1984.

29. Fisher D, Sahn D, Friedman M, et al: The mitral valve orifice method for noninvasive two-dimensional echo Doppler determinations of cardiac output. *Circulation* 67:872, 1983.

30. Valdes-Cruz L, Horowitz S, Sahn D, et al: A simplified mitral valve method for 2D echo Doppler cardiac output (abstr). *Circulation* 68(III):230, 1983.

31. Gardin J, Butman S, Olson H, et al: Limitations of the mitral valve orifice method in determination of stroke volume by Doppler echocardiography (abstr). *Clin Res* 32:6A, 1984.

32. Meijboom E, Horowitz S, Valdes-Cruz L, et al: Doppler echocardiographic method for calculating volume flow across the tricuspid valve: Correlative laboratory and clinical studies. *Circulation* 71:551, 1985.

33. Ascah K, Stewart W, Jiang L, et al: A Doppler two-dimensional echocardiographic method for quantitation of mitral regurgitation. *Circulation* 72:377, 1985.

34. Elkayam U, Gardin J, Berkley R, et al: The use of Doppler flow velocity measurements to assess the hemodynamic response to vasodilator in patients with heart failure. *Circulation* 67:377, 1983.

35. Stewart W, Dicola V, Harthorne J, et al: Doppler ultrasound measurement of cardiac output in patients with physiologic pacemakers. *Am J Cardiol* 54:308, 1984.

36. Labovitz A, Williams G, Redd R, Kennedy H: Noninvasive assessment of pacemaker hemodynamics by Doppler echocardiography: Importance of left atrial size. *J Am Coll Cardiol* 6:196, 1985.

37. Schuster A, Nanda N: Doppler echocardiography in cardiac pacing. *Pace* 5:607, 1982.

38. Zugibe F, Nanda N, Barold S, et al: Usefulness of Doppler echocardiography in cardiac pacing: Assessment of mitral regurgitation, peak aortic flow velocity and atrial capture. *Pace* 6:1350, 1983.

39. Bryg R, Labovitz A, Mehdirad A, et al: Effect of coronary artery disease on Doppler-derived parameters of aortic flow during upright exercise. *Am J Cardiol* 58:14, 1986.

40. Mehdirad A, Williams G, Labovitz A, et al: Evaluation of left ventricular function during upright exercise: Correlation of exercise Doppler with post-exercise two-dimensional echocardiography. *Circulation* 75:413, 1987.

CHAPTER 12

Evaluation of Diastolic Cardiac Function

BASIC CONCEPTS AND CLINICAL CORRELATES

Cardiac output depends not only on the ability of the heart to eject blood at each systole, but also on its capacity to fill at each diastole. Diastolic function is the ability of the ventricular myocardium to relax after ejection and accept inflow of blood. It is now well established that myocardial relaxation is an active, energy-requiring process.[1,2] At the cellular level, calcium must move away from the myofilaments in order for relaxation to occur. Adenosine triphosphate (ATP) is hydrolyzed to fuel active transport of calcium ions from the myofilaments to the sarcoplasmic reticulum where they are sequestered. It is estimated that 15 percent of the heart's total energy output is accounted for in this active process of relaxation.[2] Thus diastolic myocardial function, like systolic myocardial function, may be expected to deteriorate in the diseased heart.

In the intact organ, many descriptors of diastolic function have been developed and explored. The operative compliance, the change in volume with a given change in pressure (dV/dP), is one useful way to characterize diastolic function.[3] The dV/dP depends on both the diastolic pressure-volume curve characteristics (modulus of chamber stiffness) and the ventricular filling pressure. Operative compliance is a complex parameter that tends to vary inversely with both diastolic filling pressure and modulus of chamber stiffness. Decreased operative compliance occurs in conditions in which the modulus of chamber stiffness rises, such as ventricular hypertrophy, scarring, or infiltration. In compensated chronic volume overload without severe ventricular hypertrophy or fibrosis, the modulus of chamber stiffness falls, and operative compliance can be greater than normal.[1,3]

Disease processes that might be expected to produce changes in diastolic function are listed in Table 12–1. First, those diseases that produce

TABLE 12–1. Disease Processes with Potential to Produce Diastolic Function Changes

Pathophysiology	Pure Pressure Overload	Pure Volume Overload	Mixed Pressure and Volume Overload	Primary or Secondary Myocardial Disease
Expected Effect	↑ Stiffness	↓ Stiffness	↑ or ↓ Stiffness	↑ Stiffness
Examples				
LV	Systemic Htn	MR	AS/AR	Ischemia
	AS	AR		Hypertrophic,
		VSD		restrictive, or dilated CM
	Coarctation	PDA		Constrictive
	Pulmonary Htn	TA		pericarditis
RV	Pulmonary Htn	ASD	PS/PR	Ischemia
		APVR		Hypertrophic
	PS	TR		restrictive, or dilated CM
		PR		Constrictive pericarditis

NOTE: APVR = anomalous pulmonary venous return; AR = aortic regurgitation; AS = aortic stenosis; ASD = atrial septal defect; CM = cardiomyopathy; Htn = hypertension; LV = left ventricle; MR = mitral regurgitation; PDA = patent ductus arteriosus; PR = pulmonic regurgitation; PS = pulmonic stenosis; RV = right ventricle; TA = tricuspid atresia; TR = tricuspid regurgitation; VSD = ventricular septal defect.

ventricular hypertrophic or fibrotic changes solely due to pressure overload have been shown to decrease operative compliance.[3–8] Specific diseases in which this occurs and in which left ventricular diastolic function may be affected include systemic hypertension and aortic stenosis. Analogous pathophysiology can also affect the right side of the heart (see Table 12–1). Second, pure volume overload conditions may increase compliance until and unless hypertrophic or fibrotic changes occur in the ventricle.[3,4] Atrial septal defect, anomalous pulmonary venous return, and tricuspid or pulmonary regurgitation, therefore, may be expected to produce right ventricular compliance changes. Third, chronic volume and pressure overload may combine to produce either an increase or a decrease in compliance.[3,4] Decreased compliance under these circumstances may have implications in the long-term prognosis of patients with chronic aortic stenosis and regurgitation or of patients with pulmonic stenosis and regurgitation after tetralogy of Fallot repair. Fourth, primary or secondary myocardial disease has been shown to decrease compliance.[1,3,9–12]

CLINICAL MEASURES OF DIASTOLIC FUNCTION

Classically, the clinical evaluation of diastolic function has relied on invasive ventricular pressure measurements and contrast angiographic demonstration of ventricular volume changes with time.[4,13–15] These methods have provided parameters such as the diastolic time derivative of pressure ($-dP/dt$) and rates of diastolic inflow (including early diastolic filling rate, peak filling rate, and filling fractions). Recently, radionuclide angiographic techniques have been developed that yield rates of diastolic ventricular inflow, peak filling rate, filling fraction, and time-to-peak filling.[16–18] Echocardiographic techniques, particularly computer-assisted digitized echocardiography, have been used to estimate diastolic ventricular volume changes.[19–21] M-mode echocardiography also has been used to establish the timing of diastolic events that relate indirectly to diastolic ventricular function.[22,23] However, neither pressure or volume determinations nor timing of events alone provide direct measurement of operative compliance. Synthesis of all three is possible,[24] but can be complicated, particularly for routine clinical application.

DOPPLER EVALUATION OF LEFT VENTRICULAR DIASTOLIC FUNCTION

More recently, several investigators[7,10,12,25–33] have attempted to indirectly assess left ventricular diastolic function by using different measurements obtained from PD ultrasound mitral flow velocity recordings. In normal subjects and patients with a variety of cardiac diseases, evaluation of left ventricular filling patterns by Doppler echocardiography has compared favorably with both angiographic[26] and radionuclide[25,27] techniques.

Several different indexes of left ventricular diastolic function have been derived from the mitral valve inflow Doppler tracing. For this technique, a range-gated PD examination of the left ventricular inflow tract is performed. From the apical four-chamber view, the Doppler cursor line and sample volume are placed in the mitral valve orifice at an angle as nearly parallel to flow as possible (Fig. 12–1). Color flow imaging (CFI) is helpful in positioning the sample volume in the direction of left ventricular inflow. The sample volume position is adjusted to record the maximum

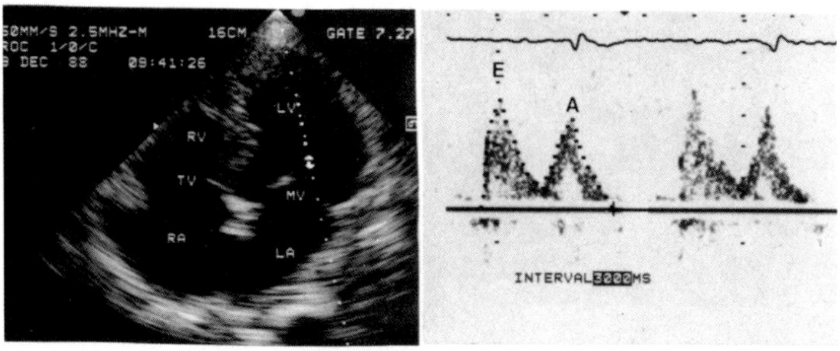

Figure 12–1. Technique used to record the mitral valve inflow Doppler tracing for evaluation of left ventricular diastolic filling. The apical four-chamber view (left) shows the position of the sample volume near the tips of the mitral valve leaflet. The Doppler tracing (right) demonstrates the peak velocities at rapid filling (peak E) and during atrial contraction (peak A). LA = left atrium, LV = left ventricle, MV = mitral valve, RA = right atrium, RV = right ventricle, TV = tricuspid valve. (Scale marks = 20 cm/s)

velocity through the mitral valve. This point is usually found just distal to the anulus near the tips of the mitral valve leaflets. The position of the sample volume is critical in order to obtain standardized results. An adequate mitral valve Doppler examination consists of clear identification of the opening and closure points of the mitral valve and the peak velocities at rapid ventricular filling (the peak E velocity) and during atrial contraction (the peak A velocity). The proportion of filling accounted for by the A wave is variable and may vary inversely with ventricular compliance.

Diastolic Time Intervals

From the mitral valve Doppler tracing, several types of indexes of left ventricular diastolic filling can be calculated (Fig. 12–2). First, diastolic time intervals reflecting the time course of relaxation can be calculated. The isovolumic relaxation time can be measured from the aortic closing component of the second heart sound to the onset of the diastolic flow velocity, and requires a phonocardiogram to be recorded simultaneously with the mitral valve Doppler tracing. This isovolumic relaxation time is 75 ± 11 ms in normal subjects and is prolonged in patients with impaired left ventricular relaxation.[25] The time from the onset of diastolic flow to the peak E velocity (acceleration time) can be measured and is 100 ± 10 ms in normal adults.[33] The duration of the early diastolic flow period can be measured from the onset of diastolic flow to the time when the Doppler curve returns from peak E velocity to the baseline (E area). This time

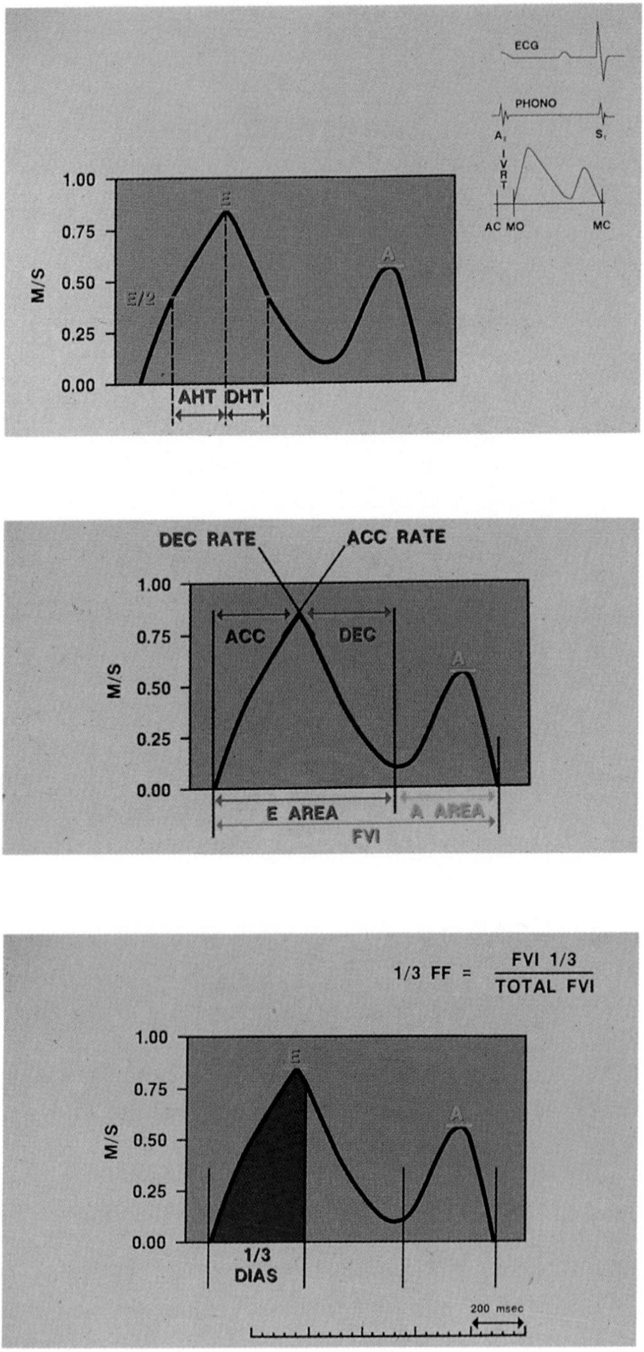
ECG
PHONO
A2
S1
IVRT
AC MO
MC
1.00
0.75
0.50
0.25
0.00
M/S
E
E/2
A
AHT
DHT
DEC RATE
ACC RATE
ACC
DEC
E AREA
A AREA
FVI
1/3 FF = FVI 1/3 / TOTAL FVI
1/3
DIAS
200 msec

Figure 12-2.

period is 214 ± 26 ms in normal subjects and has been reported to be prolonged in patients with left ventricular outflow obstruction.[25,34] Finally, the acceleration and deceleration half-times of early diastolic rapid inflow have been used to describe the time course of relaxation.[12] These time periods are measured as the intervals between the peak E velocity and 50 percent of the peak E velocity on the ascending limb (acceleration half-time) and the descending limb (deceleration half-time) of early diastolic inflow.

Acceleration and deceleration half-times of the transmitral inflow velocity have been reported to be prolonged in patients with myocardial infarction (acceleration half-time >73 ms, deceleration half-time >100 ms) compared to normal subjects (acceleration half-time = 62 ± 18 ms, deceleration half-time = 73 ± 24 ms).

Indexes of Velocity and Acceleration

A second type of diastolic parameter that has been measured from the mitral valve Doppler tracings are indexes of velocity and acceleration (Fig. 12–2). For subjects in the age range of 21 to 40 years, peak velocities are 67 ± 9 cm/s for the E component, and 40 ± 7 cm/s for the A component, of left ventricular inflow. For subjects in the age range of 51 to 70 years, peak velocities are 50 ± 10 cm/s for the E component and 54 ± cm/s for the A component.[35] These findings seem to reflect the changes in left ventricular diastolic properties that occur with aging (i.e., increases in left ventricular wall thickness). The ratio of the peak A to peak E velocities (A/E ratio) has been used to describe the pattern of left ventricular diastolic filling. Values for the A/E ratio in normal adults have ranged from 0.44 ± 0.2 to 0.66 ±

Figure 12–2. Diagrammatic representation of the various Doppler parameters of left ventricular diastolic function and how they are measured. *Top*: Characteristic transmitral flow velocity recording demonstrating early diastolic (E) and late diastolic (A) velocities, as well as acceleration (AHT) and deceleration (DHT) half-times. The schematic in the upper corner illustrates the electrocardiogram (ECG), phonocardiogram (PHONO) and left ventricular isovolumic relaxation time interval (IVRT) from aortic valve closure (AC) to mitral valve opening (MO). MC = mitral valve closure. *Middle*: Representation of the method used to trace the area under E velocity (E area) and the area under A velocity (A area). The area under the entire mitral diastolic velocity curve is the flow velocity integral (FVI). Acc = acceleration, Dec = deceleration. *Bottom*: The $\frac{1}{3}$ filling fraction (FF) corresponds to the area of the FVI encompassed by $\frac{1}{3}$ diastole (DIAS) divided by the total FVI.

0.2.[12,28,30] The deceleration of early diastolic flow can be measured as the slope of a straight line drawn between the peak E velocity and the point where peak E decreases to peak E/2 on the descending limb of the early diastolic inflow. In normal adults, values for the deceleration have ranged from 355 ± 67 cm/s^2 to 399 ± 110 cm/s^2.[28,30]

Markedly different flow velocity patterns can be seen in patients with impaired left ventricular relaxation.[10] One pattern consists of one or more of the following findings: a prolonged left ventricular isovolumic relaxation time, a decreased peak early mitral flow velocity but normal or increased mitral flow velocity at atrial contraction, an increased A/E ratio, and a prolonged mitral deceleration time (Figs. 12–3 and 12–4). This pattern, most frequently seen in patients with coronary artery disease who have normal or only slightly increased left atrial pressure, appears to occur when there is impaired left ventricular relaxation. Assuming that left atrial pressure at the time of mitral valve opening remains constant, a slower rate (reduced slope) of fall of left ventricular isovolumic pressure would result in a later mitral valve opening, longer interval from aortic closure to mitral valve opening (isovolumic relaxation time), reduced early diastolic transmitral pressure gradient, and a resultant decrease in peak early flow velocity.

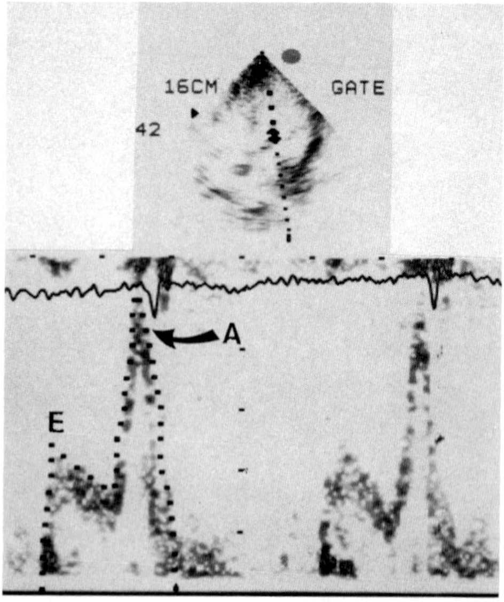

Figure 12–3. Transmitral flow in a patient with a previous myocardial infarction. Left ventricular filling is altered as demonstrated by the reduced early peak flow velocity (E), relatively greater atrial (A) contribution, and an increased A/E velocity ratio. (Scale marks = 20 cm/s)

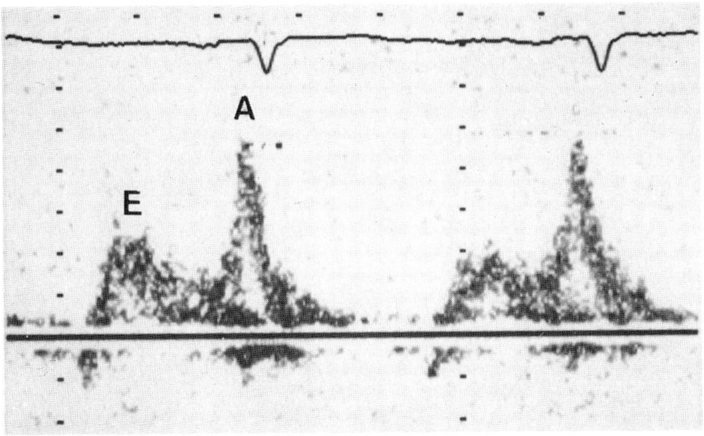

Figure 12–4. Transmitral flow in a patient with left ventricular hypertrophy and dilated globally hypokinetic ventricle. There is decreased peak early mitral flow velocity (E), increased velocity at atrial contraction (A), an increased A/E ratio, and a prolonged mitral deceleration time. (Scale marks = 20 cm/s)

With less filling in early diastole, the percent of left ventricular filling with atrial contraction would likely be increased as a compensatory mechanism, perhaps aided by atrial hypertrophy or enhanced atrial systolic function. The long mitral deceleration time frequently seen in these patients may reflect a prolonged fall in left ventricular pressure associated with the impaired relaxation and the low early diastolic ventricular filling rates. This mitral flow velocity pattern is also seen in some patients with dilated cardiomyopathy who have normal or slightly increased pulmonary wedge pressure.[10]

A second pattern is characterized by one or more of the following findings: a short left ventricular isovolumic relaxation time, a normal or increased peak mitral flow velocity in early diastole, a normal or decreased mitral velocity at atrial contraction, and a short mitral deceleration time (Fig. 12–5). This pattern is seen in patients who are more symptomatic, and it appears to indicate the presence of increased filling pressures. The patients with coronary artery disease and dilated cardiomyopathy who have this pattern also have impaired left ventricular relaxation. However, the normal or short left ventricular isovolumic relaxation time and normal or increased peak mitral flow velocity in early diastole in these patients suggests that an elevated left atrial pressure has normalized or increased the early diastolic transmitral pressure gradient and masked the expected effect of the relaxation abnormality on this gradient and the

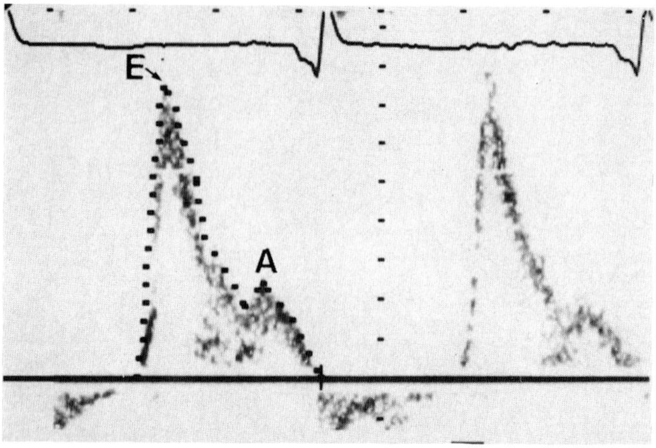

Figure 12 – 5. Mitral flow velocity in a patient with coronary artery disease. The flow velocity in early diastole (E) is much larger than flow velocity at atrial contraction (A). There is shortening of the deceleration time, and an increase in the ratio of peak early velocity to that at atrial contraction. At cardiac catheterization the left ventricular end-diastolic pressure was elevated, at 30 mmHg. (Scale marks = 20 cm/s)

Doppler variables. Most patients with this pattern have left atrial enlargement and a decrease in mitral flow velocity at atrial contraction. This decrease in velocity may be related to systolic atrial dysfunction, perhaps as a result of a long-standing increase in atrial afterload from an elevated left ventricular pressure or increased viscous forces[36] or of an elevated left ventricular pressure present at the time of atrial contraction.

Some or all of the above abnormal flow velocity patterns have been reported in patients with coronary artery disease, patients with hypertension, and patients with hypertrophic and dilated cardiomyopathy. Kitabatake and co-workers[28] found that the peak E velocity and deceleration were significantly reduced in patients with hypertension, hypertrophic cardiomyopathy, and myocardial infarction. They concluded that early diastolic filling was impaired in all three disease states and was accompanied by a compensatory increase in filling during atrial contraction in patients with hypertension and myocardial infarction. In patients with hypertrophic cardiomyopathy, the compensatory mechanism seemed to be a prolongation of rapid filling rather than an increased filling during atrial contraction. Takenaka et al[30] reported different Doppler patterns of left ventricular diastolic filling in different subgroups of patients with hypertrophic cardiomyopathy. In patients with hypertrophic cardiomyopathy and systolic anterior motion of the mitral valve, no significant differences were observed in peak E velocity, peak A velocity, A/E velocity ratio, or deceleration, compared to normal subjects. Patients with hypertrophic cardiomyopathy and no systolic anterior motion of the mitral valve, however, had decreased peak E velocity, increased A/E velocity ratio, and reduced deceleration of early diastolic flow compared to normal subjects. Mitral regurgitation was detected in all patients with systolic anterior motion of the mitral valve and in only 33 percent of patients without systolic anterior motion of the mitral valve. The authors postulated that increased left ventricular early diastolic filling caused by mitral regurgitation or a less extensive myopathic process, reported previously to occur in patients with systolic anterior motion, accounted for the differences in left ventricular diastolic filling observed in subgroups of patients with hypertrophic cardiomyopathy. In a similar study, Takenaka and co-workers[31] compared mitral valve Doppler recordings from patients with dilated cardiomyopathy, with and without mitral regurgitation, to recordings from normal subjects. Cardiomyopathy patients without mitral regurgitation had a reduced peak E velocity and an increased A/E velocity ratio compared to normal subjects. Cardiomyopathy patients with mitral regurgitation had normal peak E and peak A velocities and normal A/E velocity ratios, but shortened deceleration half-times (Fig. 12–6). These findings suggest that mitral regurgitation can mask filling abnormalities on the mitral valve Doppler examination in patients with dilated cardiomyopathy.

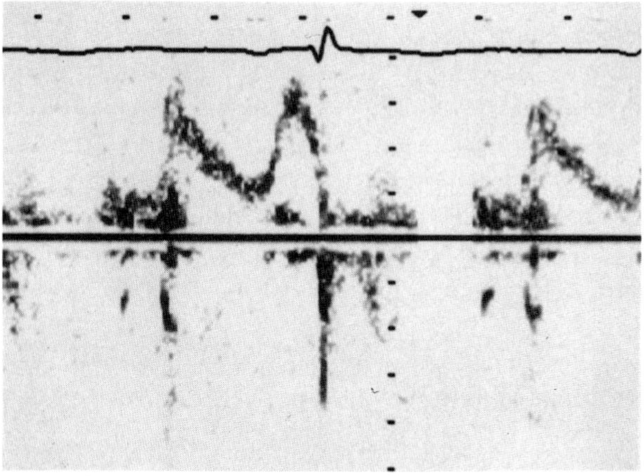

Figure 12 – 6. Mitral flow velocity in a patient with dilated cardiomyopathy and mitral regurgitation. The "normalization" of the flow velocity pattern is thought to result from a greater transmitral pressure gradient due to increased atrial blood volume during ventricular systole. (Scale marks = 20 cm/s)

Doppler Area Fractions

A third type of diastolic parameters that have been used to describe the patterns of left ventricular filling are the Doppler area fractions or filling fractions[29] (Fig. 12–2). The Doppler area fractions describe the percentage of the mitral valve Doppler envelope that is present in the various phases of diastole. Because the mitral valve cross-sectional area changes throughout diastole, calculation of the absolute volumetric flow is done by taking the product of the flow velocity integral (the integrated area under the Doppler curve) and the mitral valve cross-sectional area. Approximate values for the fraction of filling of the left ventricle in the different phases of diastole are obtained by measuring several areas under the Doppler curve and dividing these areas by the total area under the Doppler curve, or the total flow velocity integral. Using this method, the area or filling fractions in the first one-third of diastole during early diastolic inflow (E area fraction) and atrial contraction (A area fraction) can be calculated. Normal values: for E area/total area, 0.62 ± 0.07; for A area/total area, 0.26 ± 0.07; and for one-third diastole/total area, 0.53 ± 0.06.

Mitral valve Doppler area fractions have been used to detect abnormalities in left ventricular filling in a variety of disease states.[27,29,33,37–39] The Doppler patterns of left ventricular diastolic filling have been evaluated in a group of patients with coronary artery disease and normal global systolic function, and compared with the corresponding patterns of a group of age-matched normal adults.[33] The coronary artery disease patients had a decreased percentage of the mitral valve Doppler area occurring during rapid filling and an increased percentage of the Doppler area occurring in late diastole, suggesting that such patients have impaired left ventricular early diastolic filling. These diastolic filling abnormalities were unimproved 24 h after successful coronary angioplasty. Similar findings have been reported for treated hypertensive patients.[7] Furthermore, it appears that abnormalities of late left ventricular filling may be independent of left ventricular hypertrophy and may persist despite effective blood pressure control.[7]

Factors Affecting Mitral Flow Velocity Measurements

A number of factors may affect Doppler transmitral flow velocity measurements. The Doppler time intervals and peak velocities vary with cardiac cycle lengths. Peak velocities also vary with age and ventricular preload. The peak E and A velocity tend to decrease and to increase, respectively, with aging, and the A/E velocity ratio accordingly shows a significant increase with aging[40] (Fig. 12–7). Also, the peak A velocity and the A/E veloc-

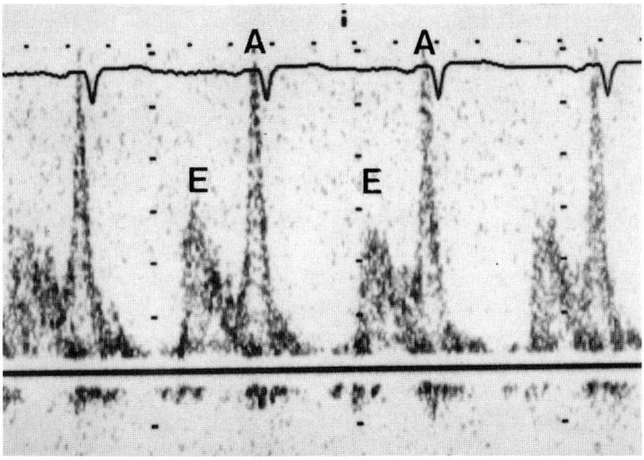

Figure 12–7. Mitral flow velocity in a normal 80-year-old subject. The peak A velocity and the A/E velocity ratio are increased. (Scale marks = 20 cm/s)

ity ratio tend to be increased in the fetus in utero and in the first few days after birth.[41] The position of the sample volume can alter the mitral valve Doppler tracing. Gardin and colleagues[42] compared Doppler tracings obtained from the left atrium just proximal to the mitral valve with Doppler tracings obtained at the tips of the mitral valve leaflets. They found that the peak E velocity was 25 percent lower, and the peak A velocity 22 percent lower, in the tracing obtained from the left atrial side. The A/E velocity ratio was the same at both sites. In addition, the mitral valve Doppler indexes vary with the phases of respiration; complexes should be measured at end-expiration to eliminate these variations.

During tachycardia, the early and late diastolic portions of the mitral flow curve progressively fuse and may become indistinguishable. When this occurs it is very difficult, if not impossible, to use the Doppler flow curve to evaluate left ventricular function. Finally, early diastolic left ventricular filling is affected not only by left ventricular relaxation properties but also by the left atrial pressure at the onset of left ventricular filling.[43] Factors that increase left atrial pressure will alter left ventricular diastolic filling patterns. For example, mitral regurgitation increases left atrial pressure and causes an increase in mitral valve flow velocity, left ventricular filling rate, and mitral volumetric flow.

Several investigators have reported alterations in mitral flow velocity curves during constrictive pericarditis and cardiac tamponade.[44–47] In constrictive pericarditis, the peak early diastolic flow velocity and the rate of early diastolic deceleration are markedly increased when compared to normal. Furthermore, in cardiac tamponade, the mitral peak flow velocities in both early and late diastole are reduced during inspiration, a reflection of decreased filling of the left side of the heart during inspiration. Marked variations in Doppler transvalvular flow velocity integrals of more than 30 to 40 percent during respiration should aid in the diagnosis of cardiac tamponade.

Figure 12–8 summarizes in diagrammatic form the various patterns of left ventricular filling as reflected by transmitral flow.

DOPPLER EVALUATION OF RIGHT VENTRICULAR DIASTOLIC FUNCTION

Little information currently is available on the use of Doppler echocardiography to assess right ventricular diastolic function. Using the tricuspid valve inflow Doppler tracing, peak velocities during early and late diastolic filling, peak filling rates, and filling fractions of the right ventricle can be calculated.

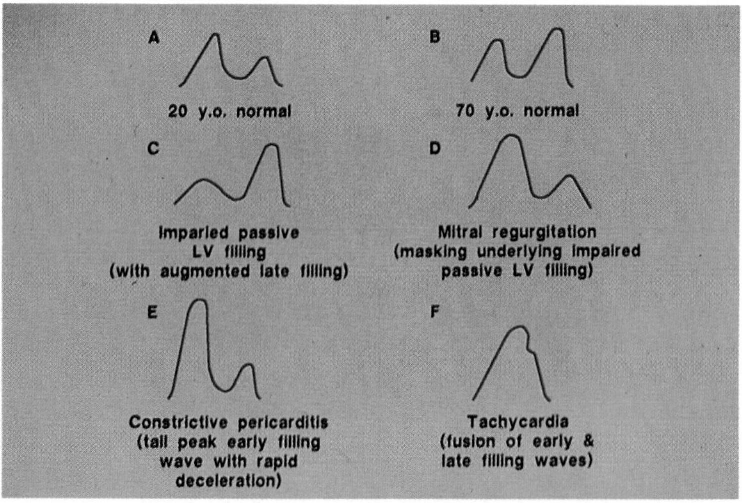

Figure 12–8. Diagrams of left diastolic filling as reflected by transmitral flow velocity recordings in younger (A) and older (B) normal subjects and in patients with decreased left ventricular compliance (C), mitral regurgitation (D), constrictive pericarditis (E), and sinus tachycardia (F).

Impaired diastolic filling of the right ventricle compensated by enhanced right atrial contraction has been reported in patients with coronary heart disease and myocardial infarction.[12] Our laboratory has also recorded increased A/E velocity ratios of transtricuspid inflow velocities in patients with pulmonary hypertension and right ventricular hypertrophy, again indicating reduced right ventricular compliance.

REFERENCES

1. Grossman W, McLaurin L: Diastolic properties of the left ventricle. *Ann Intern Med* 84:316, 1976.
2. Langer G: Ionic movement and the control of contraction, in Langer GA, Brady AJ (eds): *The Mammalian Myocardium*. New York, Wiley, 1974.
3. Gaasch W, Levine H, Quinones A, et al: Left ventricular compliance: Mechanisms and clinical implications. *Am J Cardiol* 38:645, 1976.
4. Sandor G, Olley P: Determination of left ventricular diastolic chamber stiffness and myocardial stiffness in patients with congenital heart disease. *Circulation* 38:935, 1976.
5. Hess O, Ritter M, Scheider J, et al: Diastolic function in aortic valve disease: Techniques of evaluation and pre-/postoperative changes. *Herz* 9:288, 1984.
6. Louie E, Rich S, Brundage B: Doppler echocardiographic assessment of impaired left ventricular filling in patients with right ventricular pressure overload due to primary pulmonary hypertension. *J Am Coll Cardiol* 8:1298, 1986.
7. Phillips R, Coplan N, Krakoff L, et al: Doppler echocardiographic analysis of left ventricular filling in treated hypertensive patients. *J Am Coll Cardiol* 9:317, 1987.
8. Sasson Z, Hatle L, Appleton C, et al: Intraventricular flow during isovolumic relaxation: Description and characterization by Doppler echocardiography. *J Am Coll Cardiol* 10:539, 1987.
9. Visner M, Arentzen C, Parrish D, et al: Effects of global ischemia on the diastolic properties of the left ventricle in the conscious dog. *Circulation* 71:619, 1985.
10. Appleton C, Hatle L, Popp R: Relation of transmitral flow velocity patterns to left ventricular diastolic function: New insights from a combined hemodynamic and Doppler echocardiographic study. *J Am Coll Cardiol* 12:426, 1988.
11. Iliceto S, Amico A, Marangelli V, et al: Doppler echocardiographic evaluation of the effect of atrial pacing–induced ischemia on left ventricular filling in patients with coronary artery disease. *J Am Coll Cardiol* 11:953, 1988.
12. Fujii J, Yazaki Y, Sawada H, et al: Noninvasive assessment of left and right ventricular filling in myocardial infarction with a two-dimensional Doppler echocardiographic method. *J Am Coll Cardiol* 5:1155, 1985.
13. Hammermeister K, Warbasse J: The rate of change of left ventricular volume in man II. Diastolic events in health and disease. *Circulation* 49:739, 1974.

14. Fioretti P, Brower R, Meester G, et al: Interaction of left ventricular relaxation and filling during early diastole in human subjects. *Am J Cardiol* 46:197, 1980.
15. Sasayama S, Nonogi H, Miyazaki S: Changes in diastolic properties of the regional myocardium during pacing-induced ischemia in human subjects. *J Am Coll Cardiol* 5:599, 1985.
16. Benow R, Bacharach S, Green M, et al: Impaired left ventricular diastolic filling in patients with coronary artery disease: Assessment with radionuclide angiography. *Circulation* 64:315, 1981.
17. Mancini G, Slutsky R, Norris S, et al: Radionuclide analysis of peak filling rate, filling fraction, and time to peak filling rate. *Am J Cardiol* 51:43, 1983.
18. Gewirtz H, Ohley W, Walsh J: Ischemia-induced impairment of left ventricular relaxation: Relation to reduced diastolic filling rates of the left ventricle. *Am Heart J* 105:72, 1983.
19. Goldberg S, Feldman L, Reinecke C, et al: Echocardiographic determination of contraction and relaxation measurements of the left ventricular wall in normal subjects and patients with muscular dystrophy. *Circulation* 62:1061, 1980.
20. Fujii J, Watanabe H, Koyama S, et al: Echocardiographic study on diastolic posterior wall movement and left ventricular filling by disease category. *Am Heart J* 98:144, 1979.
21. Upton M, Gibson D: The study of left ventricular function from digitized echocardiograms. *Prog Cardiovasc Dis* 20:359, 1978.
22. Ferro G, Giunta A, Maione S, et al: Diastolic time intervals during dynamic exercise: Echocardiographic assessment. *J Cardiovasc Ultra* 1:33, 1982.
23. Sanderson J, Traill T, Sutton M, et al: Left ventricular relaxation and filling in hypertrophic cardiomyopathy, an echocardiographic study. *Br Heart J* 40:596, 1978.
24. Magorien D, Shaffer P, Bush C, et al: Assessment of left ventricular pressure volume relations using gated radionuclide angiography, echocardiography, and micromanometer pressure recordings. *Circulation* 67:844, 1983.
25. Spirito P, Maron B, Bonow R: Noninvasive assessment of left ventricular diastolic function: Comparative analysis of Doppler echocardiographic and radionuclide angiographic techniques. *J Am Coll Cardiol* 7:518, 1986.
26. Rokey R, Kuo L, Zoghbi W, et al: Determination of parameters of left ventricular diastolic filling with pulsed Doppler echocardiography: Comparison with cineangiography. *Circulation* 71:543, 1985.
27. Friedman B, Drinkovic N, Miles H, et al: Assessment of left ventricular diastolic function: Comparison of Doppler echocardiography and gated blood pool scintigraphy. *J Am Coll Cardiol* 8:1348, 1986.
28. Kitabatake A, Inoue M, Asao M, et al: Transmitral blood flow reflecting diastolic behavior of the left ventricle in health and disease: A study by pulsed Doppler technique. *Jpn Circ J* 46:92, 1982.
29. Snider A, Gidding S, Rocchini A, et al: Doppler evaluation of left ventricular diastolic filling in children with systemic hypertension. *Am J Cardiol* 56:921, 1985.

30. Takenaka K, Dabestani A, Gardin J, et al: Left ventricular filling in hypertrophic cardiomyopathy: A pulsed Doppler echocardiographic study. J *Am Coll Cardiol* 7:1263, 1986.

31. Takenaka K, Dabestani A, Gardin J, et al: Pulsed Doppler echocardiographic study of left ventricular filling in dilated cardiomyopathy. *Am* J *Cardiol* 58:143, 1986.

32. Iwase M, Sotobata I, Takagi S, et al: Effects of diltiazem on left ventricular diastolic behavior in patients with hypertrophic cardiomyopathy: Evaluation with exercise pulsed Doppler echocardiography. J *Am Coll Cardiol* 9:1099, 1987.

33. Wind B, Snider R, Buda A, et al: Pulsed Doppler assessment of left ventricular diastolic filling in coronary artery disease before and immediately after coronary angioplasty. *Am* J *Cardiol* 59:1041, 1987.

34. Spirito P, Maron B, Bellotti P, et al: Noninvasive assessment of left ventricular diastolic function: Comparative analysis of pulsed Doppler ultrasound and digitized M-mode echocardiography. *Am* J *Cardiol* 58:837, 1986.

35. Gardin J, Dabestani A, Rohan M, et al: Noninvasive studies of ventricular filling with Doppler echocardiography: Effects of aging on early and late transmitral flow. J *Am Coll Cardiol* 3:613, 1984.

36. Van de Werf R, Boel A, Geboers J, et al: Diastolic properties of the left ventricle in normal adults and in patients with third heart sounds. *Circulation* 69:1070, 1984.

37. Pearson A, Schiff, M, Mrosek D, et al: Left ventricular diastolic function in weight lifters. *Am* J *Cardiol* 58:1254, 1986.

38. Gidding S, Snider A, Rocchini A, et al: Left ventricular diastolic filling in children with hypertrophic cardiomyopathy: Assessment with pulsed Doppler echocardiography. J *Am Coll Cardiol* 8:310, 1986.

39. Shaffer E, Snider A, Rocchini A, et al: Diastolic filling in left ventricular outflow obstruction pre and post balloon angioplasty (abstr). J *Am Coll Cardiol* 9(Suppl A):130A, 1987.

40. Mujatake K, Okamoto M, Kinoshita N, et al: Augmentation of atrial contribution to left ventricular inflow with aging as assessed by intracardiac Doppler flowmetry. *Am* J *Cardiol* 53:586, 1984.

41. Reed K, Sahn D, Scagnelli S, et al: Doppler echocardiographic studies of diastolic function in the human fetal heart: Changes during gestation. J *Am Coll Cardiol* 8:391, 1986.

42. Gardin J, Dabestani A, Takenaka K, et al: Effect of imaging view and sample volume location on evaluation of mitral flow velocity by pulsed Doppler echocardiography. *Am* J *Cardiol* 57:1335, 1986.

43. Ishida Y, Meisner J, Tsujioka K, et al: Left ventricular filling dynamics: Influence of left ventricular relaxation and left atrial pressure. *Circulation* 74:187, 1986.

44. King S, Pandian N, Gardin J: Doppler echocardiographic findings in pericardial tamponade and constriction. *Echocardiography* 5:361, 1988.

45. Dabestani A, Takenaka K, Allen B, et al: Effects of spontaneous respiration on diastolic left ventricular filling assessed by pulsed Doppler echocardiography. *Am J Cardiol* 61:1356, 1988.
46. Pandian N, Wang S, McInerney K, et al: Doppler echocardiography in cardiac tamponade. Abnormalities in tricuspid and mitral flow response to respiration in experimental and clinical tamponade. *J Am Coll Cardiol* 5:485, 1985.
47. Appleton C, Hatle L, Popp R: Central venous flow velocity patterns can differentiate constrictive pericarditis from restrictive cardiomyopathy (abstr). *J Am Coll Cardiol* 9(suppl A):119A, 1987.

CHAPTER 13

Assessment of Intracardiac and Pulmonary Artery Pressures

In the past, assessment of pressures within the heart and great vessels could only be performed by means of cardiac catheterization. Although cardiac catheterization provides accurate and clinically useful information, it is an expensive technique and involves some risk to the patient. Therefore, a reliable noninvasive method of estimating intracardiac and pulmonary artery pressures would be most desirable, particularly in the assessment of valvular heart disease, congenital abnormalities, and left ventricular dysfunction.

Doppler echocardiography provides a noninvasive technique by which blood flow in cardiac chambers and vessels can be characterized, and the timing and direction of flow determined. Transvalvular pressure gradients can be quantified noninvasively by Doppler echocardiography. Combined two-dimensional (2D) imaging and Doppler investigation allow quantification of volume flow rates. Intracardiac pressures and cardiac function can be evaluated by combining such measurements with observations from the physical examination.

Recently, several approaches have been taken to obtain quantitative estimates of intracardiac and pulmonary artery pressures by Doppler echocardiography. Calculations of certain intracardiac pressures have been performed in patients with valvular regurgitation and stenosis by virtue of the ability to estimate the pressure drop across valves using the modified Bernoulli equation (discussed in Chap 2):

$$\Delta P = 4V^2$$

The assessment of Doppler velocity time intervals has also offered a reliable and clinically useful means for indirect evaluation of pulmonary artery pressures.

The objectives of this chapter will be to describe the various Doppler techniques used in estimating right ventricular, pulmonary artery, left ventricular, and left atrial pressures, and to enumerate their advantages and limitations. Because estimation of pulmonary artery pressure is most useful and least prone to error, it is discussed first.

RIGHT HEART PRESSURES

Because pulmonary artery and right ventricular systolic pressures are nearly equal in the absence of disease involving the right ventricular outflow tract, pulmonic valve, or supravalvular region, pulmonary artery systolic pressure is commonly estimated by techniques that measure right ventricular systolic pressure. The most common method involves using tricuspid regurgitation to calculate the right ventricular–to–right atrial pressure gradient. Pulmonary artery systolic pressure can also be calculated directly by noting the timing of the peak pulmonary artery pressure. Both approaches are clinically useful.

Pulmonary Artery Systolic Pressure from Tricuspid Regurgitation

Doppler echocardiographic evidence of tricuspid regurgitation is common in patients with pulmonary hypertension.[1–4] The Doppler signals characteristic of tricuspid regurgitation can be recorded by placing the transducer at the cardiac apex and obtaining a four-chamber view or from a parasternal short axis view at the level of the tricuspid valve. The ultrasound beam is directed through the tricuspid valve and aligned parallel to the high-velocity jet between the right ventricle and the right atrium. Careful adjustment of the transducer location and the ultrasound beam is essential to ensure a small Doppler angle and accurate quantification of actual velocity. Color flow imaging (CFI) is useful in detecting tricuspid regurgitation, estimating the severity of regurgitation, and aligning the ultrasound beam parallel to the jet. Using CW Doppler echocardiography, the flow velocity spectral recording in the setting of tricuspid regurgitation and pulmonary hypertension demonstrates retrograde flow of high velocity into the right atrium during systole (Fig. 13–1). Accordingly, the pressure drop, or gradient, between the right ventricle and right atrium during systole can be estimated using the maximal retrograde flow velocity and the modified Bernoulli equation. Thus, the maximal velocity of the regurgitant jet (V) is measured, and is inserted into the Bernoulli equation:

$$\Delta P = 4V^2$$

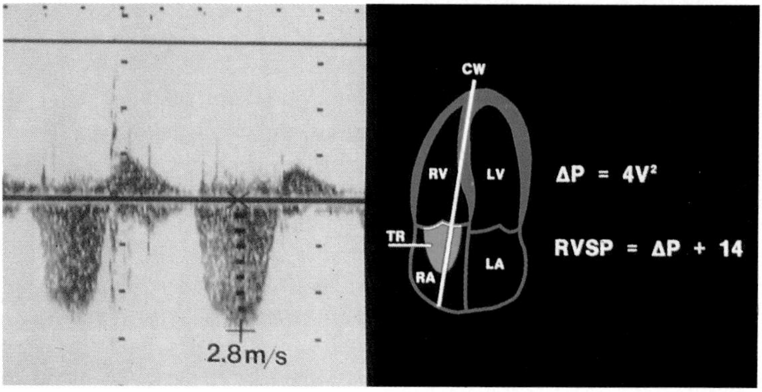

Figure 13–1. Schema for the method of estimating right ventricular systolic pressure (RVSP) from tricuspid regurgitation (TR). The CW Doppler ultrasound beam is directed across the tricuspid valve as indicated by the cursor. The transtricuspid gradient (ΔP, in mmHg) is calculated by use of the modified Bernoulli equation, $\Delta P = 4V^2$, where V represents the maximum velocity of the regurgitant jet in meters per second (left). The RVSP is then estimated by adding the estimated right atrial pressure, or 14 mmHg ($RVSP = \Delta P + 14$).

Once the transvalvular gradient (ΔP) is determined, adding the estimated or measured right atrial pressure during systole to the Doppler-derived pressure gradient allows an estimation of right ventricular systolic pressure by the equation (Fig. 13–1):

$$RVSP = \Delta P + RAP$$

where ΔP is the transtricuspid gradient, RAP is the right atrial pressure, and RVSP is the right ventricular systolic pressure. In the absence of right ventricular outflow or pulmonary artery obstruction, right ventricular systolic pressure should be equivalent to pulmonary artery systolic pressure; a mechanism thereby exists to evaluate for the presence of pulmonary hypertension (Figs. 13–2 and 13–3). Using this technique, there has been excellent correlation between Doppler and invasive measurements of right ventricular and pulmonary artery systolic pressures.[1–4]

Several methods exist for determining right atrial pressure. If a central venous catheter is present, right atrial pressure can be measured directly. An estimation of right atrial pressure can be made by inspecting the jugular venous pulse. The height of the jugular venous pulse above the sternal angle (second intercostal space) plus 5 cm, which is the average distance from the right atrium to the sternal angle, provides an estimated right atrial pressure in centimeters of blood. Dividing by 1.3 converts this value

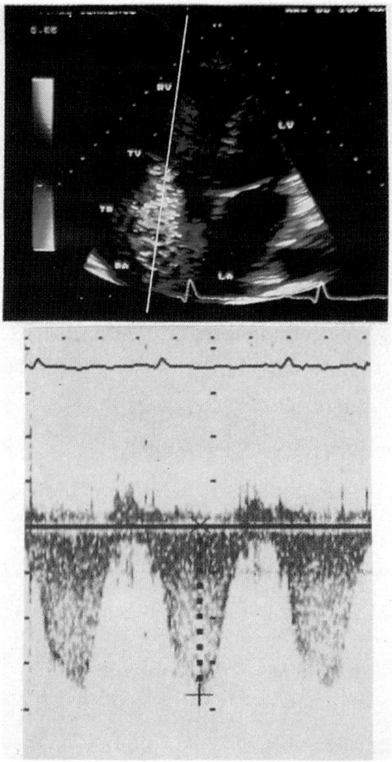

Figure 13–2. Tricuspid regurgitation in a patient with pulmonary hypertension, apical four-chamber view. *Top*: Color flow image during systole displaying severe tricuspid regurgitation (TR) with image-guided continuous wave Doppler beam aligned parallel to flow (straight solid line). LA = left atrium, LV = left ventricle, RA = right atrium, RV = right ventricle, TV = Tricuspid valve. *Bottom*: Spectral recording of tricuspid regurgitation jet showing a velocity of 3.5 m/s. The calculated pressure gradient between right ventricle and right atrium ($\Delta P = 4V^2$) is 49 mmHg. Adding a right atrial pressure of 14 mmHg to the transtricuspid gradient results in a right ventricular systolic pressure of 63 mmHg. (Scale marks = 1 m/s)

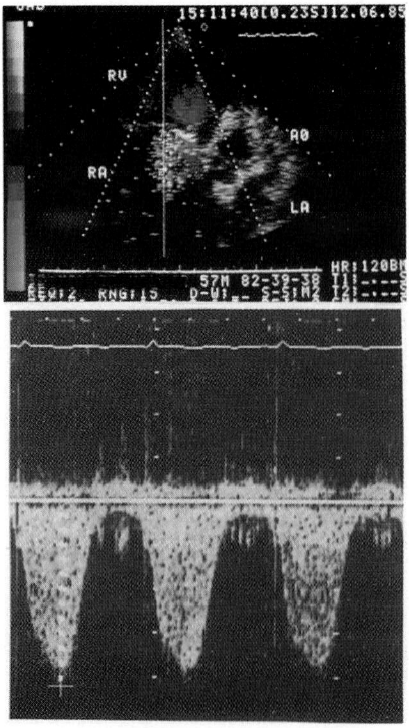

Figure 13–3. Tricuspid regurgitation in a patient with severe pulmonary hypertension, parasternal short axis view. *Top*: The blue jet in the right atrium (RA) is due to tricuspid regurgitation. Color Doppler imaging can be used to align the continuous wave Doppler beam (straight solid line) parallel to the regurgitant jet. AO = aorta, LA = left atrium, RV = right ventricle. *Bottom*: Spectral recording of peak regurgitant velocity of 4 m/s, and a calculated transtricuspid gradient of 64 mmHg. The estimated right ventricular systolic pressure is 78 mmHg. (Scale marks = 1 m/s)

to millimeters of mercury. Since the clinical estimation of right atrial pressure is often difficult and most patients do not have central venous catheters, an alternate method for estimation of right ventricular systolic pressure between the right atrium and right ventricle has been developed. Right atrial pressure is generally of substantially lesser magnitude than the gradient between the right atrium and right ventricle. Therefore, the absolute deviation estimated from true right atrial pressure is generally a small value, and its effect on right ventricular pressure estimation is diluted. Because of this, some investigators have found that adding 14 mmHg to the transtricuspid gradient allows accurate estimation of right ventricular systolic pressure[2,3]:

$$RVSP = \Delta P + 14$$

Berger et al[1] simplified this approach by regressing the right ventricular–to–right atrial gradient derived by Doppler study against the pulmonary artery systolic pressure measured at catheterization. Berger's regression equation allows direct calculation of pulmonary artery systolic pressure (PASP) without determination or estimation of right atrial pressure:

$$PASP = 4.9V^2 - .09 \text{ mmHg}$$

Pulmonary Artery Systolic Pressure from Ventricular Septal Defect

In patients with ventricular septal defect, right ventricular systolic pressure can be estimated using a CW Doppler recording of the peak velocity (V) across the septum. Peak systolic pressure gradient between the right and left ventricles (ΔP) is calculated using the Bernoulli equation (Figs. 13–4 and 13–5):

$$\Delta P = 4V^2$$

In the absence of aortic stenosis, left ventricular systolic pressure equals systolic blood pressure (brachial artery sphygmomanometer pressure). Thus, subtracting the systolic gradient between right and left ventricles (ΔP) from the systolic blood pressure (SBP), one obtains the right ventricular systolic pressure (RVSP):

$$RVSP = SBP - \Delta P$$

If right ventricular outflow obstruction is also absent, right ventricular systolic pressure is nearly equal to pulmonary artery systolic pressure. Thus, this approach allows detection of pulmonary hypertension in patients with

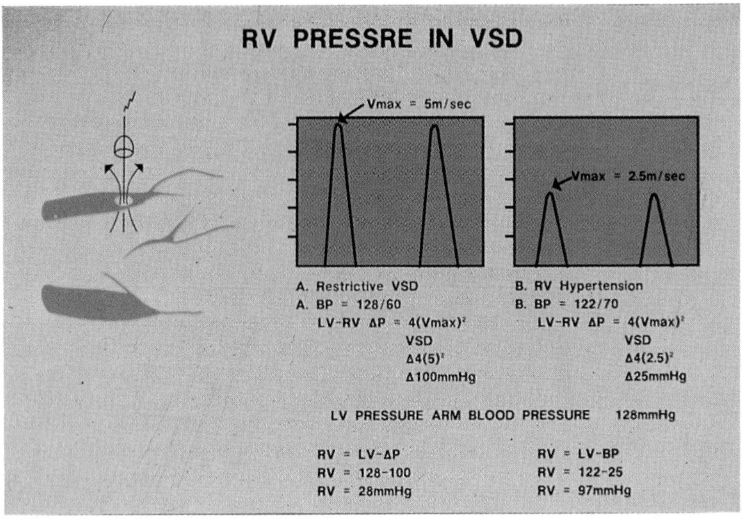

Figure 13–4. Schematic outline of the use of the ventricular septal defect (VSD) jet for calculation of right ventricular (RV) pressures. Two examples are given, one of a small restrictive VSD with normal RV pressures, and the other of a larger VSD with RV hypertension. In either case, continuous wave Doppler investigation is used to measure the velocity of the jet, which is usually oriented anteriorly in perimembranous septal defects. In the left panel, the maximum velocity is 5 m/s, from which a left ventricular–right ventricular pressure gradient of 100 mmHg can be calculated. The difference between the systolic blood pressure (BP) (determined by blood pressure cuff) and this gradient is the RV pressure (in this example, 28 mmHg). In the case of RV hypertension (right panel), a lower-velocity jet of 2.5 m/s is seen, allowing calculation of a pressure gradient between the left and right ventricles of 25 mmHg and calculation of a RV systolic pressure of 97 mmHg.

ventricular septal defect and absence of left or right ventricular outflow tract obstruction. Using this approach, several investigators have reported excellent correlations between Doppler- and catheterization-determined right ventricular systolic pressures ($r = 0.93$–95).[5,6]

Technically, the examination requires a CW Doppler system capable of recording high velocities, and parallel alignment of velocity vectors through the septal defect and the ultrasound beam. Although multiple ultrasound windows are used to ensure the smallest possible Doppler angle, the left parasternal and subcostal windows provide the highest Doppler frequency shifts. In general, the jet through perimembranous ventricular septal defects is directed anteriorly and to the right; therefore the transducer is placed at the mid-left sternal border and aimed posteri-

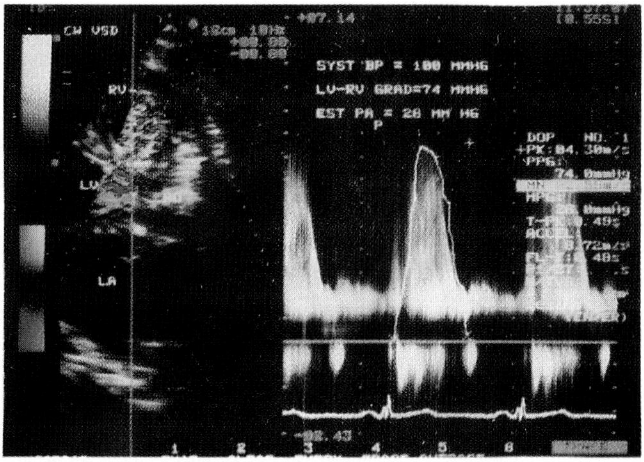

Figure 13–5. Continuous wave Doppler estimation of pulmonary artery pressure from a patient with a ventricular septal defect, parasternal long axis view. Color flow imaging is used to direct the continuous wave Doppler signal through the eccentric ventricular septal defect jet (straight solid line). The peak gradient is estimated to be 74 mmHg, and the systolic blood pressure 100 mmHg; the peak systolic pulmonary artery pressure is therefore 26 mmHg (normal). AO = aorta, LA = left atrium, LV = left ventricle, RV = right ventricle.

orly, leftward, and inferiorly.[5] Muscular ventricular septal defects are usually more easily interrogated from a subcostal or apical window. Direct visualization of the jet with 2D CFI can be helpful to align the ultrasound beam parallel to the jet or to measure the Doppler angle (Fig. 13–5).

Pulmonary Artery Mean and Diastolic Pressure from Pulmonic Regurgitation

The incidence of pulmonary regurgitation is greater in patients with pulmonary hypertension than in patients without pulmonary hypertension.[7] Quantification of diastolic velocities in patients with pulmonary regurgitation is helpful in calculating pulmonary artery mean and end-diastolic pressures. It should be remembered that the degrees of severity of pulmonary regurgitation, pulmonary hypertension, and right ventricular function all affect the end-diastolic pressure gradient across the pulmonic valve. In the presence of mild pulmonic regurgitation, normal right ventricular end-diastolic pressure, and low pulmonary artery diastolic pressure, pulmonic regurgitation Doppler velocities return to the baseline at end-diastole.[8,9] The low end-diastolic velocity indicates a low end-diastolic pulmonary artery–to–right ventricle pressure gradient. Unfortunately, as illustrated in Fig. 13–6, low end-diastolic velocities can also be detected in patients with severe pulmonic regurgitation and elevation of right ventricular end-diastolic pressure. In individuals with elevated pulmonary artery systolic and diastolic pressures and less-than-severe pulmonary regurgitation, the end-diastolic pulmonic regurgitation remains elevated (Fig. 13–7).

Despite these limitations, Masuyama and coworkers[10] showed that mean and end-diastolic pulmonary artery pressures can be calculated accurately using pulmonary regurgitant velocities. Using the Bernoulli equation and the peak pulmonary regurgitant velocity at end-diastole (V), they calculated the diastolic pressure gradient between the pulmonary artery and the right ventricle (ΔP):

$$\Delta P = 4V^2$$

Comparisons between catheterization and Doppler estimates were good $r = 0.94$; SEE = 3 mmHg).

Calculation of pulmonary artery diastolic pressure (PADP) is possible if right atrial diastolic pressure (RAP) is known or estimated (Fig. 13–8):

$$PADP = \Delta P + RAP$$

Velocity Time Intervals in Estimating Pulmonary Hypertension

In patients in whom tricuspid regurgitation and ventricular septal defect are absent, or in those with such pathology in whom confirmatory evi-

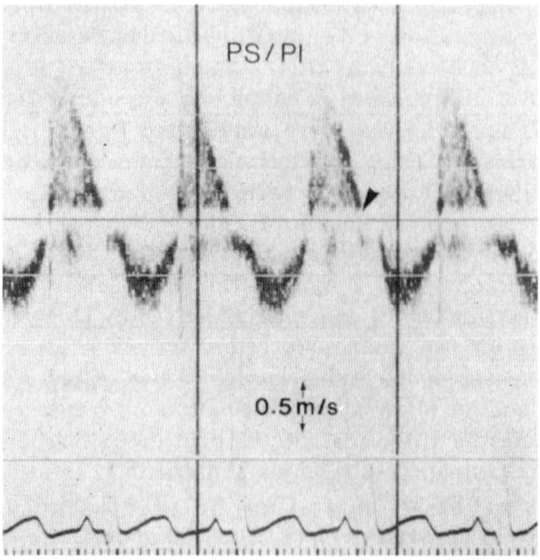

Figure 13–6. Continuous wave Doppler tracing from a patient with significant pulmonary insufficiency and elevated right ventricular end-diastolic pressure. The Doppler signal from the PI jet returns to baseline (black arrow) before the end of diastole because of equalization of right ventricular and pulmonary artery pressures in late diastole. PS = pulmonary stenosis.

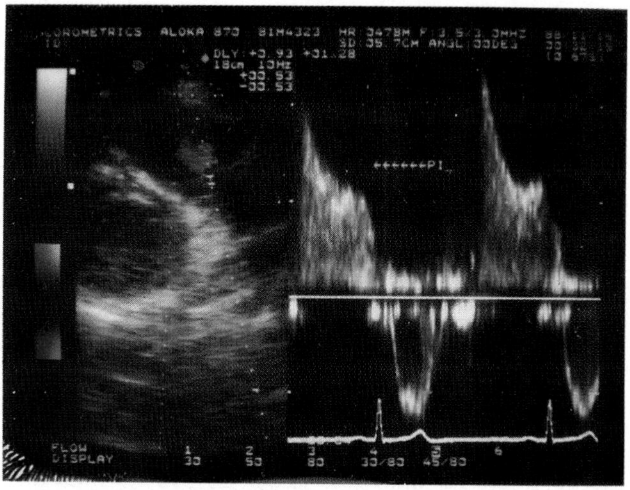

Figure 13–7. Pulmonary regurgitation in a patient with pulmonary hypertension, parasternal short axis view. *Left*: Color flow imaging displays mild pulmonic insufficiency (PI) as a red jet emanating from the pulmonic valve. *Right*: Pulsed Doppler recording demonstrating PI sustained throughout diastole.

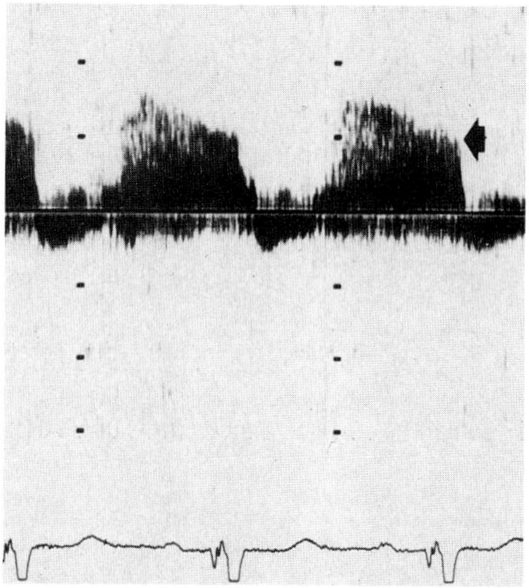

Figure 13–8. Pulmonary flow velocity profile of the pulmonary valve of a patient with pulmonary regurgitation. The end-diastolic velocity (arrow) measures 2 m/s, which by the Bernoulli equation estimates a 16 mmHg end-diastolic gradient. On the assumption that right ventricular end-diastolic pressure was equal to the right atrial mean pressure, estimated at 14 mmHg, the pulmonary artery diastolic pressure was estimated at 30 mmHg. The catheter-measured pulmonary artery diastolic pressure was 32 mmHg.

dence of pulmonary hypertension is required, Doppler pulmonary artery velocity estimates can be helpful. (See Chap.3, Fig. 3–13, for pulsed Doppler recording of pulmonary artery flow illustrating the Doppler velocity time intervals used in the assessment of pulmonary artery pressure.) Hatle et al[11] and Kitabatake and coworkers[12] have suggested that Doppler study tracings from the pulmonary valve orifice in patients in whom pulmonary outflow tract obstruction is absent can be used to identify patients with pulmonary hypertension. Kitabatake and associates[12] noted that acceleration time (the time from onset to peak pulmonary velocity) is shortened in patients with pulmonary hypertension. In their study, patients with mean pulmonary artery pressure < 20 mmHg had acceleration times of 137 ± 24 ms. Those with mean pulmonary artery pressure > 20 mmHg had acceleration times of 97 ± 20 ms. The ratio of acceleration time to right ventricular ejection time correlated well with the log of the mean pulmonary artery pressure ($AT/ET = 0.45 \pm 0.05$ in normal subjects and 0.30 ± 0.06 in patients with pulmonary hypertension). Other studies suggest the usefulness of acceleration time alone, or of acceleration time/ejection time.[13–15]

In patients with pulmonary hypertension, the flow velocity pattern is changed in either of two ways.[12] One pattern, resembling a triangle, is characterized by rapid acceleration of flow velocity—with earlier appearance of its sharp peak than is seen in patients with normal pulmonary artery pressure—followed by a rapid deceleration. In some patients, the deceleration curve has a concave form. Another pattern is represented by a rapid rise of the flow velocity to its peak level, followed by deceleration,

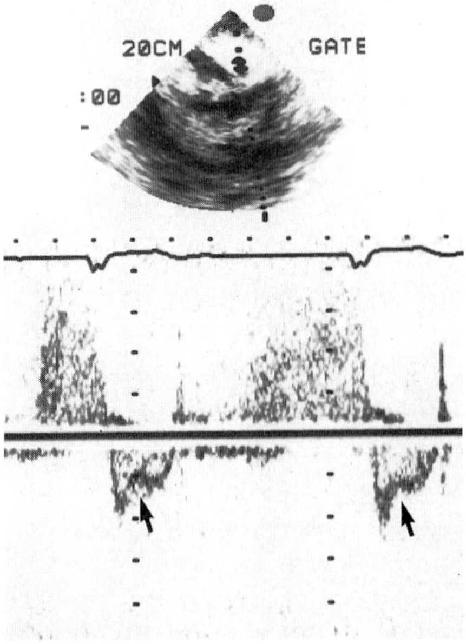

Figure 13–9. Pulsed Doppler recording at the level of the pulmonic valve demonstrating many of the features of pulmonary hypertension: (1) pulmonary regurgitation sustained throughout diastole, (2) early acceleration time (80 ms) and early systolic peak, and (3) midsystolic notching (arrows). (Scale marks = 20 cm/s)

and then another slow deceleration of flow velocity, producing a notch in midsystole (Fig. 13–9).

Isobe and coworkers[16] recently noted that the ratio of right ventricular preejection period (Q wave to onset of pulmonary artery flow) divided by acceleration time was the best predictor of pulmonary hypertension. Ratios >1.1 were found in 93 percent of his patients with pulmonary hypertension, whereas 97 percent of normal subjects had ratios of <1.1. Since factors other than mean pulmonary artery pressure (such as age, heart rate, right ventricular preload and function) can alter the Doppler time intervals, pulmonary artery pressure based on these measurements should be interpreted with caution.[17]

Table 13–1 summarizes the Doppler echocardiographic methods for estimating pulmonary artery pressure. The Doppler method using pulmonary closure to tricuspid opening, acceleration time, or ratio of acceleration time to right ventricular ejection time appears to have better utility in estimating pulmonary artery pressure in children and adults. An acceleration time of less than 100 ms identifies a patient group with abnormal pulmonary artery pressure with a predictive value of 97 percent.[20]

The mean pulmonary artery pressure (PAP) can be estimated using the regression equation proposed by Mahan et al,[18] which involves acceleration time (AcT):

$$\text{Mean PAP} = -0.5\ \text{AcT} + 80$$

Prediction of mean pulmonary artery pressure was found to be unsatisfactory ($r = 0.65$) but improved ($r = 0.85$) when only patients with heart rates between 60 and 100 beats/min were considered.[2]

TABLE 13–1. Correlation Coefficient of Doppler Methods Estimating Pulmonary Artery Pressure

RVEP/RVET	Pc–To	AcT	AcT/RVET	Reference
—	0.89	—	—	11
—	—	−0.88[a]	−0.90[a]	12
—	—	−0.87	−0.86	18
—	—	−0.78	—	19
0.83	—	−0.82	—	13
0.89	—	−0.88	—	16

[a]Log_{10} of mean PA.

AcT = pulmonary acceleration time; Pc–To = pulmonary closure to tricuspid opening; RVEP = right ventricular preejection period; RVET = right ventricular ejection time.

LEFT HEART PRESSURES

Left ventricular systolic and diastolic pressures are calculated in the presence of aortic valve disease by using systolic stenotic and diastolic regurgitant blood velocity, the Bernoulli equation, and sphygmomanometer blood pressures.

Left Ventricular Systolic Pressure

In normal patients, left ventricular systolic pressure is estimated easily by measuring brachial systolic blood pressure. In patients with aortic stenosis, left ventricular peak systolic pressure is calculated from Doppler measurement of the peak gradient across the aortic valve in systole and the simultaneous measurement of arm systolic blood pressure. Using the Bernoulli equation, the aortic valve pressure gradient (ΔP) is determined from the peak systolic velocity across the aortic valve orifice (V):

$$\Delta P = 4V^2$$

where the pressure gradient is given in millimeters of mercury if the velocity is shown in meters per second. Peak left ventricular systolic pressure (LVSP) is calculated by adding brachial artery systolic sphygmomanometer blood pressure (SBP):

$$LVSP = \Delta P + SBP$$

Accurate determination of velocity across the stenotic orifice is essential for accurate measurement of the transvalvular pressure gradient and left ventricular systolic pressure (discussed in Chap. 4).

Four possible sources of error should be considered. First, the pressure gradient can be underestimated if the Doppler record is obtained from a site other than the high-velocity jet in the valve orifice, or if the Doppler angle is greater than 25°. Second, brachial artery systolic pressure overestimates central aortic pressure. Therefore the use of brachial artery pressure, rather than central aortic pressure, would overestimate left ventricular systolic pressure. Third, the sphygmomanometer can lead to over- or underestimation of true brachial artery pressure by 5 to 10 mmHg. Fourth, simultaneous measurements of brachial artery pressure and the transvalvular pressure gradient is difficult; potentially, nonsimultaneous measurements can lead to over- or underestimation of the true left ventricular systolic pressure.

Left Ventricular Diastolic Pressure

Left ventricular end-diastolic pressure can be useful in assessing left ventricular function or the severity of valvular disease. In the setting of aortic regurgitation, a high-velocity retrograde flow signal during diastole will be recorded by Doppler in the left ventricular outflow tract. Using the modified Bernoulli equation, the pressure gradient between the aorta and the left ventricle at end-diastole (ΔP) can be calculated from the maximal velocity at end-diastole (V) (indicated by the arrow in Fig. 13–10) recorded by CW Doppler:

$$\Delta P = 4V^2$$

Left ventricular end-diastolic pressure (LVEDP) is calculated as the difference between brachial artery diastolic pressure (DBP) and the aortic regurgitant end-diastolic pressure gradient (ΔP):

$$\text{LVEDP} = \text{DBP} - \Delta P$$

Using this method, Yock and Popp[21] reported accurate estimation of left ventricular end-diastolic pressure in only 4 of 14 patients. The dropout

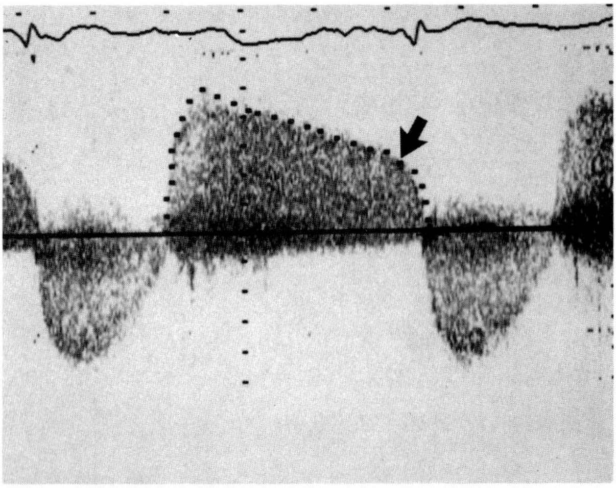

Figure 13–10. Continuous wave Doppler recording from a patient with aortic regurgitation and severe left ventricular dysfunction. The peak velocity of the aortic regurgitation jet at end-diastole (arrow) is 2.5 m/s. This predicts a pressure gradient between the aorta and the left ventricle at end-diastole (arrow) of 25 mmHg ($\Delta P = 4V^2$). The patient's arm diastolic blood pressure was 50 mmHg. Left ventricular end-diastolic pressure is, therefore, 50 minus 25, or 25 mmHg. (Scale marks = 1 m/s)

of high-velocity signals in most of their patients precluded accurate estimation of left ventricular end-diastolic pressure. Handshoe et al[22] similarly found poor correlation between the Doppler method and catheter-measured pressure, but a better correlation was found in a small subset of patients. Further analysis of this subset indicated that those patients had full spectral displays, so that at end-diastole there was little dropout of high-velocity signals. When only patients with full spectral displays were analyzed, a good correlation was found. Similar results have been reported by other investigators.[23] The data indicate that Doppler estimates of left ventricular end-diastolic pressure may be valid in aortic regurgitation when a full spectral display can be recorded.

Left Atrial Pressure

Peak systolic left atrial pressure can be calculated in patients in whom mitral regurgitation is present but aortic stenosis is absent. The peak mitral regurgitant velocity (V) is used to calculate the peak systolic pressure gradient between the left ventricle and the left atrium (ΔP) (Fig. 13–11):

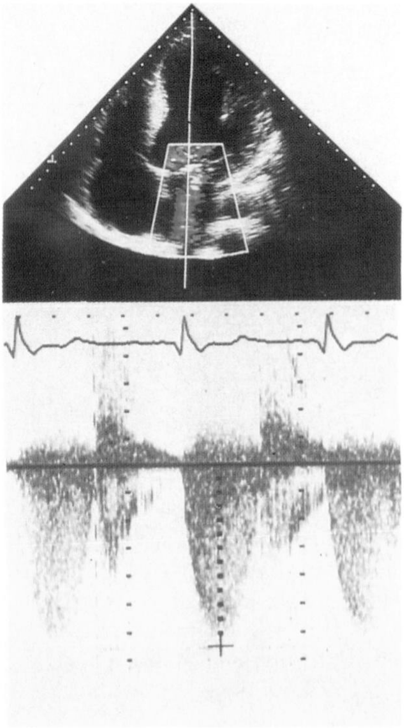

Figure 13–11. Mitral regurgitation recorded from an apical four-chamber view. *Top*: The color Doppler tracing demonstrates the blue jet of mitral regurgitation. Color Doppler imaging can be used to align the continuous wave beam (straight solid line) parallel to the regurgitant jet. *Bottom*: The peak velocity of the regurgitant jet is 6.2 m/s. This predicts a pressure gradient of 154 mmHg ($\Delta P = 4V^2$) across the mitral valve in systole. The patient's systolic blood pressure was 180 mmHg; therefore, left atrial peak pressure in systole is 180 minus 154, or 26 mmHg. (Scale marks = 1 m/s)

$$\Delta P = 4V^2$$

If it is assumed that brachial artery systolic pressure is equivalent to left ventricular peak systolic pressure, then left atrial peak systolic pressure (LAP) can be calculated as the difference between brachial systolic blood pressure (SBP) and the systolic pressure gradient across the mitral valve (ΔP):

$$LAP = SBP - \Delta P$$

The potential errors encountered in the use of this approach are similar to those noted for left ventricular diastolic pressure calculation in the presence of aortic regurgitation. Despite these limitations, the approach can be applied to patients with cardiomyopathy and mitral stenosis.[9]

REFERENCES

1. Berger M, Haimowitz A, Van Tosh A, et al: Quantitative assessment of pulmonary hypertension in patients with tricuspid regurgitation using continuous wave Doppler ultrasound. *J Am Coll Cardiol* 6:359, 1985.
2. Chan K, Currie P, Seward J, et al: Comparison of three Doppler ultrasound methods in the prediction of pulmonary artery pressure. *J Am Coll Cardiol* 9:549, 1987.
3. Currie P, Seward J, Chan K, et al: Continuous wave Doppler determination of right ventricular pressure: A simultaneous Doppler-catheterization study in 127 patients. *J Am Coll Cardiol* 6:750, 1985.
4. Yock P, Popp R: Noninvasive estimation of right ventricular systolic pressure by Doppler ultrasound in patients with tricuspid regurgitation. *Circulation* 70:657, 1984.
5. Murphy D Jr, Ludomirsky A, Huhta J: Continuous-wave Doppler in children with ventricular septal defect: Noninvasive estimation of interventricular pressure gradient. *Am J Cardiol* 57:428, 1986.
6. Silbert D, Brunson A, Schiff R, et al: Determination of right ventricular pressure in the presence of a ventricular septal defect using continuous wave Doppler ultrasound. *J Am Coll Cardiol* 8:379, 1986.
7. Waggoner A, Quinones M, Young J: Pulsed Doppler echocardiographic detection of right-sided valve regurgitation: Experimental results and clinical significance. *Am J Cardiol* 47:279, 1981.
8. Miyatake K, Okamoto M, Kinoshita N: Pulmonary regurgitation studied with the ultrasonic pulsed Doppler technique. *Circulation* 65:969, 1982.
9. Hatle L, Angelsen B: *Doppler Ultrasound in Cardiology*, 2d ed. Philadelphia, Lea & Febiger, 1985.
10. Masuyama T, Kodama K, Kitabatake A, et al: Continuous-wave Doppler echocardiographic detection of pulmonary regurgitation and its application to noninvasive estimation of pulmonary artery pressure. *Circulation* 74:484, 1986.

11. Hatle L, Angelsen B, Tromsdal A: Noninvasive estimation of pulmonary artery systolic pressure with Doppler ultrasound. *Br Heart J* 45:157, 1981.
12. Kitabatake A, Inoue M, Asao M, et al: Noninvasive evaluation of pulmonary hypertension by a pulsed Doppler technique. *Circulation* 68:302, 1983.
13. Kosturakis D, Goldberg S, Allen H, et al: Doppler echocardiographic prediction of pulmonary arterial hypertension in congenital heart disease. *Am J Cardiol* 53:1110, 1984.
14. Martin-Duran R, Larman M, Trugeda A, et al: Comparison of Doppler-determined elevated pulmonary arterial pressure with pressure measured at cardiac catheterization. *Am J Cardiol* 57:859, 1986.
15. Matsuda M, Sekiguchi T, Sugishita Y, et al: Reliability of non-invasive estimates of pulmonary hypertension by pulsed Doppler echocardiography. *Br Heart J* 56:158, 1986.
16. Isobe M, Yazaki Y, Takaku F, et al: Prediction of pulmonary arterial pressure in adults by pulsed Doppler echocardiography. *Am J Cardiol* 57:316, 1986.
17. Serwer G, Cougle A, Eckerd J, et al: Factors affecting use of the Doppler-determined time from flow onset to maximal pulmonary artery velocity for measurement of pulmonary artery pressure in children. *Am J Cardiol* 58:352, 1986.
18. Mahan G, Dabestani A, Gardin J, et al: Estimation of pulmonary artery pressure by pulsed Doppler echocardiography (abstr). *Circulation* 68(III):367, 1983.
19. Okamoto M, Miyatake K, Kinoshita N, et al: Analysis of blood flow in pulmonary hypertension with the pulsed Doppler flowmeter combined with cross sectional echocardiography. *Br Heart J* 51:407, 1984.
20. Handshoe R, DeMaria A: Doppler assessment of intracardiac pressures. *Echocardiography* 2:127, 1985.
21. Yock P, Popp R: Noninvasive estimation of ventricular pressure by Doppler ultrasound in patients with tricuspid or aortic regurgitation (abstr). *Circulation* 68(III):919, 1983.
22. Handshoe R, Handshoe S, Kwan O, et al: Value and limitations of Doppler measurement in the estimation of left ventricular end-diastolic pressure in patients with aortic regurgitation (abstr). *Circulation* 70(II):466, 1984.
23. Talano J: Doppler echocardiography in assessing intracardiac pressures, function, and flow. *Echocardiography* 3:83, 1986.

CHAPTER 14

Evaluation and Management of Ischemic Heart Disease

The practical clinical application of two-dimensional (2D) echocardiography and Doppler echocardiography in patients with ischemic heart disease is concerned with (1) the effects of ischemia on ventricular wall motion (hypokinesis, akinesis, dyskinesis) and on the evaluation of systolic and diastolic ventricular performance, (2) complications of myocardial infarction, (3) detection of left ventricular thrombi, (4) monitoring of therapeutic interventions, and (5) detection of exercise-induced changes in left ventricular function (Table 14–1). This chapter primarily addresses the use

TABLE 14–1. Two-Dimensional Echocardiography and Doppler Echo in Ischemic Heart Disease

A. Assessment of LV function

B. Diagnosis and exclusion of acute MI
   1. Location of MI
   2. Extent of MI

C. Prognosis
   1. In-hospital
   2. Long-term

D. Complications of myocardial infarction

E. Left ventricular thrombi

F. Monitoring of therapeutic interventions

G. Exercise Doppler echocardiography

NOTE: LV = left ventricle; MI = myocardial infarction

of Doppler echocardiography in the evaluation of patients with complications of myocardial infarction and its role in the assessment of global left ventricular function at rest and with exercise.

DIFFERENTIAL DIAGNOSIS OF CHEST PAIN SYNDROMES

Cardiac ultrasonography is well suited to evaluate those patients who have atypical chest pain syndromes that are difficult diagnostic and management problems. The ability to evaluate ventricular size, shape, and function (at rest and with exercise) as well as to interrogate valvular, great vessel, and pericardial structure make this technique useful in the differential diagnosis of chest pain syndromes. The demonstration of an intimal flap and dilated aorta by 2D echocardiography is diagnostic of DeBakey Type I aortic dissection (Fig. 14–1). Color flow imaging (CFI) is also useful in identifying the sites of communication between the true and false channels either directly, by visualization of flow signals moving from one lumen into the other (Fig. 14–2), or indirectly, by analyzing differences in timing of opacification of the two lumina and flow direction.[1] Additional complications such as pericardial effusion and/or tamponade and aortic regurgitation can be promptly recognized by 2D echocardiography and Doppler

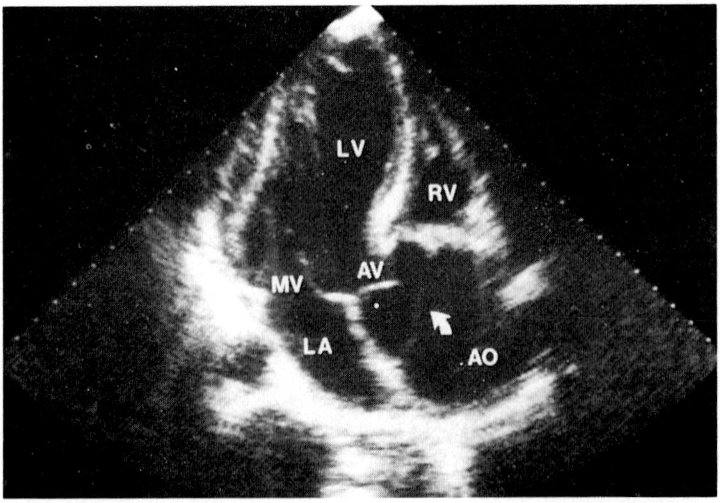

Figure 14–1. Two-dimensional apical five-chamber view in a patient with type I dissecting aneurysm of the aorta demonstrating an intimal flap (arrow). The aortic valve (AV) is seen proximally to the intimal flap and the aorta (AO) is dilated, measuring 6.5 cm. LA = left atrium, LV = left ventricle, MV = mitral valve, RV = right ventricle.

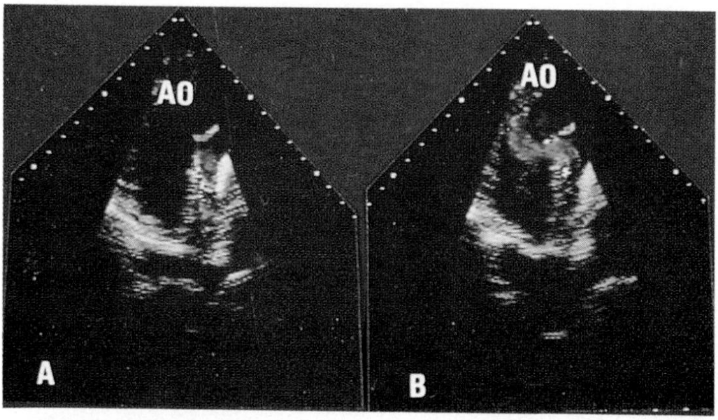

Figure 14–2. Color flow imaging in aortic dissection, suprasternal long axis view of the ascending aorta (AO). (A) In early systole, flow signals are present in the true lumen and are directed toward the transducer (red). (B) In late systole, flow signals are seen moving through the dissection flap and entering and opacifying the false lumen upward and toward the transducer (red).

techniques. Patients with these conditions should be treated promptly by surgical repair. Type III aortic dissections may be more difficult to diagnose by 2D echocardiography, and other noninvasive techniques such as CT scanning or magnetic resonance imaging may be helpful.[2] However, with the introduction of transesophageal echocardiography (discussed in Chap. 16) the aortic arch and descending thoracic aorta can be evaluated for dissection, and flow between the true and false channels can be identified with CFI.[3]

In patients with mitral valve prolapse, chest pain is not an infrequent presentation. This technique can be used, especially when coupled with Doppler echocardiography, to establish clearly the diagnosis of mitral valve prolapse as well as to determine the hemodynamic presence and severity of mitral regurgitation (Fig. 14–3). However, the ability to decide whether the pain is on the basis of mitral valve prolapse alone or on that of ischemic heart disease and coexistent mitral valve prolapse cannot always be made by the mere echocardiographic demonstration of mitral valve prolapse. In such patients, unless wall motion abnormalities are clearly demonstrated, further studies are necessary to delineate the etiology of the chest pain. Similarly, the ability to find a pericardial effusion and normal wall motion by 2D echocardiography with nonspecific ST- and T-wave changes on the electrocardiogram should alert the clinician to the possibility of pericarditis.

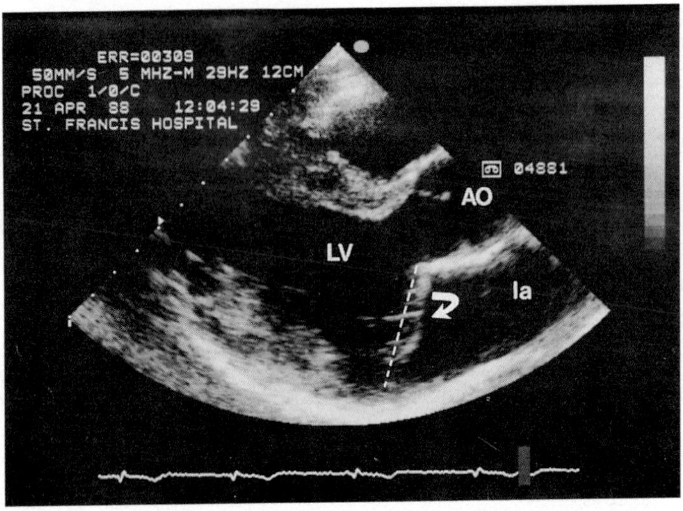

Figure 14–3. Parasternal long axis view in a patient with significant mitral valve prolapse. Both anterior and posterior leaflets (arrow) are displaced behind the plane of the mitral anulus (dotted line). AO = aorta, LA = left atrium, LV = left ventricle.

The 2D echocardiogram is well suited to determine whether hypertrophic cardiomyopathy exists in a patient presenting with chest pain. Doppler echocardiography is useful in determining subaortic gradients (discussed in Chap. 15) and in assessing diastolic function.

COMPLICATIONS OF MYOCARDIAL INFARCTION

Mitral regurgitation and ventricular septal defects are two complications of myocardial infarction that can be readily assessed by conventional Doppler echocardiography and CFI. Both are associated with new systolic murmurs and hemodynamic deterioration, and may require acute surgical intervention.

Mitral Regurgitation

Mitral regurgitation can be due to papillary muscle rupture, ischemia, or infarction; chamber enlargement and mitral anular dilatation may also be contributing factors. Two-dimensional echocardiography and CFI can be used to distinguish between these mechanisms.[4–10] The severity of mitral regurgitation can be assessed semiquantitatively using CFI.[11] Doppler echocardiography can therefore be used to study the effects of various interventions (such as drugs or intraaortic balloon pumping) on the severity of mitral regurgitation,[12] can help assess the need for valve surgery, and may assist the surgeon in deciding whether valve repair or replacement should be performed.

Mitral regurgitation is frequently observed in patients with myocardial infarction.[9] Since it develops in the absence of any lesions in the mitral valve leaflet, its pathogenesis has been explained by the concept of "papillary muscle dysfunction" proposed by Burch et al.[13] At present, papillary muscle dysfunction is thought to be a sequence of unsuccessful coordination of the whole mitral apparatus (which is composed of the anulus, leaflets, chordae tendineae, papillary muscles, and left ventricular wall), rather than a mere disorder of the papillary muscle.

Papillary muscle dysfunction is noted on the 2D echocardiogram as incomplete closure of the mitral valve together with a scarred echo-dense papillary muscle (Fig. 14–4). A recent study has shown that there are two major causative factors of mitral regurgitation accompanying myocardial infarction: (1) asynergy of the papillary muscles or the left ventricular wall, which results in mitral regurgitation located in the commisural area of the side on which the asynergy occurs, and (2) enlargement of the mitral anulus, which results in regurgitation from the central area of the orifice.[9]

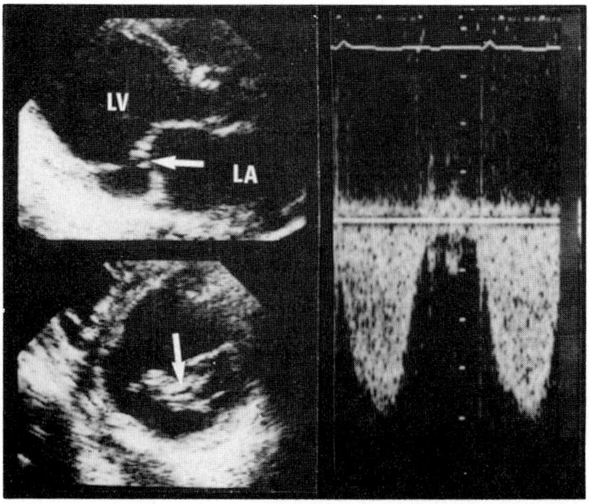

Figure 14–4. Parasternal long axis (*top*) and short axis (*bottom*) views of a patient with an inferior wall myocardial infarction. There was failure of mitral valve coaptation in systole (arrows), which produced significant mitral regurgitation (right-hand Doppler panel). LA = left atrium, LV = left ventricle.

Papillary muscle rupture is rare and has been reported to occur in about 1 percent of patients after acute myocardial infarction. The clinical presentation may be dramatic, with the sudden development of pulmonary edema, shock, and a holosystolic murmur audible at the apex. The importance of recognizing partial papillary muscle rupture is that it is a potentially treatable surgical condition. Small portions of the myocardium are affected, usually with involvement of an inferior wall infarction and the adjacent posteromedial papillary muscle.[14] In some patients with complete papillary muscle rupture there may be no audible precordial murmur;[15] such a patient may expire suddenly in an acute cardiogenic shock-like syndrome. A ruptured papillary muscle produces the characteristic 2D echocardiographic findings of a flail mitral valve with part of the valve apparatus protruding into the left atrium in systole (Fig. 14–5). The actual tip of the ruptured papillary muscle may also be seen as a small mass on the flail valve. A tumor, thrombus, or vegetation can be mimicked by this condition. Flail mitral leaflet with mitral valve prolapse may have similar echocardiographic findings. With the onset of acute and severe mitral regurgitation, and a large 'V' wave, the Doppler maximum regurgitant velocity decreases rapidly from early to late systole, reflecting the rapid equilibration of the left ventricular and left atrial pressure[16] (Fig. 14–6).

Ventricular Septal Defect (VSD)

Acute rupture of the ventricular septum is an uncommon, but life-threatening, complication of myocardial infarction.[17–24] It occurs in fewer than 1

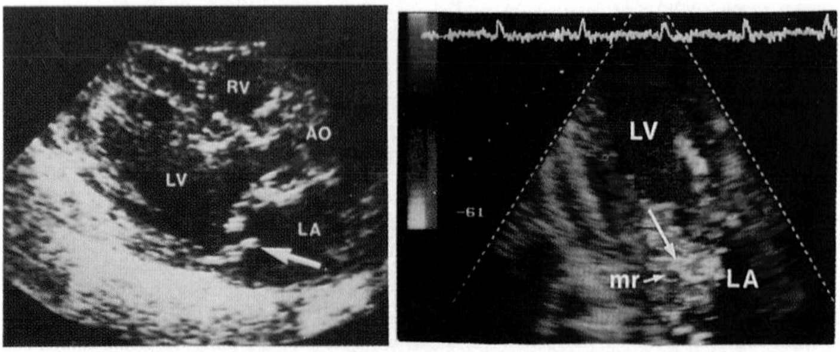

Figure 14–5. Partial papillary muscle rupture. *Left*: Parasternal long axis view demonstrating a flail posterior mitral valve leaflet (arrow) secondary to rupture of a head of the posteromedial papillary muscle. *Right*: Apical two-chamber view showing severe mitral regurgitation (*mr*) in a mosaic pattern (arrows). AO = aorta, LA = left atrium, LV = left ventricle, RV = right ventricle.

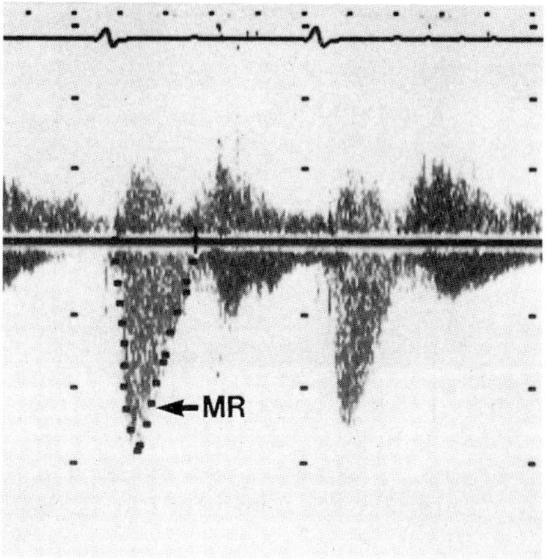

Figure 14–6. Continuous wave Doppler echocardiogram from a patient with acute mitral regurgitation (MR). The maximum velocity peaks early in systole and then decreases abruptly. This reflects the rapid equilibration of the left ventricular and left atrial pressure in mid- to late systole. (Scale marks = 1 m/s)

percent of infarcts. Ventricular septal rupture can occur in anterior as well as in inferior wall infarction.

Two-Dimensional Echocardiography. Although these defects can be seen on 2D echocardiography (Fig. 14–7), they are often difficult to visualize. Reasons for the poor visualization include small size of the defect, location in the near field of the echo sector (in the case of apical VSD), and also the fact that these defects, rather than clearcut discontinuity of the septum, are often complex channels, resulting from dissection of myocardium from intramural hematomas.[22,25] It appears that defects following anterior myocardial infarction are generally harder to visualize than defects after inferior myocardial infarction.[17,19,21]

Contrast Echocardiography. The sensitivity of 2D echocardiography is markedly enhanced by the use of contrast techniques.[24] Even though the shunt is predominantly from left to right, a small amount of right-to-left shunting is usually present. Thus, after contrast injection into a peripheral vein, some microbubbles can almost always be seen entering the left ventricle. Frequently a negative contrast effect can be observed in the right ventricle, when left ventricular blood without contrast material displaces right ventricular blood.

Although contrast echocardiography is quite sensitive in detecting VSDs, localization of the defect can be difficult.

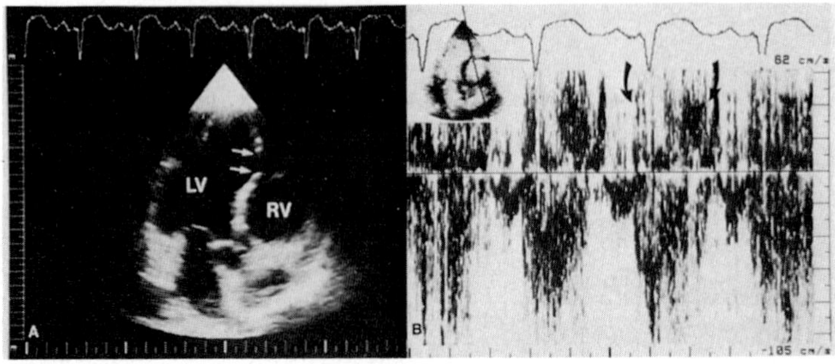

Figure 14–7. (A) Apical four-chamber view in a patient with anteroseptal myocardial infarction complicated by rupture of the interventricular septum seen in this view as a dropout of echoes (white arrows). LV = left ventricle, RV = right ventricle. (B) With pulsed Doppler echocardiography, the sample volume was positioned in the area of the suspected defect (straight arrow) and a wide systolic frequency dispersion was recorded (curved arrows). This finding was diagnostic of left-to-right shunt at the ventricular level.

Continuous Wave and Pulsed Doppler. These techniques can detect high-velocity systolic flow jets in the right ventricle (Fig. 14–7); in addition, lower-velocity diastolic flow can frequently also be seen.[18,19,26–28] The sensitivity of this method is markedly higher than that of standard 2D echocardiography, since the abnormal flow is generally easier to detect than the defect itself. As in congenital VSDs, CW Doppler echocardiography can be used to measure gradients between the ventricles, and to estimate right ventricular and pulmonary artery systolic pressure (See Chap. 13, Fig. 13–4). Calculation of left-to-right shunting in patients with acquired VSDs is possible by Doppler techniques.[29] Doppler echocardiography also can differentiate between ventricular septal rupture and acute mitral regurgitation following acute myocardial infarction, conditions with similar clinical and hemodynamic presentations.[20,30]

Color Flow Imaging. Large, high-velocity systolic flow jets can usually be readily appreciated in the right ventricle.[17,19,22] They can be seen originating on the left ventricular side of the defect and crossing the septum (Fig. 14–8). The jet location by CFI can actually be used to locate the VSD, which can frequently also be seen on 2D echocardiography after being pinpointed by CFI, even if the defect has been difficult to visualize on the initial 2D study. Furthermore, the width of the color Doppler jet appears to be useful in determining the size of the VSD.

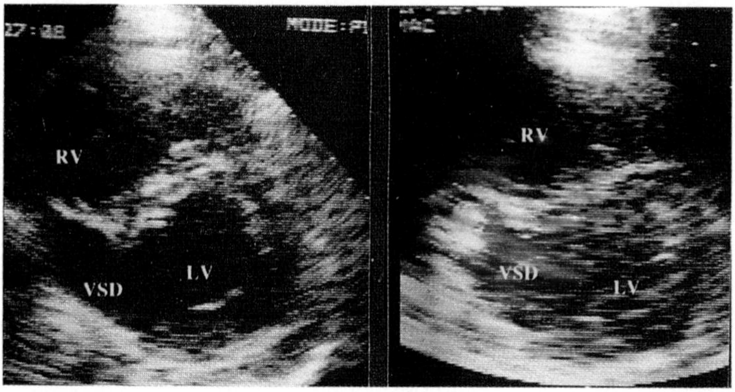

Figure 14–8. Parasternal short axis view in a patient with acute ventricular defect (VSD) secondary to an acute inferior wall myocardial infarction. *Left*: A large VSD is evident in the region of the posterior septum at mid–left ventricular level. *Right*: Color flow imaging shows a large left-to-right shunt through this region in systole. LV = left ventricle, RV = right ventricle.

Evaluation of VSD *Repair*. Conventional Doppler echocardiography and CFI both appear to be sensitive in the detection of residual shunts after VSD patch repair (Fig. 14–9). Mild early leakage, which is thought to take place through the suture line, is commonly present after VSD repair and generally appears to be self-limiting. Larger shunts, however, are normally not seen and appear to carry an adverse prognosis.

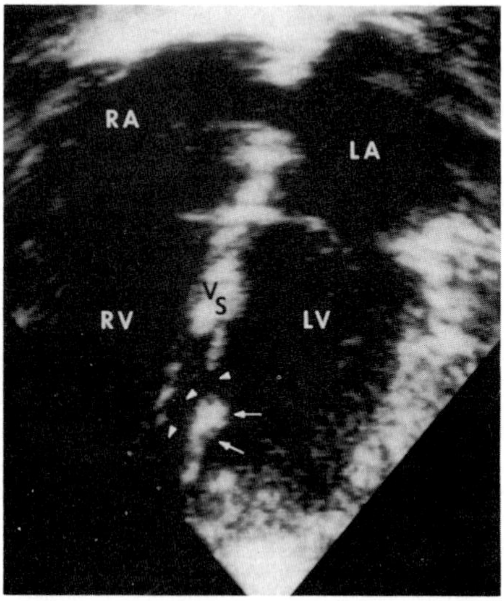

Figure 14–9. Apical four-chamber view (inverted image) of a patient with a recurrent ventricular septal defect (arrowheads) beneath the Dacron patch graft closure (arrows) of the initial ventricular septal rupture. LA = left atrium, LV = left ventricle, RA = right atrium, RV = right ventricle, VS = ventricular septum.

LEFT VENTRICULAR FUNCTION

Doppler echocardiography provides a noninvasive measurement of blood flow velocity and acceleration in the ascending aorta, and thereby provides an accurate means for assessing left ventricular function.[31,32] (See Chap. 11 for methods of measurement of flow velocity and acceleration). Studies by Sabbah et al[33] yielded good correlation between measurements of peak acceleration by Doppler ultrasonography and ejection fraction obtained by left ventriculography, indicating that peak acceleration is a sensitive measure of global left ventricular function at rest. In addition, acceleration and peak velocity have been found to be inversely related to the severity of coronary artery disease in patients undergoing cineangiography.[34,35]

Thus the acceleration and peak velocity of blood flow in the ascending aorta are related to left ventricular performance and can be measured noninvasively, at rest, during exercise, or immediately after exercise, by Doppler echocardiography. The Doppler examination is performed with the subject in the standing position, with the transducer at the suprasternal notch. A nonimaging transducer is angulated to record the maximal flow signal as defined by audio and spectral outputs. Doppler recordings are made at rest, at peak exercise, and/or immediately after exercise. A comprehensive examination combines both exercise 2D echocardiography and Doppler echocardiography. It is possible that there may be a role for just the freestanding Doppler evaluation of aortic blood flow velocity profiles with exercise as a simpler noninvasive evaluation of global left ventricular function. Harrison et al[36] reported the response of flow velocity and acceleration to exercise in normal subjects (Fig. 14–10). A progressive increase in maximal velocity, modal velocity, and acceleration occurred with increasing levels of exercise to peak exertion (0.79 ± 0.18 to 1.36 ± 0.23 m/s, 0.605 ± 0.16 to 1.22 ± 0.29 m/s, and 15.82 ± 4.14 to 52.73 ± 16.33 m/s^2, respectively). Velocity (maximal and modal) decreased slightly in the immediate postexercise period, while acceleration continued to increase. Flow velocity integral also increased with exercise in normal subjects (from 7.98 ± 2.7 cm at rest to 9.07 ± 2.6 cm at peak exertion). However, the increase in flow velocity integral was of a lower magnitude (13.6 percent) than that of maximal velocity (74 percent) and acceleration (250 percent), and was greatest during the early stages of exercise, with a gradual diminution at peak exercise.

Doppler evaluation of aortic blood flow velocities has also been used in combination with 2D echocardiography to assess left ventricular function before and after intravenous dipyridamole stress testing for detection of coronary artery disease.[37] Both velocity and acceleration responses to

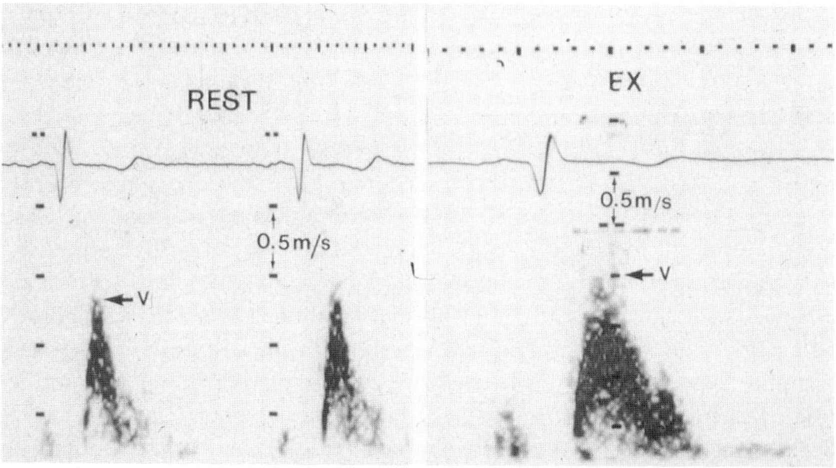

Figure 14–10. Continuous wave recording from the suprasternal notch of ascending aortic blood flow velocities at rest and immediately postexercise (EX) in a normal subject. Peak velocity (V) increased from 1.3 m/s to 2.0 m/s.

intravenous dipyridamole were found to be significantly different in individuals with normal, versus those with abnormal, thallium perfusion. However, only the percent change in acceleration after intravenous dipyridamole was significantly different between subjects with and without coronary artery disease. Patients without significant coronary artery disease had a 57-percent increase in acceleration after intravenous dipyridamole, compared with only a 7-percent increase in those with significant coronary artery disease. The addition of Doppler evaluation of aortic blood flow velocities to standard 2D electrocardiographic imaging appears to add significantly to the sensitivity of this technique.[37]

Exercise Doppler echocardiography has been used to evaluate the effects of propranolol and verapamil on aortic blood flow velocity and acceleration.[38] In that study verapamil had no effect on flow velocity or acceleration, which implies that the primary antiischemic action of this agent involves mechanisms other than reduced myocardial oxygen demand. Conversely, propranolol was accompanied by a reduction in flow acceleration and an augmentation of integrated flow velocity, implying decreased inotropy and increased stroke volume induced by enhanced preload.

In light of these recent studies, exercise Doppler flow velocity recordings have the potential for increasing application in clinical cardiology. This noninvasive technique has the potential to enhance our understanding of disease processes and therapeutic agents and permit targeted therapy of individual patients. Table 14–2 summarizes the advantages, requirements, and markers of an abnormal exercise 2D/Doppler echocardiographic examination.

Several studies addressing the use of exercise Doppler echocardiography to detect manifestations of ischemic heart disease have recently been reported. Harrison and coworkers[36] compared the exercise response of 28 normal subjects and 74 patients referred for exercise thallium perfusion scintigraphy for the evaluation of chest pain. Patients with coronary artery disease manifested by abnormal thallium perfusion scintigraphy had a reduced peak velocity and acceleration in response to exercise, compared to that achieved by healthy volunteers. Furthermore, a reduction in peak acceleration measurements to $< 30\ m/s^2$ in the absence of β-adrenergic blocking medications was of value in detecting patients with advanced stages of coronary artery disease (Fig. 14–11). Bryg et al[39] compared peak flow velocities achieved with treadmill exercise in young clinically normal subjects with those obtained in patients with coronary artery disease. Patients with severe coronary artery disease having left ventricu-

TABLE 14–2. Exercise Two-Dimensional/Doppler Echocardiography in Ischemic Heart Disease

A. Advantages
   1. Portable—office based
   2. Good global-segmental LV/RV function
   3. Good resolution (2–3 mm)
   4. No radiation
   5 Lower cost than nuclear imaging

B. Requirements
   1. Dedicated physician—Technician time
   2. Offline analysis system (cine loop)

C. Markers of an abnormal test
   1. 2D echocardiography
      a. New systolic wall motion abnormality
      b. Fall in global ejection fraction
   2. Doppler echocardiography
      a. Reduced peak velocity
      b. Reduced acceleration
      c. Unchanged or decreased stroke volume
      d. Unchanged or increased LV ejection time

NOTE: LV = left ventricle; RV = right ventricle

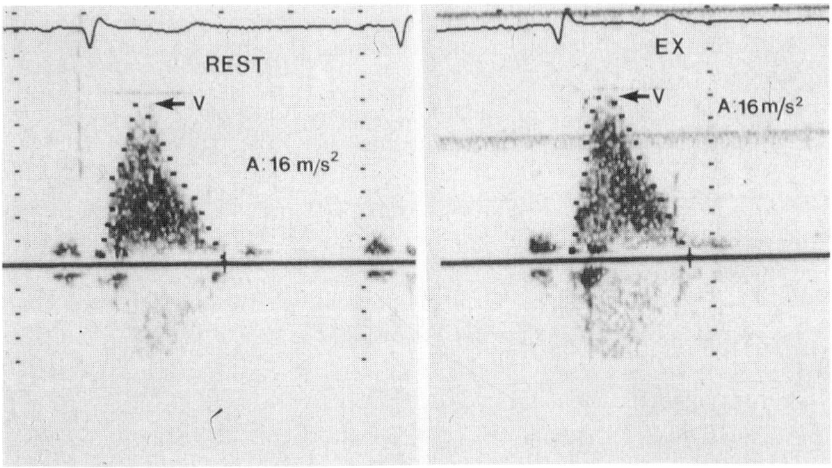

Figure 14–11. Continuous wave Doppler velocities from the suprasternal notch of blood flow in the ascending aorta at rest and immediately postexercise (EX) in a patient with ischemic heart disease. Peak velocity (V) and acceleration (A) of flow did not increase normally with exercise. (Scale marks = 20 cm/s).

lar dysfunction at rest either failed to achieve an 80-percent increase from baseline values, comparable with that observed in normal subjects, or actually experienced a decrease in peak velocity. In a preliminary report, Teague et al[40] suggested that peak flow velocities at maximal exercise failed to rise, or actually fell, in patients with advanced degrees of coronary artery disease.

A recent study compared the results of exercise Doppler echocardiography to those of radionuclide angiography in a group of 38 patients undergoing evaluation for suspected coronary artery disease.[41] Exercise-induced changes in peak velocity and acceleration tended to mirror changes in ejection fraction, and could be used to identify patients with exercise-induced ischemia and left ventricular dysfunction.

REFERENCES

1. Iliceto S, Nanda N, Rizzon P, et al: Color Doppler evaluation of aortic dissection. *Circulation* 75:748, 1987.
2. Goldman A, Kotler M, Scanlon M, et al: The complementary role of magnetic resonance imaging, Doppler echocardiography and computed tomography in the diagnosis of dissecting thoracic aneurysms. *Am Heart* J 111:970, 1986.

3. Seward J, Khanderia B, Oh J, et al: Transesophageal echocardiography: Technique, anatomic correlations, implementation, and clinical applications. *Mayo Clin Proc* 63:649, 1988.

4. Loperfido F, Biasucci L, Pennestri F, et al: Pulsed Doppler echocardiographic analysis of mitral regurgitation after myocardial infarction. *Am J Cardiol* 58:692, 1986.

5. Tei C, Sakamaki T, Shah P, et al: Mitral valve prolapse in short-term experimental coronary occlusion: A possible mechanism of ischemic mitral regurgitation. *Circulation* 68:183, 1983.

6. Ogawa S, Hubbard F, Mardelli T, et al: Cross-sectional echocardiographic spectrum of papillary muscle dysfunction. *Am Heart J* 97:312, 1979.

7. Godley R, Wann L, Rogers E, et al: Incomplete mitral leaflet closure in patients with papillary muscle dysfunction. *Circulation* 63:565, 1981.

8. Kinney E, Frangi M: Value of two-dimensional echocardiographic detection of incomplete leaflet closure. *Am Heart J* 109:87, 1985.

9. Izumi S, Miyatake K, Beppu S, et al: Mechanism of mitral regurgitation in patients with myocardial infarction: A study using real-time two-dimensional Doppler flow imaging and echocardiography. *Circulation* 76:777, 1987.

10. Mintz G, Victor M, Kotler M, et al: Two-dimensional echocardiographic identification of surgically correctable complications of acute myocardial infarction. *Circulation* 64:91, 1981.

11. Helmcke F, Nanda N, Hsiung M, et al: Color Doppler assessment of mitral regurgitation with orthogonal planes. *Circulation* 75:175, 1987.

12. Czer L, Maurer G, Bolger A, et al: Intraoperative evaluation of mitral regurgitation by Doppler color flow mapping. *Circulation* 76(III):108, 1987.

13. Burch G, DePasquale N, Phillips J: The syndrome of papillary muscle dysfunction. *Am Heart J* 75:399, 1968.

14. Kotler M, Mintz G, Segal B: Operable complication of MI: Noninvasive diagnosis. *J Cardiovasc Med* 7:1070, 1982.

15. Come P, Riley M, Weintraub R, et al: Echocardiographic detection of complete and partial papillary muscle rupture during acute myocardial infarction. *Am J Cardiol* 56:787, 1985.

16. Hatle L, Angelsen B: *Doppler Ultrasound in Cardiology*, 2d ed. Philadelphia, Lea & Febiger, 1985.

17. Zachariah Z, Hsiung M, Nanda N, Camarano G: Diagnosis of rupture of the ventricular septum during acute myocardial infarction by Doppler color flow mapping. *Am J Cardiol* 59:162, 1987.

18. Bhatia S, Plappert T, Theard M, Sutton M: Transseptal Doppler flow velocity profile in acquired ventricular septal defect in acute myocardial infarction. *Am J Cardiol* 60:372, 1987.

19. Miyatake K, Okamoto M, Kinoshita N, et al: Doppler echocardiographic features of ventricular septal rupture in myocardial infarction. *J Am Coll Cardiol* 5:182, 1985.

20. Eisenberg P, Barzilai B, Perez J: Noninvasive detection by Doppler echocardiography of combined ventricular septal rupture and mitral regurgitation in acute myocardial infarction. *J Am Coll Cardiol* 4:617, 1984.

21. Chandraratna P, Balachandran P, Shah P, Hodges M: Echocardiographic observations on ventricular septal rupture complicating acute myocardial infarction. *Circulation* 51:506, 1975.

22. Hodsden J, Nanda N: Dissecting aneurysm of the ventricular septum following acute myocardial infarction: Diagnosis by real time two-dimensional echocardiography. *Am Heart J* 101:671, 1981.

23. Bishop H, Gibson R, Stamm R, et al: Role of two-dimensional echocardiography in the evaluation of patients with ventricular septal rupture postmyocardial infarction. *Am Heart J* 102:965, 1981.

24. Drobac M, Gilbert B, Howard R, et al: Ventricular septal defect after myocardial infarction: Diagnosis by two-dimensional contrast echocardiography. *Circulation* 67:335, 1983.

25. Panidis I, Mintz G, Goel I, et al: Acquired ventricular septal defect after myocardial infarction: Detection by combined two-dimensional and Doppler echocardiography. *Am Heart J* 111:427, 1986.

26. Keren G, Sherez J, Roth A, et al: Diagnosis of ventricular septal rupture from acute myocardial infarction by combined 2-dimensional and pulsed Doppler echocardiography. *Am J Cardiol* 53:1202, 1984.

27. Come P: Doppler detection of acquired ventricular septal defect. *Am J Cardiol* 55:586, 1985.

28. Goldman A, Kotler M, Goldberg S, et al: The uses of two-dimensional Doppler echocardiographic techniques preoperatively and postoperatively in a ventricular septal defect caused by penetrating trauma. *Ann Thorac Surg* 40:625, 1985.

29. Barron J, Sahn D, Valdes-Cruz L, et al: Clinical utility of two-dimensional Doppler echocardiographic techniques for estimating pulmonary to systemic blood flow ratios in children with left to right shunting atrial septal defect, ventricular septal defect or patent ductus arteriosus. *J Am Coll Cardiol* 3:169, 1984.

30. Pandian N, Isner J, McInerney K, et al: Noninvasive assessment of the complicated myocardial infarction: Use of Doppler and two-dimensional echocardiography to differentiate ventricular septal rupture from rupture of mitral apparatus. *Echocardiography* 2:329, 1985.

31. Stein P, Sabbah H, Albert D, Snyder J: Blood velocity and acceleration. Comparison of continuous wave Doppler with electromagnetic flowmetry (abstr). *Fed Proc* 44:1565, 1985.

32. Bennet E, Barclay S, Davis A, et al: Ascending aortic blood flow velocity and acceleration using Doppler ultrasound in the assessment of left ventricular function. *Cardiovasc Res* 18:632, 1984.

33. Sabbah H, Khaja F, Brymer J, et al: Noninvasive evaluation of left ventricular performance based on peak aortic blood acceleration measured with a continuous-wave Doppler velocity meter. *Circulation* 76:232, 1986.

34. Bennett E, Else W, Miller G, et al: Maximum acceleration of blood from the left ventricle in patients with ischemic heart disease. *Clin Sci Mol Med* 46:49, 1974.

35. Mehta N, Bennet D, Mannering D, et al: Usefulness of non-invasive Doppler measurement of ascending aortic blood velocity and acceleration in detecting impairment of the left ventricular functional response to exercise three weeks after acute myocardial infarction. *Am J Cardiol* 58:879, 1986.

36. Harrison M, Smith M, Friedman B, DeMaria A: Uses and limitations of exercise Doppler echocardiography in the diagnosis of ischemic heart disease. *J Am Coll Cardiol* 10:809, 1987.

37. Labovitz A, Pearson A, Chaitman B, et al: Doppler and two-dimensional echocardiographic assessment of left ventricular function before and after intravenous dipyridamole stress testing for detection of coronary artery disease. *Am J Cardiol* 62:1180, 1988.

38. Harrison M, Smith M, Nissen S, et al: Use of exercise Doppler echocardiography to evaluate cardiac drugs: Effects of propranolol and verapamil on aortic blood flow velocity and acceleration. *J Am Coll Cardiol* 11:1002, 1988.

39. Bryg R, Labovitz A, Mehdirad A, et al: Effect of coronary artery disease on Doppler-derived parameters of aortic flow during upright exercise. *Am J Cardiol* 58:14, 1986.

40. Teague S, Mark D, Radford M, et al: Doppler velocity profiles reveal ischemic exercise responses (abstr). *Circulation* 70(II):185, 1984.

41. Daley P, Sagar K, Collier D, et al: Detection of exercise induced changes in left ventricular performance by Doppler echocardiography. *Br Heart J* 58:447, 1987.

CHAPTER 15

Cardiomyopathies

Primary cardiomyopathies are diseases of the heart muscle of unknown etiology. These diseases comprise a significant and important group of cardiac pathologic processes. The primary cardiomyopathies are classified into three major groups[1,2] (Table 15–1): (1) Dilated cardiomyopathy, the most common cardiomyopathic process, characterized by dilatation of the left ventricle with impaired systolic ventricular function and usually associated with congestive heart failure; (2) hypertrophic cardiomyopathy, characterized by disproportionate hypertrophy of the left ventricle typically involving the septum and anterolateral free wall (but often with variable

TABLE 15–1. Classification and Echocardiographic Features of the Cardiomyopathies

Echocardiographic Features	Dilated	Hypertrophic	Restrictive
Diastolic LV cavity size	Increased	Decreased	Normal/decreased
LV wall thickness to radius ratio	Normal/decreased	Markedly increased	Increased
LV systolic function	Severly decreased	Increased	Normal/decreased
LA size relative to LV size	Increased in proportion to LV size	Increased out of proportion to LV size	Markedly increased out of proportion to LV size
LV outflow tract	Increased in size	Decreased in size	Normal
LV inflow tract	Normal	Decreased in size	Decreased in size

NOTE: LV = left ventricle; LA = left atrium

distribution of hypertrophy—the left ventricular cavity size is usually small, intraventricular gradients are common in the obstructive type, and systolic function is normal or hyperdynamic); and (3) restrictive cardiomyopathy, the least common, which can be divided into infiltrative and storage disorders (the latter characterized by an increase in ventricular wall thickness caused by infiltration or deposition of pathologic substances).

The above-mentioned pathologic features of primary cardiomyopathies can be well characterized by 2D echocardiography (Table 15–1). Additionally, hemodynamic information as well as insight into diastolic dysfunction can be obtained by use of conventional Doppler examinations. Recently, CFI has been shown to be a sensitive method for determining blood flow direction and velocity. It can effectively determine the location, size, and number of regurgitant lesions and identify areas of obstruction and turbulent flow.[3] This chapter will review the role of Doppler echocardiography in the evaluation of patients with cardiomyopathy.

DILATED CARDIOMYOPATHY

Dilated cardiomyopathy is characterized by reduced systolic ventricular function and chamber dilatation. These abnormalities produce a fairly characteristic color flow pattern which is commonly seen in patients with a dilated and poorly functioning left ventricle. Although on 2D echocardiography stagnant swirling of intracardiac blood flow occasionally may be visualized, CFI is the best method by which to accurately and vividly delineate this particular abnormal flow pattern.

When imaging with the transducer at the cardiac apex (flow directed toward the transducer), a distinctive pattern of the blood flow entering the left ventricle is visualized. This is characterized as a series of short boluses of flow during diastole giving the appearance of "puffs of smoke." Because of the low output state, the velocity of flow is relatively low; thus the usual color flow image of ventricular inflow is composed of darker shades of red on a velocity map. As diastole progresses, swirling of flow is visualized in a clockwise direction medially toward the ventricular septum. In the process of completion of this semicircular motion, the flow direction changes at the apical and midventricular levels so that the flow direction is away from the transducer. This is depicted as darker blue color on the velocity flow map (Fig. 15–1).

Ventricular dilatation, a common occurrence in dilated cardiomyopathy, is frequently associated with atrioventricular valvular regurgitation.[4–7] Thus, mitral and/or tricuspid regurgitation is commonly present in patients with this condition (Fig. 15–2). Although valvular regurgitation is generally

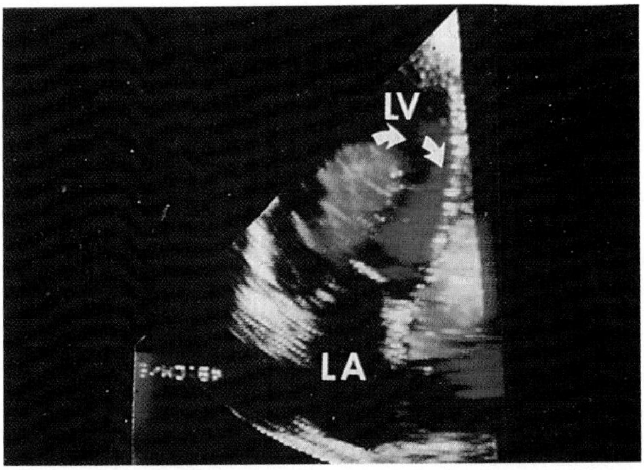

Figure 15 – 1. Color flow imaging in dilated cardiomyopathy. The characteristic low-velocity intraventricular swirling blood is seen in a dilated, poorly contractile left ventricle (LV). The darker red color depicts low-velocity blood flow toward the transducer. This blood flow "swirls" counterclockwise (arrows) at the apical and midventricular levels. This reversal of flow at these levels is seen as dark blue color, indicating low-velocity flow away from the transducer. LA = left atrium.

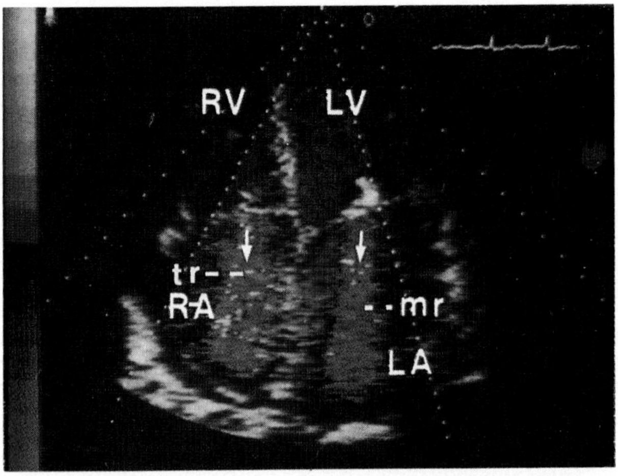

Figure 15 – 2. Apical four-chamber view showing severe mitral and tricuspid regurgitation in a patient with dilated cardiomyopathy. Greenish-blue jets in the left (MR) and right atria (tr) (arrows) represent regurgitant flow. LA = left atrium, LV = left ventricle, RA = right atrium, RV = right ventricle.

mild or moderate, it may be severe in some patients. Meese et al[4] demonstrated a very high incidence of atrioventricular valvular regurgitation in patients with dilated cardiomyopathy. Mitral regurgitation was noted in all patients (100 percent), and tricuspid regurgitation was present in 91 percent.

Although the reasons for development of mitral regurgitation remain uncertain, it is thought that left ventricular dilatation plays a major factor. As the chamber dilates, the left ventricular cavity is displaced downward and laterally; as a consequence, the valve leaflets are displaced inferiorly with resultant valvular incompetence (Fig. 15–3). In addition, the mitral anulus may be dilated, and its dilatation appears to be related to the presence of mitral regurgitation.[8] The complex geometric interaction between changes in anular circumference, total leaflet area, and derangements of the subvalvular apparatus may result in ineffective valve closure and mitral regurgitation.[5]

Although tricuspid regurgitation is commonly associated with right ventricular dilatation, its pathogenic mechanisms have been less rigorously studied. It has been demonstrated that tricuspid anular size, measured by 2D echocardiographic analysis of multiple tricuspid inflow views, is significantly enlarged in patients with functional tricuspid regurgitation.[9]

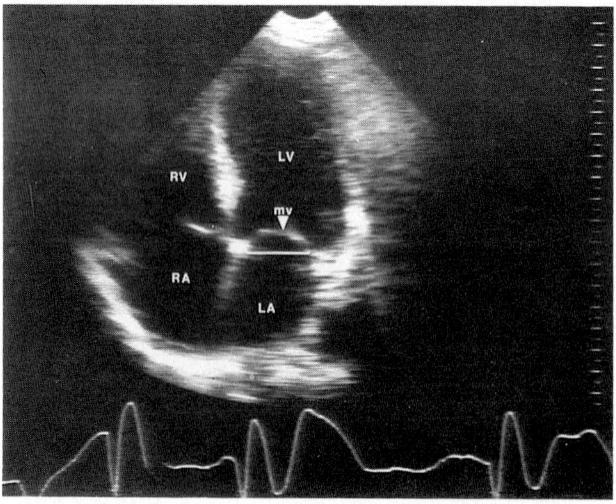

Figure 15–3. Apical four-chamber view in systole of dilated cardiomyopathy. The left ventricle (LV) is diffusely hypokinetic. There is incomplete closure of the mitral valve (MV). The closed leaflets fail to reach the plane of the mitral anulus (horizontal line). LA = left atrium, RA = right atrium, RV = right ventricle.

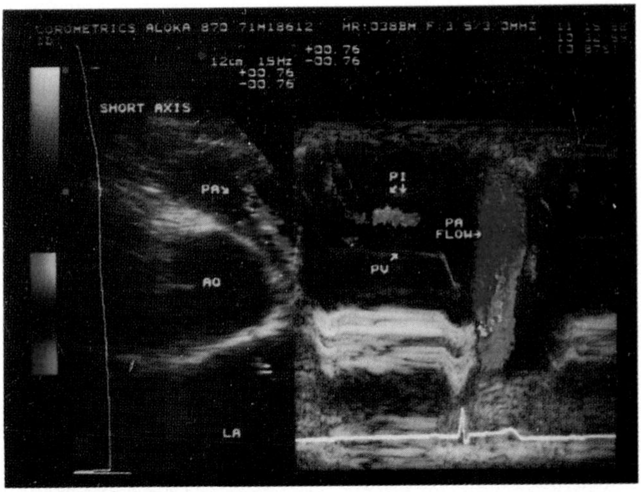

Figure 15–4. Pulmonic insufficiency (PI) in a patient with dilated cardiomyopathy and pulmonary hypertension. *Left*: Parasternal short axis view demonstrating a red jet of PI emanating from the pulmonary artery (PA). AO = aorta, LA = left atrium. *Right*: Color M-mode tracing showing both diastolic regurgitant signals (PI) and pulmonary artery (PA) systolic flow (blue jet with red in center, due to aliasing). PV = pulmonic valve.

This may serve as a major mechanism of tricuspid regurgitation in dilated cardiomyopathy.

Pulmonary and aortic valvular regurgitation occur less often. Missri et al[10] found that pulmonary regurgitation was present in 20 percent and aortic regurgitation was present in 40 percent of the patients with dilated cardiomyopathy. The pulmonic valve regurgitation is best visualized in the parasternal short axis view. From this orientation, pulmonic regurgitation is characterized as a yellow-orange "flamelike" jet directed toward the transducer (Fig. 15–4). The development of passive pulmonary hypertension in patients with chronic mitral regurgitation and severe dilated cardiomyopathy may contribute to insufficiency of the pulmonic valve, but this has not been proven. The reasons for the 40-percent prevalence of aortic regurgitation are less clear. In a preliminary report from our laboratory on patients with dilated cardiomyopathy, there was significant aortic anular dilatation in patients with aortic regurgitation versus those patients without aortic regurgitation.[10] These findings suggest that aortic anular size, as well as dilatation of the left ventricular outflow tract, is a major contributing factor in the development of aortic regurgitation.

Doppler techniques are helpful in accurate determination of the presence and severity of pulmonary hypertension in patients with dilated cardiomyopathy (see Chap. 13). The systolic pulmonary artery pressure can be calculated from the peak tricuspid regurgitant velocity obtained by CFI-guided CW Doppler examination. This calculation can be made by adding the determined transtricuspid systolic gradient to the calculated or assumed right atrial pressure. Similarly, the peak end-diastolic pulmonary regurgitant velocity can be used to determine the pulmonary artery diastolic pressure.

The flow velocity profile of the left ventricular outflow or ascending aorta has been used to evaluate systolic left ventricular function in dilated cardiomyopathy.[11] Patients with dilated cardiomyopathy exhibit a decrease in peak flow velocity, ejection time, and area under the curve (flow velocity integral, FVI), which reflects a reduction in stroke volume. The time to peak acceleration of the aortic flow pulse shows progressive prolongation with decreasing pump function.

Serial analysis of the Doppler-derived aortic flow velocity profile has been performed in patients with dilated cardiomyopathy undergoing afterload reduction with vasodilator therapy.[12,13] The reproducibility of these measurements has been analyzed by Gardin et al,[11] who suggest that differences of 10 percent in FVI, 11 percent in ejection time, 13 percent in peak flow velocity, and 17 percent in acceleration time would constitute significant hemodynamic changes. A good correlation between Doppler-derived estimates of cardiac output and cardiac output measured by thermodilution during such vasodilator interventions ($r = 0.88$) suggests that noninvasive monitoring of the efficacy of vasodilator therapy is feasible.[13] Similarly, other investigators have found that the percent increase in the Doppler-derived aortic FVI correlated well with the percent increase in stroke volume measured by thermodilution ($r = 0.88$), and that the percent increase in peak aortic flow velocity correlated well with the percent decrease in systemic vascular resistance ($r = 0.89$) during vasodilator therapy of patients with dilated cardiomyopathy.[12]

The Doppler-derived mitral flow velocities have also proved useful in the evaluation of diastolic function in dilated cardiomyopathy. Takenaka et al[14] have analyzed the mitral flow velocity waveforms in patients with dilated cardiomyopathy. In contrast to normal individuals, patients with dilated cardiomyopathy (without mitral regurgitation) had increased peak flow velocity during atrial systole with respect to the peak flow velocity during early diastolic filling. In this study, fractional mitral FVIs were not measured; however, the inversion of peak velocities in late and early diastole suggests that the proportion of the FVI falling in the last half of diastole is increased in these patients. These findings suggest an increased dependence on atrial systole for diastolic filling. In this same study, patients with dilated cardiomyopathy and mitral regurgitation had peak velocities during rapid diastolic filling that were similar to those in normal subjects. This observation probably reflects the increased left atrial–to–left ventricular pressure gradient in early diastole secondary to the "V" pressure wave of mitral regurgitation (see Chap. 12, Fig. 12–6).

HYPERTROPHIC CARDIOMYOPATHY

Hypertrophic cardiomyopathy is characterized by idiopathic hypertrophy of the heart, with or without obstruction to left ventricular outflow. There are few conditions in which cardiac ultrasound has played so critical a role in defining the disorder, understanding its pathophysiology, quantitating its severity, and assessing the effects of medical or surgical therapy. The condition was first recognized pathologically by Teare,[15] who showed asymmetric hypertrophy of the heart involving the ventricular septum, and sometimes extending to the anterolateral free wall, in young adults who had had sudden death.

Cardiac ultrasonography has contributed significantly to our understanding of the disorder. Two-dimensional and M-mode echocardiography allowed better definition of the site and variable extent of hypertrophy and the relationship of the extent of hypertrophy to symptoms and prognosis.[16–20] Unusual sites of hypertrophy localized to the apex[21–24] or causing midventricular obstruction[19] were also recognized. Pulsed wave Doppler (PD) echocardiography allowed us to better characterize abnormal left ventricular and aortic ejection dynamics and to focus attention on the importance of diastolic abnormalities.[25–28] Continuous wave (CW) Doppler studies made it possible to more precisely quantitate the left ventricular outflow pressure gradient.[3,29] Finally, CFI[30,31] has made important contributions to our understanding of the pathophysiology of the obstruction and to quantitating the degree of associated mitral regurgitation. As medical and surgical therapy have evolved and improved, echocardiographic and Doppler studies have played an invaluable role in assessing the benefits of therapy.

Echocardiographic Diagnosis

The diagnosis of hypertrophic cardiomyopathy is established by characteristic echocardiographic features (Table 15–2). These include asymmetric septal hypertrophy (ASH), systolic anterior motion (SAM) of the mitral valve apparatus, and normal or small left ventricular cavity size with usually hyperdynamic systolic function (Fig. 15–5). However, there may be several different patterns of left ventricular hypertrophy present consist-

TABLE 15–2. Echocardiographic Diagnosis of Hypertrophic Cardiomyopathy

A. Left ventricular hypertrophy
   1. Asymmetrical hypertrophy
      a. Ventricular septal
      b. Midventricular
      c. Apical
      d. Posteroseptal and/or lateral wall
   2. Symmetrical (concentric hypertrophy)

B. Right ventricular hypertrophy

C. Systolic anterior motion of the mitral valve apparatus

D. Small left ventricular cavity and hyperdynamic systolic function

E. Decreased ventricular septal thickening

F. Partial closure of aortic valve in mid-systole (with obstruction)

G. Ground-glass appearance of hypertrophied myocardium

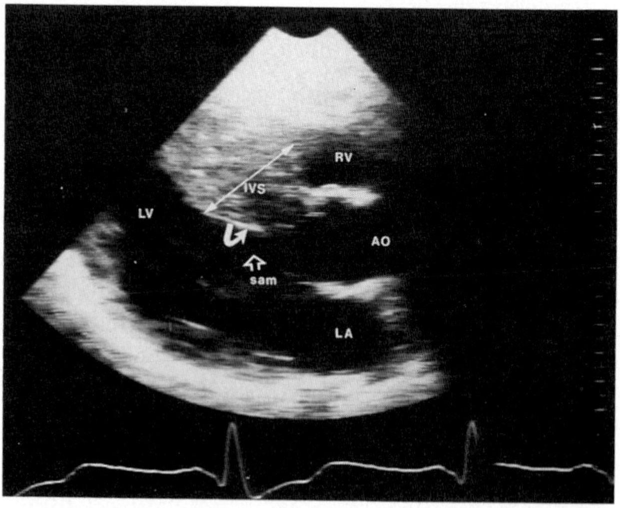

Figure 15–5. Parasternal long axis view in systole of obstructive hypertrophic cardiomyopathy. There is marked septal hypertrophy (IVS), and a ground-glass appearance of the abnormal septum. An endocardial plaque is visible on the septal surface (curved arrow), and there is systolic anterior motion (SAM) of the mitral valve. AO = aorta, LA = left atrium, LV = left ventricle, RV = right ventricle.

ing of concentric hypertrophy or of asymmetric hypertrophy of the ventricular septum, the free wall, or the ventricular apex.[17,23,24]

The specificity of ASH has been increased by better definition of the septum by 2D echocardiography and the use of a septal to posterior wall ratio of 1.5:1. Although minor degrees of SAM can occur in other conditions, usually because of anterior bowing of chordae, the presence of prolonged SAM septal contact always correlates with a dynamic outflow tract pressure gradient. Occasionally this is seen in the absence of ASH, and almost always in conditions in which there are hyperdynamic left ventricular wall motion and a narrowed left ventricular outflow tract.

In addition to the hypertrophy and presence of SAM of the mitral valve, other echocardiographic features of hypertrophic cardiomyopathy include: (1) ground-glass appearance of the hypertrophied myocardium, especially of the interventricular septum; (2) hypokinetic septal motion with reduced systolic thickening of the septum; (3) generally normal or increased motion of the posterior wall; (4) partial closure of the aortic valve in midsystole in those patients with obstruction to left ventricular outflow; and (5) left atrial enlargement, especially in patients with resting obstruction.[19]

Doppler Assessment of Left Ventricular Ejection Dynamics and Obstruction

Hypertrophic cardiomyopathy can be obstructive or nonobstructive. Obstruction can be present at rest, or may be latent. With latent obstruction no resting pressure gradient is present, but one can be provoked with maneuvers or agents that decrease afterload or increase contractility. Systolic anterior motion and midsystolic closure of the aortic valve often indicate a resting gradient.

Doppler techniques identify subaortic obstruction and allow precise measurement of the pressure gradient.[29,32,33] In normal ventricles, there is gradual flow velocity acceleration from the left ventricular apex toward the aortic valve during systole. Maximum velocity in the left ventricular outflow tract is usually 1 m/s or less; it may be slightly greater in high output states. Pulsed Doppler echocardiography, used in the setting of hypertrophic cardiomyopathy with obstruction, shows increased systolic flow velocity at the site or immediately distal to SAM, usually accompanied by aliasing of the pulsed wave signal (Fig. 15–6). Velocities then decrease in the left ventricular outflow tract just below the aortic valve, as the flow area increases.

The CW Doppler recording across the left ventricular outflow tract in hypertrophic obstructive cardiomyopathy displays a distinctive signal

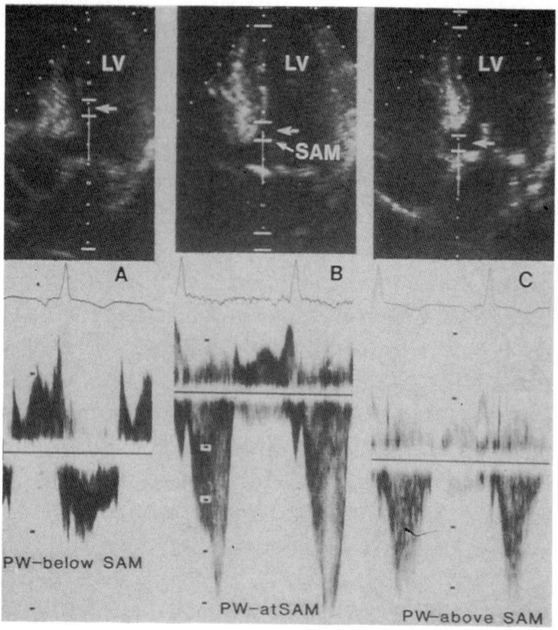

Figure 15–6. Pulsed wave (PW) mapping of left ventricular (LV) outflow jet, taken in apical four-chamber view, from a patient with obstructive hypertrophic cardiomyopathy with SAM. (A) Low-velocity flow before SAM septal contact. (B) High-velocity jet at region of SAM septal contact (using high PRF). (C) Velocities decrease in outflow tract above level of SAM septal contact.

(Fig. 15–7) with a characteristic early- to mid-systolic acceleration of the flow velocity that peaks in late systole, which is consistent with the dynamic temporal evolution of the gradient. The subaortic pressure gradient can be accurately measured using a modified Bernoulli equation ($\Delta P = 4V^2$).[3] Some patients exhibit obstruction at the midventricular level rather than at the outflow. Midventricular narrowing can be detected by 2D echocardiography and the gradient measured by Doppler echocardiography.

When CW tracings are recorded, care must be taken to distinguish the outflow tract jet from that of mitral regurgitation, since they have similar directions and, when the gradient is severe, similar velocities. The outflow jet starts after the QRS wave (later than mitral regurgitation), often has a low-velocity presystolic outflow signal, and usually has a characteristic change in acceleration velocity (see Chap. 4, Fig. 4–7).

Color flow imaging of the left ventricular outflow tract in patients with hypertrophic cardiomyopathy shows a normal-velocity laminar flow during early systole. As ejection progresses, velocities accelerate in the midventricular region and result in aliasing with resultant color reversal in this region. This is followed by intraventricular obstruction as a result of SAM of the mitral apparatus. Left ventricular outflow tract obstruction is manifested in the flow map as a mosaic of color within this area (Figs. 15–8 and 15–9). Late in systole, as velocities decrease toward normal, laminar flow is again visualized.[30] Once the areas of increased flow velocity and turbulence have been identified by CFI, then CW Doppler examination guided by the flow image will permit determination of the intraventricular pressure gradient.

Aortic Flow Velocity

Aortic flow velocity waveforms in patients with obstructive hypertrophic cardiomyopathy are distinctly abnormal and differ markedly from those in patients with nonobstructive hypertrophic cardiomyopathy or of normal subjects.[34,36] A "bifid" flow velocity pattern (notching in midsystole) is present in the majority of patients with the obstructive component, with the second peak constituting a relatively small fraction of the overall forward flow velocity.

Studies of ascending aortic blood flow in patients with obstructive hypertrophic cardiomyopathy have demonstrated that midsystolic flow

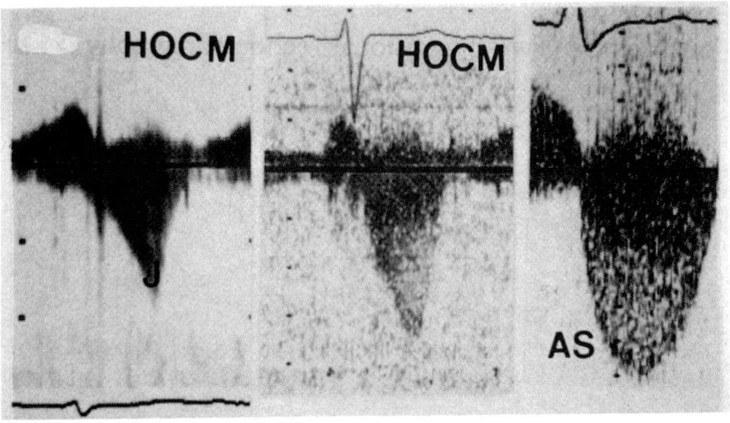

Figure 15–7. Continuous wave Doppler tracing of the left ventricular outflow tract recorded from the apex from two patients with hypertrophic obstructive cardiomyopathy (HOCM) (*left* and *middle*) and from a patient with valvular aortic stenosis (AS) (*right*). In HOCM, the rise in velocity during early systole is gradual, but then the dynamic obstruction causes a steep rise to a maximum in late systole, giving a characteristic dagger-shaped flow velocity profile different from that seen in AS.

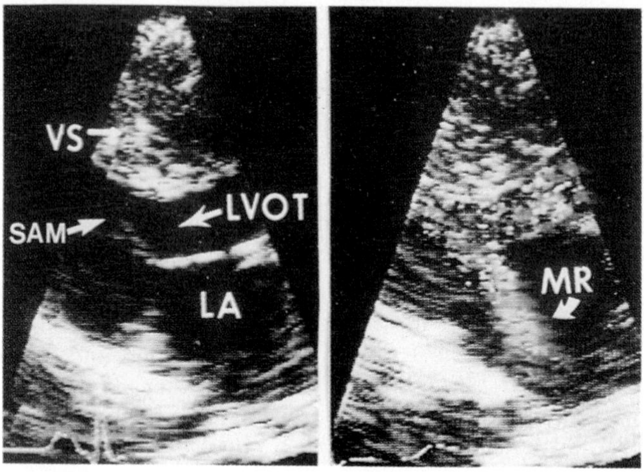

Figure 15–8. Two-dimensional echocardiogram and CFI in a patient with obstructive hypertrophic cardiomyopathy, parasternal long axis view. *Left*: 2D echocardiogram showing asymmetrical septal hypertrophy (VS) and systolic anterior motion (SAM) of the anterior mitral leaflet contributing to left ventricular outflow tract (LVOT) obstruction. The left atrium (LA) is enlarged. *Right*: Turbulent flow (mosaic pattern) is seen in the LVOT, and mitral regurgitation (MR) directed toward posterior LA atrial wall.

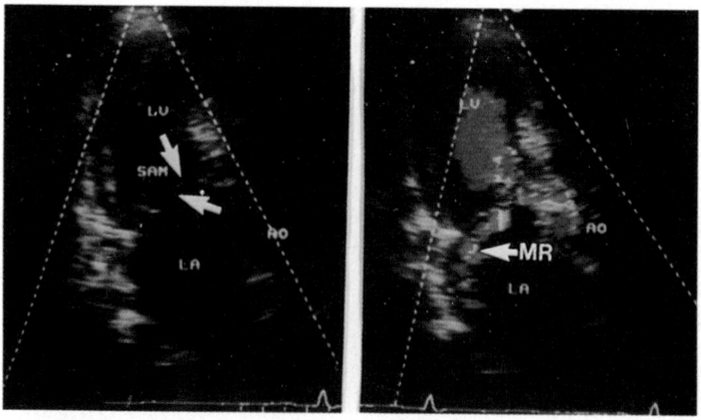

Figure 15–9. Two-dimensional echocardiogram and CFI in a patient with obstructive hypertrophic cardiomyopathy. *Left*: Two arrows indicate site of SAM septal contact with marked narrowing of outflow tract. *Right*: Color flow imaging showing acceleration of flow at the approach to the site of SAM septal contact, with blue outflow becoming brighter and finally aliasing. At the site of SAM septal contact, the outflow jet is narrowed; then it diverges into two turbulent high-velocity jets, one directed toward the posterior outflow tract and the other an eccentric posteriorly directed jet of mitral regurgitation (MR). AO = aorta, LA = left atrium, LV = left ventricle.

does not cease but rather is inhomogeneous, with more flow in the anterior portion of the aorta. Flow in the posterior portion of the aorta is reduced or absent, or may even demonstrate flow reversal.[37] Thus, when flow across the aorta is not uniform, it follows that a single flow velocity signal may not be representative of true aortic flow and therefore must be interpreted with caution.

Mitral Regurgitation

Mitral regurgitation occurs in almost all patients with obstructive cardiomyopathy, as shown by angiographic,[19,38] indicator dilution,[19,38] and Doppler[3,26,30,32,39] techniques. Because the pressure gradient correlates directly with the severity of SAM, it follows that the mitral regurgitation is caused by systolic anterior displacement of the mitral apparatus, which results in abnormal leaflet coaptation. Further evidence for this can be seen from color flow assessment of the eccentric nature of the mitral regurgitation jet, as shown in Figs. 15–8 and 15–9. The mitral leaflets in systole are directly anteriorly toward the ventricular septum, creating a funnel on their left atrial side that results in a posteriorly directed mitral regurgitation jet. Because of the eccentric nature of the jet, its severity can be underestimated by PD mapping alone. Although mitral regurgitation starts in early systole, it is maximal after the onset of SAM.[30]

In patients without obstruction of the left ventricular outflow tract, Doppler evidence of mitral regurgitation is present in only about 35 percent of cases[39] and is usually mild. In these patients the mitral regurgitation is likely caused by a more anterior position of the mitral apparatus,[40] mitral anular calcification, or other leaflet abnormalities.

Diastolic Filling Abnormalities

Most patients with obstruction at rest or severe hypertrophy have evidence of impaired diastolic left ventricular filling on Doppler examination.[25–28] When left ventricular filling is impaired, abnormalities may include prolongation of the isovolumic relaxation time, as well as delayed and reduced early diastolic filling with reduced early diastolic velocity (E) and flow, decreased half-time and half-filling fraction, shortened diastasis, and increased atrial systolic velocity (A) and flow,[25–28] as shown in Fig. 15–10. There is, however, significant variability; some patients with marked hypertrophy and obstruction have perfectly normal left ventricular filling parameters.[41] This variability is likely caused by such factors as loading conditions, the degree of mitral regurgitation, age, heart rate, and treatment.

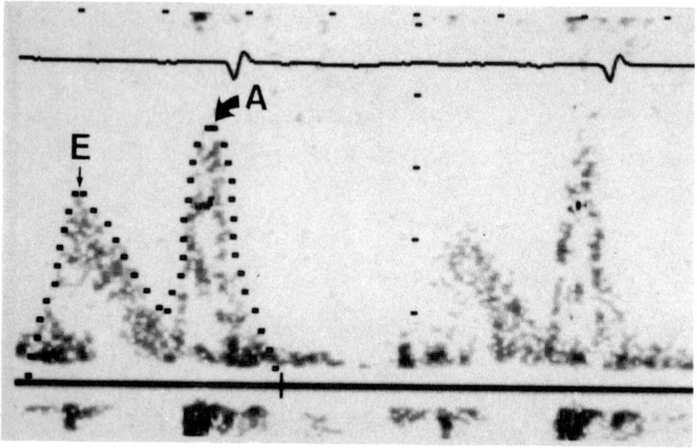

Figure 15–10. Pulsed wave Doppler study showing the characteristic diastolic filling abnormalities in obstructive hypertrophic cardiomyopathy. Exaggerated atrial systolic flow (A) is present, with reduced early diastolic velocity (E), and shortened diastasis, suggesting impaired left ventricular relaxation. (Scale marks = 20 cm/s)

Doppler Echocardiographic Evaluation of Therapy

Echocardiography and Doppler studies are useful in monitoring and evaluating the results of medical and surgical therapy, as listed in Table 15–3. Decreased or abolished left ventricular outflow obstruction, improved diastolic function, and decrease or abolition of mitral regurgitation are specific therapeutic goals that are readily evaluated by combined 2D echocardiography, conventional Doppler echocardiography, and CFI examination.

RESTRICTIVE CARDIOMYOPATHY

The restrictive cardiomyopathies are the least common of the three major categories of cardiomyopathic disorders seen in Western countries.[2,42] The restrictive cardiomyopathies are characterized by a primary abnormality of diastolic ventricular function (decreased distensibility) with normal to near-normal systolic function and normal ventricular internal dimensions.[43,44] Generally, diastolic ventricular function in the restrictive cardiomyopathies can be primarily impaired in the absence of morphologically detectable myocardial or endomyocardial disease (idiopathic restrictive cardiomyopathy), because of (1) extracellular (interstitial) infiltration of abnormal substances; (2) intracellular accumulation of abnormal sub-

TABLE 15–3. Echocardiographic and Doppler Assessment of Efficacy of Medical and Surgical Treatment

A. Decreased or abolished obstruction
   1. Decrease or abolition of SAM
   2. Decrease of LVOT velocity
   3. Disappearance of systolic aortic notching
   4. Normalized aortic systolic flow pattern

B. Decrease or abolition of mitral regurgitation

C. Improved diastolic function
   1. Increased LV filling during early diastole
   2. Lower atrial LV filling velocity
   3. Longer diastasis
   4. Shortening of the isovolumic relaxation time

NOTE: LV = left ventricle; LVOT = left ventricular ourflow tract; SAM = systolic anterior motion

stances; or (3) disease of endomyocardium (Table 15–4). This section will focus on some of the most common restrictive cardiomyopathies.

Cardiac Amyloidosis

Echocardiography is the procedure of choice for noninvasive detection of cardiac amyloidosis.[45,46] The constellation of findings of a small or normal left cavity size and markedly increased thickness of the ventricular walls,

TABLE 15–4. Classification of the Restrictive Cardiomyopathies

A. Myocardial
   1. Noninfiltrative
      a. Idiopathic
      b. Scleroderma
   2. Infiltrative
      a. Amyloid
      b. Sarcoid
      c. Gaucher's disease
      d. Hurler's disease
   3. Storage diseases
      a. Hemochromatosis
      b. Fabry's disease
      c. Glycogen storage diseases

B. Endomyocardial
   1. Endomyocardial fibrosis
   2. Hypereosinophilic syndrome
   3. Carcinoid
   4. Metastatic malignancies
   5. Radiation
   6. Anthracycline toxicity

associated with a highly abnormal texture, make up the characteristic 2D echocardiographic appearance of cardiac amyloidosis. The ventricular septum, left and right ventricular walls, atrial septum, papillary muscles, and cardiac valves show increased thickness (Fig. 15–11). The ventricular septum may be thicker than the free wall; this may lead to asymmetric hypertrophy of the left ventricle. Global left ventricular systolic function is variable—often normal in the early stages, and reduced in the more advanced stages. The atria are usually enlarged, and pericardial effusions are common.[45–47] The granular sparkling appearance of the thickened ventricular walls is presumably due to the tissue characteristics imparted by amyloid deposits[47] (Fig. 15–11).

Pulsed Doppler echocardiography and CFI in cardiac amyloidosis frequently reveal mitral and tricuspid regurgitation (Fig. 15–12), much less commonly aortic and pulmonic regurgitation—all usually mild.[48] Right ventricular pressure can be assessed by CW Doppler interrogation of the tricuspid regurgitant jet.

The stage of amyloid infiltration determines diastolic ventricular function as assessed by Doppler. Early cardiac amyloidosis (mean ventricular wall thickness $<$15 mm) reveals an abnormal relaxation pattern[48,49] characterized by decreased early E diastolic ventricular inflow velocities and a prolonged deceleration time ($>$240 ms), increased A velocities (thus an increased A/E ratio), and a prolonged isovolumic relaxation time ($>$86 ms).[50–52] The advanced state of cardiac amyloidosis (mean ventricular wall thickness $\geq$15 mm) manifests a typical restrictive pattern characterized by increased early E diastolic ventricular inflow velocities with short-

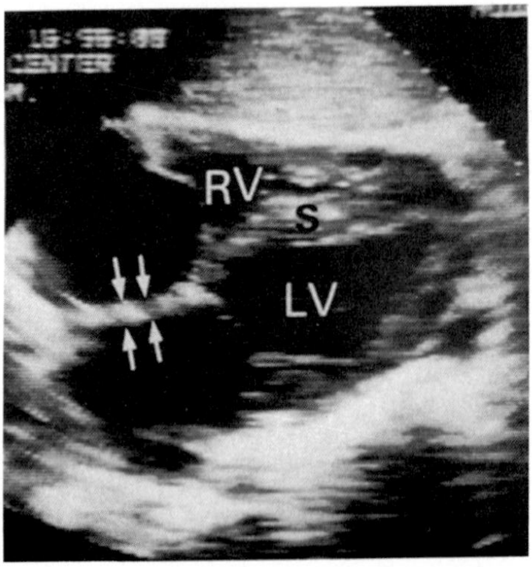

Figure 15–11. Two-dimensional subcostal view in cardiac amyloidosis reveals biatrial enlargement and a thickened interatrial septum (dual white arrows). Note the thickened ventricular walls and septum (S) and small right (RV) and left (LV) ventricular cavities. The increased echogenicity of the ventricular septum (S) is apparent.

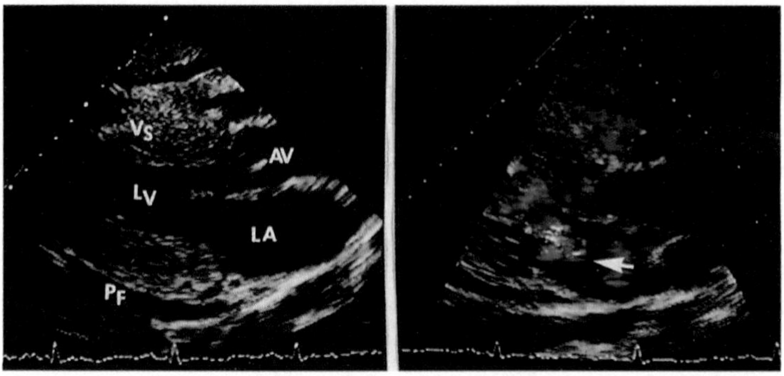

Figure 15-12. Two-dimensional echocardiogram and CFI, parasternal long axis view. *Left*: The left ventricular (LV) cavity size is normal, with markedly thickened ventricular walls and its characteristic granular sparkling appearance. A small pericardial effusion (PF) is also present. AV = aortic valve, LA = left atrium, VS = ventricular septum. *Right*: CFI shows mild mitral regurgitation (arrow).

ened deceleration times (<160 ms), decreased A velocities (with a decreased A/E ratio), and a normal isovolumic relaxation time.[48,49] In brief, Doppler diastolic filling patterns in cardiac amyloidosis reflect not only the presence, but also the degree, of infiltration of the myocardium. Accordingly, normal, early, intermediate, and advanced stages have been identified.[48]

Cardiac Sarcoidosis

Sarcoidosis is a multisystem granulomatous disease that involves the heart.[53] Granulomas are found at autopsy in the myocardial interstium in 25 percent of patients with sarcoidosis.[54] Two-dimensional echocardiography may detect focal areas of myocardial involvement or aneurysm formation (the latter often a consequence of corticosteroid therapy[55]). Color flow imaging is utilized in evaluating valvular regurgitation which results from granuloma deposits in the papillary muscles.[48,55] Rarely, there may be evidence of restrictive hemodynamics with extensive myocardial involvement.[56]

Hemochromatosis

Echocardiography is a useful noninvasive technique in the assessment of hemochromatosis, since it can detect clinically occult heart involvement, do follow-up on patients sequentially, and assess left ventricular function after phlebotomy.[57]

There is a wide spectrum of echocardiographic findings in patients with primary hemochromatosis. These features include left ventricular dilatation as well as normal systolic wall thickness, impaired systolic function, and left atrial enlargement.[48]

Doppler echocardiography demonstrates a spectrum of right and left ventricular diastolic function abnormalities. Some patients have demonstrated a restrictive pattern, whereas other patients have shown an abnormal relaxation pattern.[48] Color flow imaging has also been useful in the semiquantitation of valvular regurgitation in this condition (Fig. 15–13).

Carcinoid Endocardial Disease

Carcinoid syndrome results in cardiac involvement as a late complication in 50 percent of cases.[58] Endocardial involvement of the pulmonic and tricuspid valves with stenosis and regurgitation dominates the clinical picture,[58,59] but a restrictive cardiomyopathy has been described.[60] Accurate diagnosis of cardiac involvement is important because of the potential for surgical treatment.[61] Two-dimensional echocardiography identifies thickened, stiff, and retracted pulmonic and tricuspid valves.[62–65] Doppler interrogation reveals increased pulmonic systolic velocities and increased tricuspid diastolic velocities with an increased pressure gradient half-time (stenosis of each valve), in addition to pulmonic and tricuspid regurgitation.[62–65] Detection of coexistent endocardial restriction is difficult.

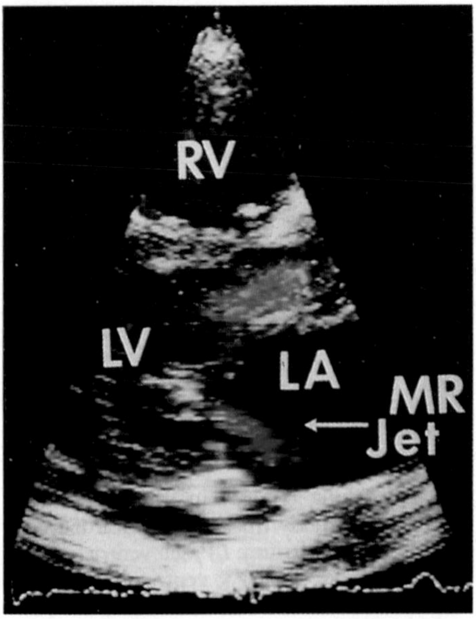

Figure 15–13. CFI in a patient with primary hemochromatosis. There is mild mitral regurgitation (MR) depicted by the eccentric blue jet in the left atrium (LA). LV = left ventricle, RV = right ventricle.

REFERENCES

1. Goodwin J: The frontiers of cardiomyopathy. *Br Heart J* 48:1, 1982.
2. Brandenberg R, Chazov E, Cherion G, et al: Report of the WHO/ISFC task force on definition and classification of cardiomyopathies. *Circulation* 64:437A, 1981.
3. Hatle L, Angelsen B: *Doppler Ultrasound in Cardiology*, 2d ed. Philadelphia, Lea & Febiger, 1985.
4. Meese R, Adams D, Kisslo J. Assessment of valvular regurgitation by conventional and color flow Doppler in dilated cardiomyopathy. *Echocardiography* 3:505, 1986.
5. Boltwood C, Tei C, Wong M, et al: Quantitative echocardiography of the mitral complex in dilated cardiomyopathy: The mechanism of functional mitral regurgitation. *Circulation* 68:498, 1983.
6. Ballester M, Jajoo J, Rees S, et al: The mechanism of mitral regurgitation in dilated left ventricle. *Clin Cardiol* 6:333, 1983.
7. Pollick C, Pittman M, Filly K, et al: Mitral and aortic valve orifice area in normal subjects and in patients with congestive cardiomyopathy: Determination by two-dimensional echocardiography. *Am J Cardiol* 49:1191, 1982.
8. Frankl W, Brest A: *Valvular Heart Disease: Comprehensive Evaluation and Management*. Philadelphia, FA Davis, 1986.
9. Tei C, Pilgrim J, Shah P, et al: The tricuspid valve annulus: Study of size and motion in normal subjects and in patients with tricuspid regurgitation. *Circulation* 66:665, 1982.
10. Missri J, Hognason J, Tenet W, et al: Functional multivalvular regurgitation in dilated cardiomyopathy detected by Doppler echocardiography (abstr), in *Proceedings of the X World Congress of Cardiology*. Washington, DC, 1986.
11. Gardin J, Seri L, Elkayam U, et al: Evaluation of dilated cardiomyopathy by pulsed Doppler echocardiography. *Am Heart J* 10:1057, 1983.
12. Elkayam V, Gardin J, Berkley R, et al: The use of Doppler flow-velocity measurement to assess the hemodynamic response to vasodilators in patients with heart failure. *Circulation* 67:377, 1983.
13. Rose J, Nanna M, Rahimtoola S, et al: Accuracy of determination of changes in cardiac output by transcutaneous continuous wave Doppler computer. *Am J Cardiol* 54:1099, 1984.
14. Takenaka K, Dabestani A, Gardin J, et al: Pulsed Doppler echocardiographic study of left ventricular filling in dilated cardiomyopathy. *Am J Cardiol* 58:143, 1986.
15. Teare R: Asymmetrical hypertrophy of the heart in young adults. *Br Heart J* 20:1, 1958.
16. Martin R, Rakowski H, French J, et al: Idiopathic hypertrophic subaortic stenosis viewed by wide angle phased-array echocardiography. *Circulation* 59:1206, 1979.

17. Maron B, Gottdiener J, Epstein S: Patterns and significance of distribution of left ventricular hypertrophy in hypertrophic cardiomyopathy. *Am J Cardiol* 48:418, 1981.

18. Shapiro L, McKenna W: Distribution of left ventricular hypertrophy in hypertrophic cardiomyopathy: A two-dimensional echocardiographic study. *J Am Coll Cardiol* 2:437, 1983.

19. Wigle E, Sasson Z, Henderson M, et al: Hypertrophic cardiomyopathy: The importance of the site and extent of hypertrophy. A review. *Prog Cardiovasc Dis* 28:1, 1985.

20. Rakowski H, Fulop J, Wigle E: The role of echocardiography in the assessment of hypertrophic cardiomyopathy. *Postgrad Med J* 62:557, 1986.

21. Sakamoto T, Tei C, Muramaya M, et al: Giant negative T-wave inversion as a manifestation of asymmetric apical hypertrophy (AAH) of the left ventricle. Echocardiographic and ultrasonocardiotomographic study. *Jpn Heart J* 17:611, 1976.

22. Yamaguchi H, Ishimura T, Nishiyama S, et al: Hypertrophic non-obstructive cardiomyopathy with giant negative T-waves (apical hypertrophy): Ventriculographic and echocardiographic features in 30 patients. *Am J Cardiol* 44:401, 1979.

23. Keren G, Belhassen B, Sherez J, et al: Apical hypertrophic cardiomyopathy: Evaluation by non-invasive and invasive technique in 23 patients. *Circulation* 71:45, 1985.

24. Louie E, Maron B: Apical hypertrophic cardiomyopathy: Clinical and two-dimensional echocardiographic assessment. *Ann Intern Med* 106:663, 1987.

25. Bryg R, Pearson A, Williams G, Labovitz A: Left ventricular systolic and diastolic flow abnormalities determined by Doppler echocardiography in obstructive hypertrophic cardiomyopathy. *Am J Cardiol* 59:925, 1987.

26. Takenaka K, Dabestani A, Gardin J, et al: Left ventricular filling in hypertrophic cardiomyopathy: A pulsed Doppler echocardiographic study. *J Am Coll Cardiol* 7:1263, 1986.

27. Gidding S, Snider A, Rocchini A, et al: Left ventricular diastolic filling in children with hypertrophic cardiomyopathy: Assessment with pulsed Doppler echocardiography. *J Am Coll Cardiol* 8:310, 1986.

28. Maron B, Arce J, Bonow R, et al: Non-invasive assessment of left ventricular relaxation and filling by pulsed echocardiography in hypertrophic cardiomyopathy (abstr). *Circulation* 70:18, 1984.

29. Sasson Z, Yock P, Hatle L, et al: Doppler echocardiographic determination of the pressure gradient in hypertrophic cardiomyopathy. *J Am Coll Cardiol* 11:752, 1988.

30. Nishimura R, Tajik A, Reeder G, Seward J: Evaluation of hypertrophic cardiomyopathy by Doppler color flow imaging: Initial observations. *Mayo Clin Proc* 61:631, 1986.

31. Stewart W, Schiavone W, Salcedo E, et al: Intraoperative Doppler echocardiography in hypertrophic cardiomyopathy: Correlations with the obstructive pressure gradient. *J Am Coll Cardiol* 10:327, 1987.

32. Yock P, Hatle L, Popp R: Patterns and timing of Doppler detected intracavitary and aortic flow in hypertrophic cardiomyopathy. *J Am Coll Cardiol* 8:1047, 1986.

33. Rakowski H, Sasson Z, Wigle E: Echocardiographic and Doppler assessment of hypertrophic cardiomyopathy. *J Am Soc Echo* 1:31, 1988.

34. Gardin J, Dabestani A, Glasgow G, et al: Echocardiographic and Doppler flow observations in obstructed and non-obstructed hypertrophic cardiomyopathy. *Am J Cardiol* 56:614, 1985.

35. Maron B, Gottdiener J, Arce J, et al: Dynamic subaortic obstruction in hypertrophic cardiomyopathy analysis by pulsed Doppler echocardiography. *J Am Coll Cardiol* 6:1, 1985.

36. Cogswell T, Sagar K, Wann L: Left ventricular ejection dynamics in hypertrophic cardiomyopathy and aortic stenosis: Comparison with the use of Doppler echocardiography. *Am Heart J* 113:110, 1987.

37. Vieli A, Jenni R, Anliker M: Spatial velocity distributions in the ascending aorta of healthy humans and cardiac patients. *IEEE Trans Biomed Eng* 33:32, 1986.

38. Wigle E, Adelman A, Auger P, et al: Mitral regurgitation in muscular subaortic stenosis. *Am J Cardiol* 24:698, 1969.

39. Prieur T, Fulop J, Sasson Z, et al: The relationship between mitral regurgitation and left ventricular outflow in hypertrophic cardiomyopathy. *Circulation* 72:156, 1985.

40. Gilbert G, Pollick C, Adelman A, Wigle E: Hypertrophic cardiomyopathy: The subclassification by M-mode echocardiography. *Am J Cardiol* 45:861, 1980.

41. Sasson Z, Hatle L, Appleton C, Popp R: Doppler ultrasound assessment of diastolic function in hypertrophic cardiomyopathy (abstr). *Circulation* 74:228, 1986.

42. Abelman W: Classification and natural history of primary myocardial disease. *Prog Cardiovasc Dis* 27:73, 1984.

43. Child J, Shah P: Restrictive and infiltrative cardiomyopathies. In Pohost G, O'Rourke R (eds): *Cardiac Imaging*. Boston, Little, Brown, 1988.

44. Seward J, Tajik A: Restrictive cardiomyopathies. *Curr Opin Cardiol* 2:499, 1987.

45. Cueto-Garcia L, Tajik A, Kyle R, et al: Serial echocardiographic observation in patients with primary systemic amyloidosis: An introduction to the concept of early (asymptomatic) amyloid infiltration of the heart. *Mayo Clin Proc* 59:589, 1984.

46. Cueto-Garcia L, Reeder G, Kyle R, et al: Echocardiographic findings in systemic amyloidosis: Spectrum of cardiac involvement and relation to survival. *J Am Coll Cardiol* 6:737, 1985.

47. Siqueira-Filho A, Cunha L, Tajik A, et al: M-mode and two-dimensional echocardiographic features in cardiac amyloidosis. *Circulation* 63:188, 1981.

48. Klein A, Oh J, Miller F, et al: Two-dimensional and Doppler echocardiographic assessment of infiltrative cardiomyopathy. *J Am Soc Echo* 1:48, 1988.

49. Klein A, Luscher T, Hatle L, et al: Spectrum of diastolic function abnormalities in cardiac amyloidosis (abstr). *Circulation* 76(IV):499, 1987.

50. Labovitz A, Pearson A: Progress in cardiology. Evaluation of left ventricular diastolic function: Clinical relevance and recent Doppler echocardiographic insights. *Am Heart J* 114:836, 1987.

51. Rokey R, Kuo L, Zohgbi W, et al: Determination of parameters of left ventricular diastolic filling with pulsed Doppler echocardiography: Comparison with cineangiography. *Circulation* 71:543, 1985.

52. Spirito P, Maron B, Bonow R: Noninvasive assessment of left ventricular diastolic function: Comparative analysis of Doppler echocardiographic and radionuclide angiographic techniques. *J Am Coll Cardiol* 7:518, 1986.

53. Wenger N, Goodwin J, Roberts W: Cardiomyopathy and myocardial involvement in systemic disease, in Hurst JW (ed): *The Heart*. New York, McGraw-Hill, 1985.

54. Silverman K, Hutchins G, Bulkley B: Cardiac sarcoid. A clinicopathologic study of 84 unselected patients with systemic sarcoidosis. *Circulation* 58:1204, 1978.

55. Roberts W, McAllister H Jr, Ferrans V: Sarcoidosis of the heart. A clinicopathologic study of 35 necropsy patients (group I) and review of 78 previously described necropsy patients (group II). *Am J Med* 63:86, 1977.

56. Lorell B, Alderman E, Mason J: Cardiac sarcoidosis: Diagnosis with endomyocardial biopsy and treatment with corticosteroids. *Am J Cardiol* 42:143, 1978.

57. Olson L, Baldus W, Tajik A: Cardiac involvement in idiopathic hemochromatosis: Echocardiographic and clincial correlations. *Am J Cardiol* 60:885, 1987.

58. Roberts W, Sjoerdsma A: The cardiac disease associated with the carcinoid syndrome (carcinoid heart disease). *Am J Med* 36:5, 1964.

59. Millman S: Tricuspid stenosis and pulmonary stenosis complicating carcinoid of the intestine with metastases to the liver. *Am Heart J* 25:391, 1943.

60. McGuire M, Pugh D, Dunn M: Carcinoid heart disease: A restrictive cardiomyopathy as a late complication. *J Kansas Med Soc* 79:661, 1978.

61. Hendel N, Leckie B, Richards J: Carcinoid heart disease: Eight-year survival following tricuspid valve replacement and pulmonary valvotomy. *Ann Thorac Surg* 30:391, 1980.

62. Baker B, McNee V, Scovil J, et al: Tricuspid insufficiency in carcinoid heart disease: An echocardiographic description. *Am Heart J* 101:107, 1981.

63. Callahan J, Wroblewski E, Reeder G, et al: Echocardiographic features of carcinoid heart disease. *Am J Cardiol* 50:762, 1982.

64. Forman M, Byrd B, Oates M, et al: Two-dimensional echocardiography in the diagnosis of carcinoid heart disease. *Am Heart J* 107:492, 1984.

65. Howard R, Drobac M, Rider W, et al: Carcinoid heart disease: Diagnosis by two-dimensional echocardiography. *Circulation* 66:1059, 1982.

CHAPTER 16

Intraoperative Doppler Echocardiography

Intraoperative application of imaging ultrasound to the study of cardiac structure and function was pioneered by Johnson and colleagues in 1972.[1] Since this initial report on the utility of M-mode echocardiography for evaluation of mitral valve function, intraoperative ultrasonography has been used to assess the adequacy of repair of heart valves and of congenital heart problems,[2,3] to study myocardial perfusion,[4] to screen for the presence of intracardiac air after cardiopulmonary bypass,[5] and to detect underperfused myocardial segments.[6] More recently, Doppler ultrasound has been used during surgery to acquire complementary data on cardiac physiology.

Intraoperative echocardiography with Doppler (CFI) enables the cardiac surgeon to assess immediately the result of the operation and modify the surgical procedure if necessary. It also assures the surgeon when no residual defect is noted. Recently, Stewart and colleagues[7] reported that intraoperative echocardiography led to a change in surgical treatment in 22 of 150 (15 percent) consecutive patients. Intraoperative echocardiography can be performed using the epicardial or transesophageal approach. Transesophageal echocardiography (TEE) views are more limited than epicardial echocardiograms, but do not interfere with the surgical field. In the experience of Bolger and coworkers,[8] TEE was more informative than epicardial echocardiography regarding mitral prosthetic regurgitation, shunt flow, and aortic dissection. The image quality of TEE is often as good as, and sometimes better than, that obtainable by epicardial echocardiography. Although a brief description of the methods and techniques used for epicardial echocardiography is given, this chapter will focus primarily on the intraoperative use of TEE Doppler CFI. It should be noted that TEE is also receiving increased interest for use in the awake patient, and that many of the concepts discussed in this chapter are also applicable in the ambulatory setting.

METHODS AND TECHNIQUES

Epicardial Approach

Any commercially available ultrasound system capable of providing high-quality images is acceptable for use in the operating room. The size of the system usually is not a consideration, as the unit generally can be positioned so as not to interfere with the operating surgeon. A long connecting cable for the scanhead is required so that the sterility of the operating field can be preserved and the operator allowed freedom of motion. Finally, a monitor for displaying the ultrasound information which is clearly visible to the interpreting physician is essential. In the interest of speed, it is the surgeon who should perform the echocardiographic examination. The echocardiographer should be in attendance in the operative suite to orient and guide the surgeon in obtaining optimal images.

Imaging studies are performed with the transducer on the surface of the heart (Fig. 16–1). The images obtained correspond to the parasternal long and short axis views that are routinely recorded in the standard echocardiographic examination. Conventional Doppler echocardiography and CFI are incorporated in the same manner. Apical views are not obtainable if a standard median sternotomy and scanhead system are used, as the cardiac apex is not accessible without distortion of the anatomy. The standard imaging or Doppler transducer can also be positioned over the proximal segments of the great vessels for examination of the aortic and pulmonic valves.

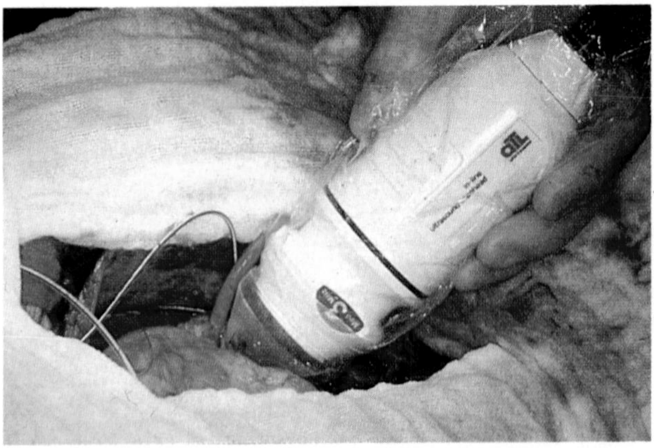

Figure 16–1. Epicardial echocardiography. A two-dimensional echocardiography transducer is placed directly on the surface of the heart.

Once the baseline echocardiographic images and Doppler examination have been obtained, the information can be used immediately to help guide therapeutic interventions in the operating room. When the operative procedure is completed, and the patient is weaned from cardiopulmonary bypass and a stable rhythm established, a repeat Doppler echocardiographic examination is obtained in the same planes used in the baseline study. Examination time varies, depending on the nature of the study, from 2 to 15 min.

Difficulties arise in ensuring scanhead sterility. Several methods are available: hot and cold gas sterilization, immersion of the scanhead in isopropyl alcohol for 24 h, radiation sterilization, and use of a sterile condom-type sheath to encase the scanhead (Fig. 16–1) and connecting cable. Hot gas and alcohol immersion are not employed, as they can alter the acoustic properties of the scanhead focusing lens. Radiation sterilization facilities are not widely available. The sterile sheaths are available as standard products from some ultrasound equipment manufacturers and are specifically designed for intraoperative application. Use of these sheaths spares one the complexities of the sterilization procedure and eliminates the need for an additional scanhead designated for intraoperative use.

Transesophageal Approach

With this new ultrasound imaging technique, transesophageal images are obtained using a transducer mounted on the end of an endoscope with the fiber optic material removed and replaced by the various wires leading to the transducer head. Figure 16–2 illustrates a 64-element, 5-MHz transducer (manufactured by Hewlett-Packard), which measures 9×12 mm and is incorporated onto the end of a flexible gastroscope. The TEE probe is best inserted by an anesthesiologist as soon as possible after induction of anesthesia and endotracheal intubation, so as to maximize its utility as a monitor during this critical time. The patient's airway must be protected to minimize the risks of aspiration of pharyngeal and gastric contents.

Relative contraindications to TEE include a history of esophageal disease or dysphagia, antecedent radiation therapy to the thorax, and acute penetrating chest trauma in which the integrity of the esophagus may be in question. In these situations one should consult an appropriate specialist (gastroenterologist, thoracic surgeon, or anesthesiologist) before performing TEE examination. If there is any difficulty in positioning the esophageal scope, the attempt should be aborted. The main prerequisite to a safe procedure is knowing when, and when not, to proceed with introduction of the transducer.[9,10]

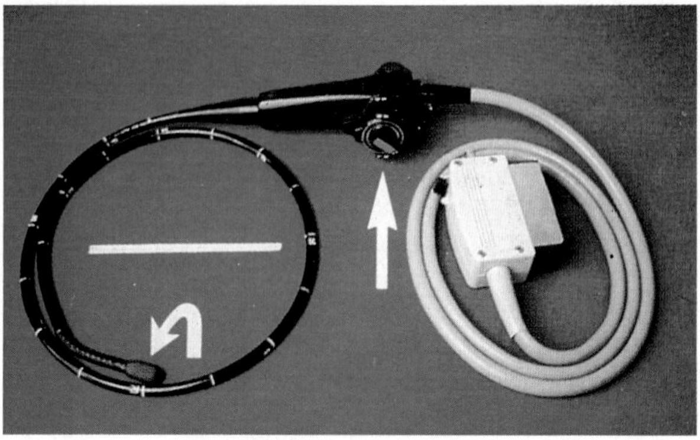

Figure 16 – 2. Transesophageal probe (manufactured by Hewlett-Packard). The 5-MHz transducer (curved arrow) is incorporated onto the end of a flexible gastroscope. The external controls for flexion/extension and sideways movement can be seen (straight arrow).

The orientation of the sector scan in current equipment is in the transverse view only. However, because it is possible to flex, extend, and bend the transducer to the right/left or up/down position as well as to rotate it within the esophagus, it is possible to obtain more than simple tomographic transverse view slicing. When the scope is advanced to approximately 25 cm from the incisors, the left atrium begins to come into view. This is the structure that is on top of the screen, since it is closest to the transducer. The right and left atrial appendage, pulmonary veins, ascending aorta, superior vena cava, and sometimes the pulmonary artery or its branches can be imaged from this position. Advancing the probe further allows imaging of the aortic valve (Fig. 16–3), which is usually seen in an oblique cut; the interatrial septum; the right atrium; portions of the tricuspid valves; and portions of the mitral valve. Further advance reveals the mitral apparatus (Fig. 16–4) in its entirety, the tricuspid apparatus, and both ventricles. Approximately 30 cm from the incisors, and sometimes with retroflexion, a four-chamber view can be obtained (Fig. 16–5). This is a modified apical projection, since the true cardiac apex may not be imaged with this modality. The scope is then introduced farther into the stomach, and the image blurs because of air in the stomach. Anterior flexion of the scope allows imaging of the short axis of the heart and the left lobe of the liver (Fig. 16–6). In this view, the posterior papillary muscle appears on top of the screen and the anterior papillary muscle in the far field. This is the position used to monitor myocardial function intraoperatively. At the end of the exam, the scope is withdrawn back into the esophagus and rotated posteriorly to image the descending thoracic aorta. Por-

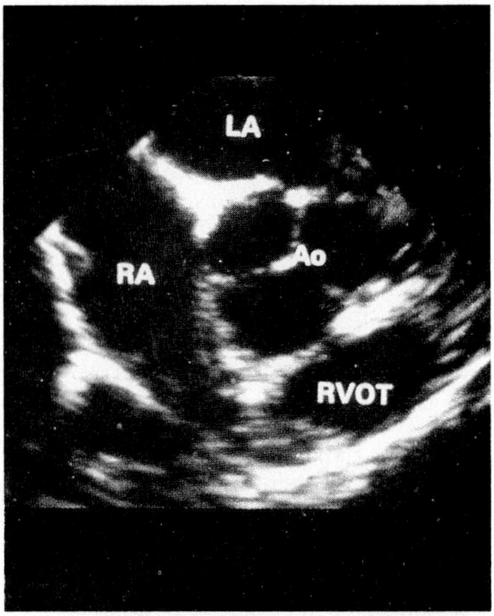

Figure 16–3. (TEE) transducer at the aortic (AO) level. The aortic valve, interatrial septum, right atrium (RA), left atrium (LA), and right ventricular outflow tract (RVOT) are imaged.

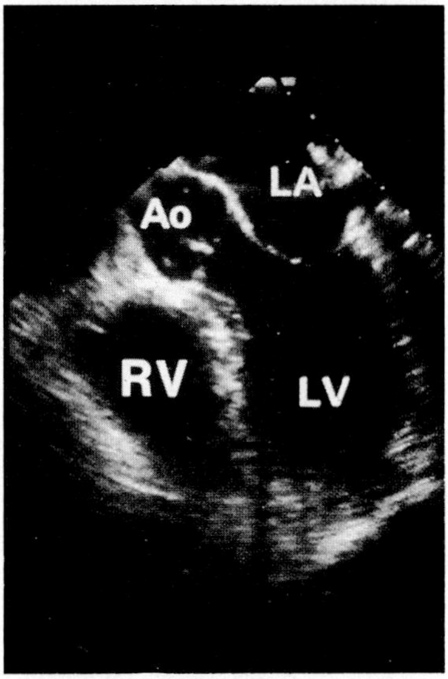

Figure 16–4. A modified TEE long axis view shows the mitral apparatus and both ventricles. AO = aorta, LA = left atrium, LV = left ventricle, RV = right ventricle.

tions of the aortic arch and the left carotid and left subclavian arteries can also be imaged through the transesophageal approach. It must be emphasized that during manipulation the probe should be in the neutral position with the locking mechanisms free, and that no force should be used.

Color display of normal cardiac flow in TEE is different from conventional transthoracic echocardiography because of the nearly opposite

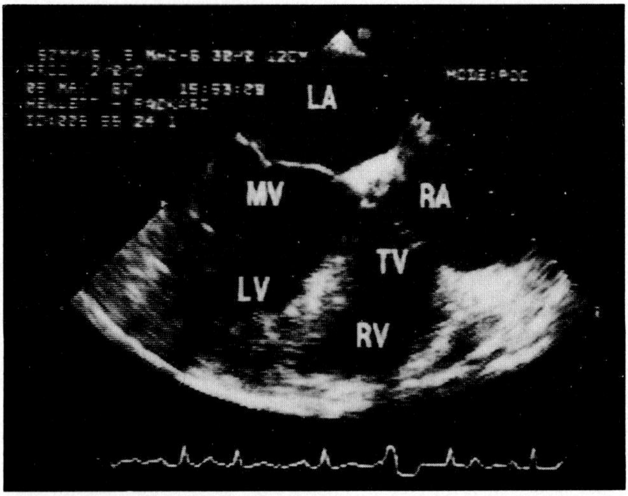

Figure 16–5. TEE four-chamber view. All four cardiac chambers are imaged simultaneously along with respective septa and atrioventricular valves, as in an apical four-chamber view. LA = left atrium, LV = left ventricle, MV = mitral valve, RA = right atrium, RV = right ventricle, TV = tricuspid valve.

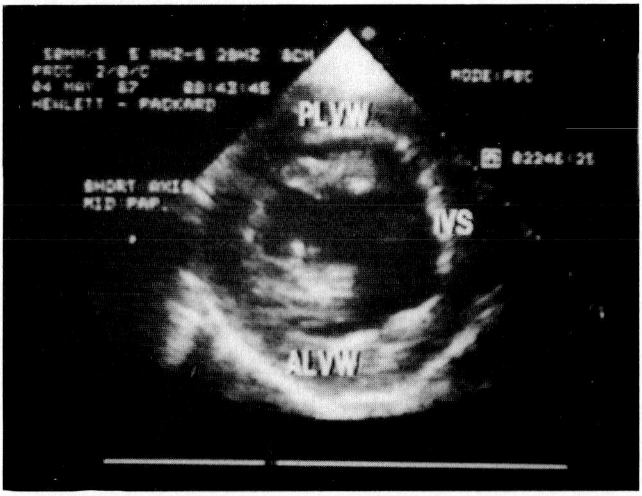

Figure 16–6. TEE short axis view at the level of the papillary muscles near the left ventricular apex. The posterior left ventricular wall (PLVW) is seen at the top of the image, and the anterior left ventricular wall (ALVW) is seen at the bottom of the image. The interventricular septum (IVS) is seen to the right. This is the standard view for monitoring left ventricular wall motion abnormalities during surgery.

transducer position. Blood flows that normally are not clearly seen by the conventional transthoracic approach (due to distance and inaccessibility) are easily visualized with TEE. Figure 16–7 demonstrates a normal Doppler CFI tracing from the four-chamber approach in diastole, and Fig. 16–8 a normal left ventricular systolic flow.

The transducer should be cleaned and inspected before and after each TEE examination.[11] The endoscope should be inspected for perforations or tears in the outer casing that would prevent proper cleaning and increase the possibility of electrical hazard. Once the test is completed, the probe is removed and rinsed promptly, then cold-sterilized in a glutaraldehyde solution (Cidex) for at least 10 min. This process destroys any bacterial and viral contaminants. The endoscope is washed with tap water and dried before storage. The instrument should not be reused for approximately 30 min. after removal from the Cidex.[9]

There is potential for complications associated with TEE, but reports of them are almost nonexistent. Laryngeal nerve damage during neurologic surgery with neck flexion[12] and esophageal mucusal burns[10] are rare potential complications. The potential for esophageal perforation exists when a disorder such as an esophageal malignancy or a congenital diverticulum are present. Because gastroscopy, inadvertent esophageal intubation, and other instrumentation of the airway and esophagus have reported complications, it can be expected that some problems will be

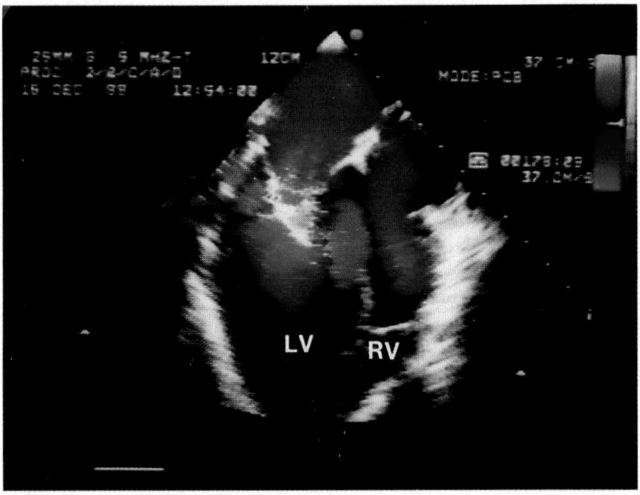

Figure 16–7. TEE Doppler color flow image of four-chamber view in diastole. The blue color represents normal transmitral and transtricuspid flow. LV = left ventricle, RV = right ventricle.

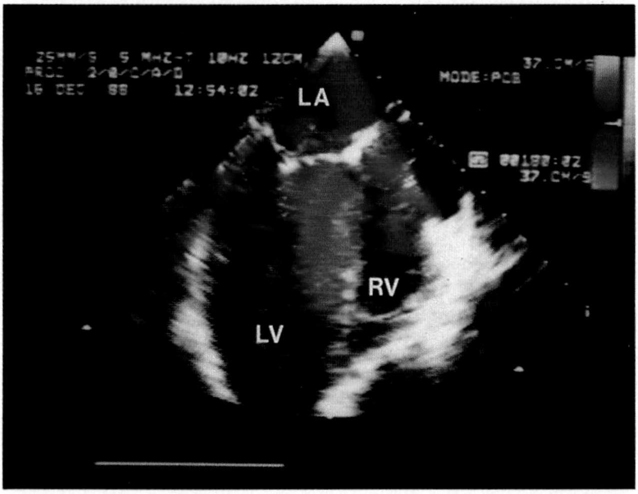

Figure 16–8. TEE Doppler color flow image from the same patient as in Fig. 16–7, showing flow in systole (red) in the left ventricular (LV) outflow tract. LA = left atrium, RV = right ventricle.

reported as availability and utilization of TEE increases.[13] Although TEE has generally been accepted as a routine clinical procedure, written informed consent from the patient is sought at most centers.

CLINICAL APPLICATIONS

TEE is especially useful as an intraoperative technique, both for diagnosis and for monitoring[14–18] (Table 16–1). Potentially, TEE combined with Doppler CFI can provide the surgeon with an intraoperative angiographic

TABLE 16–1. Indications for Transesophageal Echocardiography

Intraoperative Monitoring	Diagnosis
Coronary bypass surgery	Atrial lesions
Mitral valve repair	Intraoperative assessment of MR and AR severity
Congenital cardiac surgery	Prosthetic Valve Dysfunction
Neurosurgery in sitting position	Aortic dissection
Myectomy	LV size, function, regional wall motion, valve function

NOTE: AR = aortic regurgitation; MR = mitral regurgitation; LV = left ventricle assessment of surgical valve repair or replacement.[19,20] Surgical procedures that may be more reliably accomplished with the aid of TEE include resection of ventricular aneurysms, removal of endocardial tumors, myectomy for obstructive hypertrophic cardiomyopathy, closure of atrial or ventricular septal defects, and repair of thoracic aortic aneurysms and dissection.[17,21–27] Immediate intraoperative evaluation of a repair by ultrasound techniques allows for more precise and effective surgical results, since cardiopulmonary bypass can be reinstituted or extended and further surgery performed if necessary.

Valvular Regurgitation

TEE Doppler CFI allows rapid, accurate intraoperative assessment of the presence and severity of mitral regurgitation (Fig. 16–9 and 16–10), and is especially useful in judging the adequacy of valve repair.[28–30] This technique allows early identification of excessive residual regurgitation after valve repair or revascularization and permits remedial action before chest closure. Clinically significant mitral regurgitation appears as a mosaic of colors extending far back into the left atrium, and sometimes into the pulmonary veins.

In patients with suspected malfunction of a mitral prosthesis, TEE with Doppler CFI can provide reliable diagnostic information beyond that

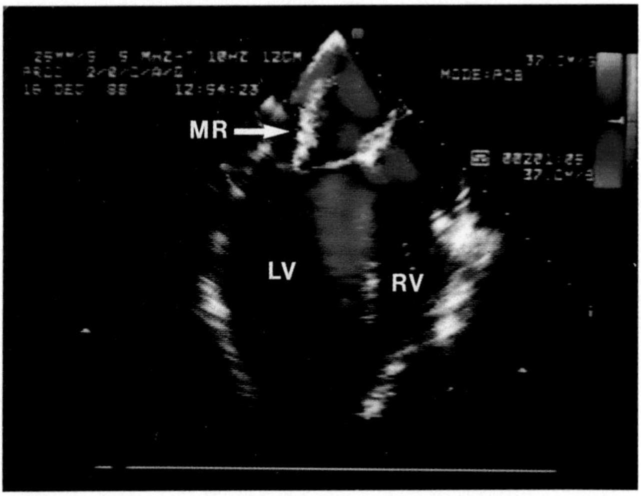

Figure 16–9. TEE Doppler color flow image showing mild mitral valve regurgitation (MR). The regurgitant jet was localized to the central point of leaflet coaptation. LV = left ventricle, RV = right ventricle.

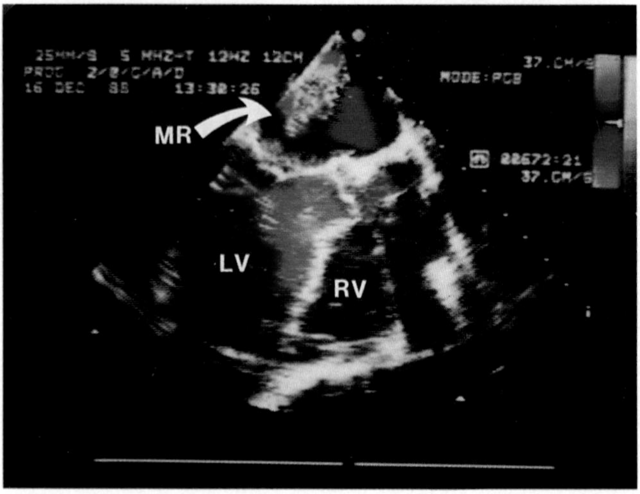

Figure 16–10. TEE Doppler color flow image showing moderate mitral regurgitation (MR). The mosaic pattern seen in the left atrium represents turbulent flow from the regurgitant jet. LV = left ventricle, RV = right ventricle.

available from the transthoracic approach, with the degree of mitral regurgitation corresponding to that found on left ventricular angiography.[31] TEE circumvents the problem of flow masking (see Chap. 10, Fig. 10–1), as the transducer is placed immediately behind the left atrium. However, because TEE causes some discomfort and is not completely free of risk, it should be performed only in selected patients in whom the transthoracic echocardiogram is of suboptimal quality and for whom the TEE study may alter management.

In addition, TEE is useful in the detection of paravalvular leaks immediately following mitral valve replacement, in which a small jet of flow may appear intermittently from the mitral valve anulus, adjacent to the prosthetic valve.[30] Such leaks, apparent immediately after surgery, have disappeared within two weeks postoperatively, suggesting that small suture-line leaks are obliterated during the healing process and do not constitute grounds for revision of the anular attachment of the valve.[32]

Aortic regurgitation may be best detected in the long axis view, where the left ventricular outflow tract is opened (Fig. 16–11). This view is similar to that used for the mitral valve. Tricuspid regurgitation is frequently seen in normal subjects and during intraoperative studies (Fig. 16–12) and is usually mild. Images of the tricuspid valve are obtained by slight clockwise rotation of the transducer.

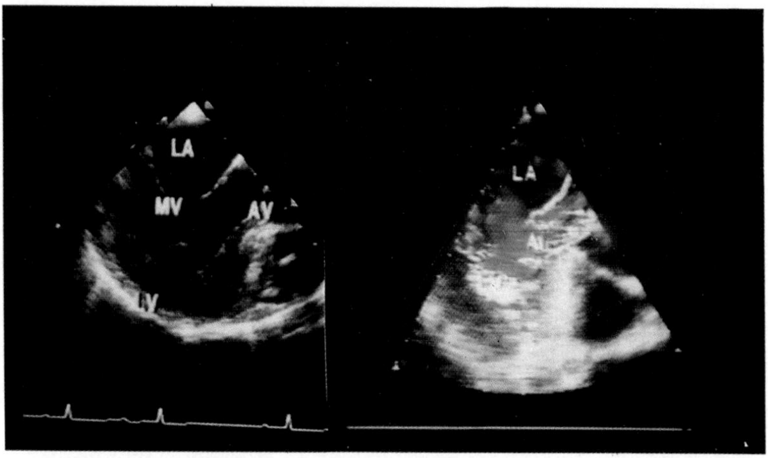

Figure 16–11. TEE image of aortic insufficiency. *Left*: Two-dimensional echocardiogram of a long axis view showing the left ventricular (LV) outflow tract, aortic valve (AV), and mitral valve (MV). LA = left atrium. *Right*: Color flow image of severe aortic insufficiency (AI). The AI jet (blue-cyan) encompasses the entire left ventricular outflow tract. Note the mitral inflow, seen as a darker blue color at the level of the mitral valve.

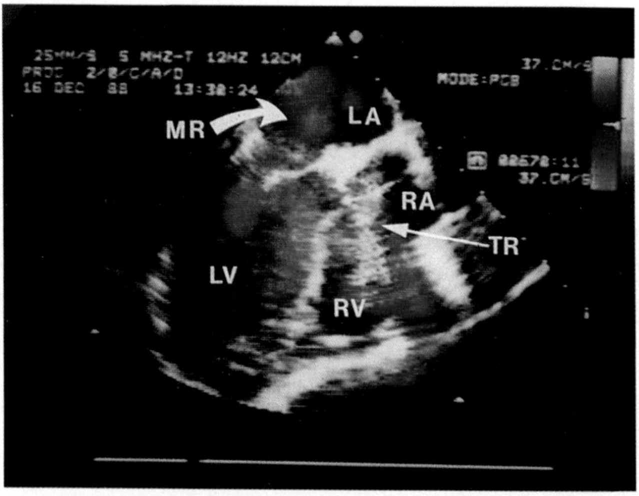

Figure 16–12. TEE Doppler color flow image of tricuspid and mitral regurgitation. The mosaic pattern seen between the right atrium (RA) and right ventricle (RV) represents turbulent flow in tricuspid regurgitation (TR). Mitral regurgitation (MR) is seen as a red color in the left atrium (LA). LV = left ventricle.

Aortic Dissection

Reports of TEEs accurate diagnosis of aortic dissection, including the localization of the entrance tear and reentry site of the false into the true lumen, has generated intense interest. Initial reports by Borner and Engberding have been extended by Takamoto, using TEE Doppler CFI.[25,27,33] These investigations applied TEE to type A and type B dissection. With the detection of flow in and out of the false lumen by CFI, the intimal tear and site of reentry were defined in nearly all patients. Difficulty in imaging the high ascending aorta may be expected with TEE, because of the air-filled trachea interposed between that portion of the aorta and the esophagus.

An oscillating intimal flap is direct evidence of dissection within the aortic wall. The intimal flap and the entry point of the flap can be readily visualized by TEE Doppler CFI (Fig. 16–13). It is not uncommon to see multiple entry points into a false lumen. Flow through these channels is seen as a discrete jet.[34]

Intraoperative Monitoring

TEE has been used most widely by cardiovascular anesthesiologists monitoring for myocardial ischemia and volume status in patients undergoing coronary bypass or vascular reconstruction surgery. For this application

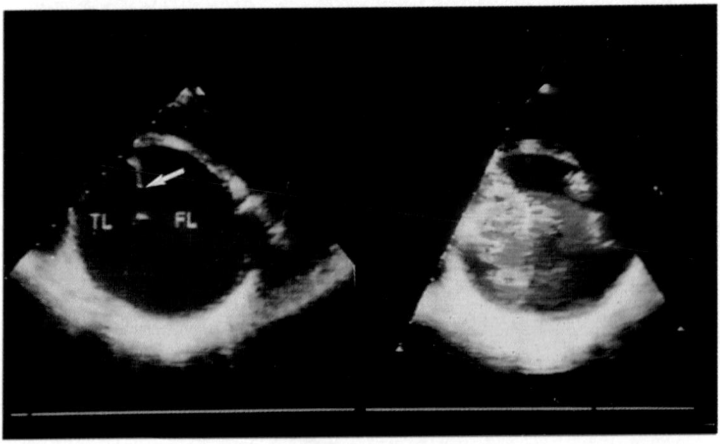

Figure 16–13. Aortic dissection. *Left*: Cross section of thoracic aorta by TEE demonstrating intimal flap (arrow) separating a true lumen (TL) from a false lumen (FL). *Right*: This color flow image shows a red jet, indicating site of intimal tear with a flow communication.

the TEE probe is positioned in the short axis view at the papillary muscle level for continuous imaging. Available reports suggest that TEE observation of new systolic wall motion abnormalities is much more sensitive than ST-segment changes for detecting intraoperative myocardial ischemia and infarction.[6,35,36] Other studies have demonstrated TEE to be a more accurate predictor of changes in left ventricular filling than flow-directed wedge catheters.[35]

During certain neurological procedures performed with the patient in a sitting position, large boluses of air may enter the central circulation because of a combination of low superior vena caval pressure and the tethering-open of intracranial veins by their attachments to the skull. The paradoxical embolization of this air may occur in the presence of a patent foramen ovale and elevated right atrial pressure. A minor risk of air embolism is also associated with other surgical procedures, including laparoscopy and cervical laminectomy. TEE is the most sensitive monitor for intracardiac air and the only effective monitoring device for parodoxical air embolism.[12,37–39]

Other Indications

Other clinical indications for TEE include the following: (1) suspected atrial source of systemic embolization, particularly the left atrial appendage;[22,40] (2) endocarditis and its complications;[41–43] (3) need for perioperative assessment of congenital heart disease;[26,44,45] (4) suspicion of intracardiac mass lesion;[46–48] and (5) need for imaging of the proximal coronary arteries.[49] The spread of these applications of TEE would be greatly accelerated by the availability of a small-diameter transducer suitable for mounting on a pediatric bronchoscope, which would permit more comfortable TEE examination.

RESEARCH AND FUTURE APPLICATIONS

In addition to its use in cardiac monitoring and diagnosis, TEE is a proven research tool. In patients undergoing cardiac surgery, Matsumoto et al.[50] used TEE to demonstrate the effects of pericardial and sternal closure on cardiac filling, causing marked reductions in left ventricular compliance. This study also established that septal thickening is normally preserved after cardiopulmonary bypass and that apparent changes in septal motion after open heart surgery are probably related to the role of the intact pericardium in maintaining synchronous filling and contraction of the ventricles.

In anesthesiology, TEE has been used to compare the effects of different anesthetics on left ventricular function and to assess the effects of positive end-expiratory pressure ventilation on right and left ventricular volumes.[51] New areas of investigation include intraoperative use of TEE coupled with intraaortic contrast to assess regional perfusion, ultrasonographic tissue characterization by TEE, and detailed study of ischemic changes in ventricular mechanics.

REFERENCES

1. Johnson M: Usefulness of echocardiography in patients undergoing mitral valve surgery. *J Thorac Cardiovasc Surg* 64:922, 1972.
2. Goldman M, Mindich B, Stavile K, et al: Intraoperative contrast two-dimensional echocardiography to assess mitral valve operations. *J Am Coll Cardiol* 4:1035, 1984.
3. Takamoto S: Intra-operative color flow mapping by real-time two-dimensional Doppler echocardiography for evaluation of valvular and congenital heart disease and vascular disease. *J Thorac Cardiovasc Surg* 90:802, 1985.
4. Goldman M, Mindich B: Intraoperative cardioplegic contrast echocardiography for assessing myocardial perfusion during open heart surgery. *J Am Coll Cardiol* 4:1021, 1984.
5. Rodigas P: Intraoperative two-dimensional echocardiography: Ejection of microbubbles from the left ventricle after cardiac surgery. *Am J Cardiol* 50:1130; 1982.
6. Smith J, Calahan M, Benefiel D, et al: Intraoperative detection of myocardial ischemia in high-risk patients: Electrocardiography versus two-dimensional transesophageal echocardiography. *Circulation* 72:1015, 1985.
7. Stewart W, Currie P, Lytle B, et al: The role of intraoperative echocardiography during cardiac valvular surgery (abstr). *J Am Coll Cardiol* 11:217A, 1988.
8. Bolger A, Czer L, Friedman A, et al: Intraoperative transesophageal color Doppler imaging: Advantages and limitations (abstr). *J Am Coll Cardiol* 11:217A, 1988.
9. Seward J, Khandheria B, Oh J, et al: Transesophageal echocardiography: Technique, anatomic correlations, implementation, and clinical applications. *Mayo Clin Proc* 63:649, 1988.
10. Mitchell M, Sutherland G, Gussenhoven E, et al: Transesophageal echocardiography. *J Am Soc Echo* 1:362, 1988.
11. Vennes J: Infectious complications of gastrointestinal endoscopy. *Dig Dis Sci* 26 (suppl):60s, 1981.
12. Cucchiara R, Nugent M, Seward J, et al: Air embolism in upright neurosurgical patients. Detection and localization by two-dimensional transesophageal echocardiography. *Anesthesiology* 60:353, 1984.

13. Johnson K, Hood D: Esophageal perforation associated with endotracheal intubation. *Anesthesiology* 64:281, 1986.

14. Cahalan M, Litt L, Botvinick E, Schiller N: Advances in noninvasive cardiovascular imaging: Implications for the anesthesiologist. *Anesthesiology* 66:356, 1987.

15. Konstadt S, Thys D, Mindich B, et al: Validation of quantitative intraoperative transesophageal echocardiography. *Anesthesiology* 65:418, 1986.

16. Kremer P, Cahalan M, Beaupre P, et al: Intraoperative monitoring by two-dimensional echocardiography. *Anaesthesist* 34:111, 1985.

17. Kyo S, Takamoto S, Matsumura M, et al: Immediate and early postoperative evaluation of results of cardiac surgery by transesophageal two-dimensional Doppler echocardiography. *Circulation* 76 (V):113, 1987.

18. De Bruijn N, Clements F: *Transesophageal Echocardiography*. The Hague, Martinus Nijhoff, 1987.

19. Dahm M, Iversen S, Schmid F, et al: Intraoperative evaluation of reconstruction of the atrioventricular valves by transesophageal echocardiography. *Thorac Cardiovasc Surg* 35 (special issue 2):140, 1987.

20. de Bruijn N, Clements F, Kisslo J: Intraoperative transesophageal color flow mapping. Initial experience. *Anesth Analg* 66:386, 1987.

21. Ezekowitz M, Smith E, Rankin R, et al: Left atrial mass: Diagnostic value of transesophagial two-dimensional echocardiography and ^{111}In platelet scintilography. *Am J Cardiol* 51:1563, 1983.

22. Aschenberg W, Schluter M, Kremer P, et al: Transesophageal two-dimensional echocardiography for the detection of left atrial appendage thrombus. *J Am Coll Cardiol* 7:163, 1986.

23. Gussenhoven E, Taams M, Roelandt J, et al: Transesophageal two-dimensional echocardiography: Its role in solving clinical problems. *J Am Coll Cardiol* 8:975, 1986.

24. Roelandt J: Colour-coded Doppler flow imaging: What are the prospects? *Eur Heart J* 7:184, 1986.

25. Takamoto S, Omoto R: Visualization of thoracic dissecting aortic aneurysm by transesophageal Doppler color flow mapping. *Herz* 12:187, 1987.

26. Hanrath P, Schluter M, Langenstein B, et al: Detection of ostium secundum atrial septal defects by transesophageal cross-sectional echocargiography. *Br Heart J* 49:350, 1983.

27. Engberdin R, Bender F, Grosse-Heitmeyer W, et al: Identification of dissection or aneurysm of the descending thoracic aorta by conventional and transesophageal two-dimensional echocardiography. *Am J Cardiol* 59:717, 1987.

28. Goldman M, Thys D, Ritter S, et al: Transesophageal real-time Doppler flow imaging: A new method for intraoperative cardiac evaluation. *J Am Coll Cardiol* 7:1A, 1986.

29. Drexler M, Oelert H, Dahm M, et al: Assessment of successful valve reconstruction by intraoperative transesophageal echocardiography. *Circulation* 74(II):390, 1986.

30. de Bruijn N, Clements F, Kisslo J: Transesophageal applications of color flow imaging. *Echocardiography* 4:557, 1987.

31. Nellessen U, Schnittger I, Appleton C, et al: Transesophageal two-dimensional echocardiography and color Doppler flow velocity mapping in the evaluation of cardiac valve prostheses. *Circulation* 78:848, 1988.

32. Omoto R: *Color Atlas of Real-Time Two-Dimensional Doppler Echocardiography*, 2d ed. Tokyo, Shindan-to-Chyrio, 1987.

33. Borner N, Erbel R, Braun B, et al: Diagnosis of aortic dissection by transesophageal echocardiography. *Am J Cardiol* 54:1157, 1984.

34. Oh J, Khandheria B, Seward J, et al: Transesophageal color flow imaging. *Echocardiography* 5:407, 1988.

35. Beaupre P, Kremer P, Cahalan M, et al: Intraoperative detection of changes in left ventricular segmental wall motion by transesophageal two-dimensional echocardiography. *Am Heart J* 107:1021, 1984.

36. Shively B, Watters T, Benefiel D, et al: The intraoperative detection of myocardial infarction by transesophageal echocardiography. *J Am Coll Cardiol* 7:2A, 1986.

37. Cucchiara R, Seward J, Nishimura R, et al: Identification of patent foramen ovale during sitting position craniotomy by transesophageal echocardiography with positive airway pressure. *Anesthesiology* 63:107, 1985.

38. Topol E, Humphrey L, Borkon A, et al: Value of intraoperative left ventricular microbubbles detected by transesophageal two-dimensional echocardiography in predicting neurologic outcome after cardiac operations. *Am J Cardiol* 56:773, 1985.

39. Furuya H, Okumura F: Detection of paradoxical air embolism by transesophageal echocardiography. *Anesthesiology* 60:374, 1984.

40. Nellessen U, Daniel W, Matheis G, et al: Impending paradoxical embolism from atrial thrombus: Correct diagnosis by transesophageal echocardiography and prevention by surgery. *J Am Coll Cardiol* 5:1002, 1985.

41. Gussenhoven E, van Herwerden L, Roelandt J, et al: Detailed analysis of aortic valve endocarditis: Comparison of precordial, esophageal and epicardial two-dimensional echocardiography with surgical findings. *J Clin Ultrasound* 14:209, 1986.

42. Geibel A. Hofmann T, Behroz A, et al: Echocardiographic diagnosis of infective endocarditis—Additional information by transesophageal echocardiography? (abstr) *Circulation* 76(IV):38, 1987.

43. Erbel R, Rohmann S, Drexler M, et al: Improved diagnostic value of echocardiography in patients with infective endocarditis by transesophageal approach: A prospective study. *Eur Heart J* 9:43, 1988.

44. Messina A, Leslie J, Gold J, et al: Passage of microbubbles associated with intravenous infusion into the systemic circulation in cyanotic congenital heart disease: Documentation by transesophageal echocardiography. *Am J Cardiol* 59:1013, 1987.

45. Schluter M, Langenstein B, Thier W, et al: Transesophageal two-dimensional echocardiography in the diagnosis of cor triatriatum in the adult. *J Am Coll Cardiol* 2:1011, 1983.

46. Engberging R, Bender F, Schulze-Waltrup N, et al: Improved ultrasonic diagnosis of peri- or paracardial tumors by transesophageal 2D-echocardiography (abstr). *Circulation* 76(IV):38, 1987.

47. Thier W, Schluter M, Krebber H-J, et al: Cysts in left atrial myxomas identified by transesophageal cross-sectional echocardiography. *Am J Cardiol* 51:1793, 1983.

48. Hofmann T, Behroz A, Koster W, Kasper W: Detection of intracardiac masses by two-dimensional transesophageal echocardiography (abstr). *Circulation* 76(IV):37, 1987.

49. Kyo S, Takamoto S, Matsumara M, et al: Color flow visualization of coronary blood flow using transesophageal transducer, in *Proceedings of the 48th Meeting of the Japan Society of Ultrasonics in Medicine.* Tokyo, 1986.

50. Matsumoto M, Oka Y, Strom J: Application of transesophageal echocardiography to continuous intraoperative monitoring of left ventricular performance. *Am J Cardiol* 46:95, 1980.

51. Terai C, Uenishi M, Sugimoto H: Transesophageal echocardiographic dimensional analysis of the four cardiac chambers during positive end-expiratory pressure. *Anesthesiology* 63:640, 1985.

CHAPTER 17

Evaluation of Congenital Heart Disease

Doppler echocardiography is a noninvasive procedure that uses ultrasound to measure intracardiac and intravascular flow velocities. These velocity measurements can be used to calculate intracardiac pressures in patients with stenotic, regurgitant, and shunt lesions. Complementary to 2D echocardiography, Doppler examination provides spatial localization of abnormal flows and thus helps identify the site of intracardiac shunting. With combined use of 2D and Doppler echocardiography, comprehensive, noninvasive evaluation of many types of congenital heart disease has been facilitated. Consequently, in some patients, cardiac catheterization may be avoided; other patients can be identified for selective use of catheterization in a goal-directed study.

The advent of high-quality 2D ultrasound with Doppler capabilities and, in particular, CFI, has greatly enhanced the ability to characterize the anatomy, architecture and pathophysiology of congenital heart defects. CFI allows the cardiologist to rapidly detect and assess abnormal intracardiac flow patterns and areas of abnormal communication. This application—rapid and sensitive detection of intracardiac shunts and regurgitant lesions—is one of the specific advantages that CFI offers the cardiologist.

Doppler examination of the patient with congenital heart disease should include the following: PD examination and CFI of all valves and septa for abnormal antegrade flow signals (where they are indications of stenosis and shunt, respectively); and PD, CW Doppler, and CFI examinations of the great vessels and branches for localized stenotic lesions or abnormal communications.

A comprehensive review of echocardiography and congenital heart disease is beyond the scope of this chapter. There are many excellent texts and articles that discuss these topics in great detail.[1–5] This chapter will focus on the use of Doppler CFI in (1) the diagnosis of commonly encountered congenital heart lesions, and (2) the evaluation of patients who have undergone repair of congenital heart lesions. Some of the newer applications, including intraoperative and fetal Doppler echocardiography, are also discussed.

SHUNT LESIONS

Atrial Septal Defects

Two-dimensional echocardiography is diagnostically reliable for atrial septal defects (ASDs) large enough to cause a shunt of 1.5:1 or greater.[6,7] Problems, however, have included questions of false-positive dropout in the fossa ovalis area, multiple ASDs, and sinus venosus defects. CFI overcomes these limitations by showing flow patterns in and around the ASD and by providing a reference for alignment of the Doppler cursor. Correct alignment allows accurate measurement of velocities and pressure gradients. Also, detection of multiple or fenestrated defects is enhanced by demonstration of multiple jets by CFI.

The best planes of imaging for ASDs include the subcostal, parasternal, and apical four-chamber views and the transverse (short axis subcostal) view. Parasternal short axis views at the level of the great vessels and left atrium also display transatrial color flow, since Doppler CFI is not as dependent on angle as is PD.

In Doppler CFI, laminar flow signals moving from the left to the right atrium generally indicate an ASD (Fig. 17–1); a large number of flow signals in the right atrium may also suggest a defect. Left-to-right shunt is manifest as a predominantly diastolic, and to a lesser extent systolic, red-orange color jet originating at the defect and extending variably into the right atrium.[8] Color aliasing is common and only a small amount of mosaic pattern is present, as a major degree of turbulence does not occur. With right-to-left shunting, the jet extends into the left atrium and is opposite (blue) in color. Pitfalls in examination mainly relate to image quality and color gain control. Because of signal attenuation, adequate gains cannot be achieved when the target is distant; for this reason the best transducer positions are subcostal and foreshortened parasternal four-chamber views. A rapid heart rate, as in infants, shortens diastole and makes visual assessment of shunt patterns more difficult. Slow-motion replay will enhance the ease of visualizing rapid color flow events.

The types of ASD are distinguished by their locations within the septum. A secundum ASD is located in the middle of the atrial septum (Figs. 17–1 and 17–2), whereas the sinus venosus ASD is located near the origin

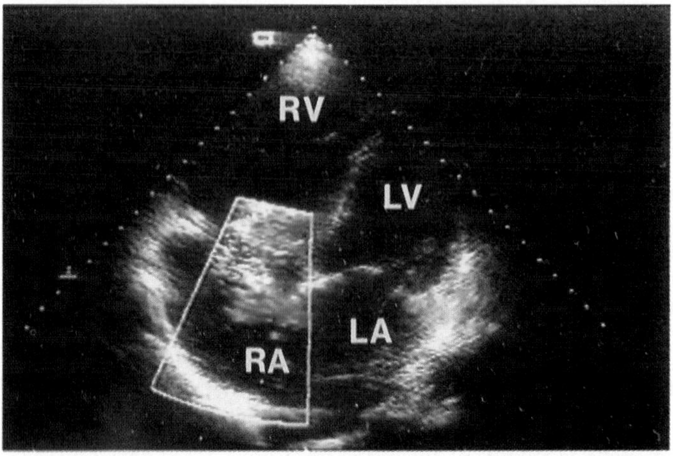

Figure 17–1. Atrial septal defect: Ostium secundum type. Apical four-chamber view. The red-orange flow from the left atrium (LA) to the right atrium (RA) is noted on the 2D color flow image. A small amount of mosaic pattern is present. The right atrium and right ventricle are dilated. LV = left ventricle, RV = right ventricle.

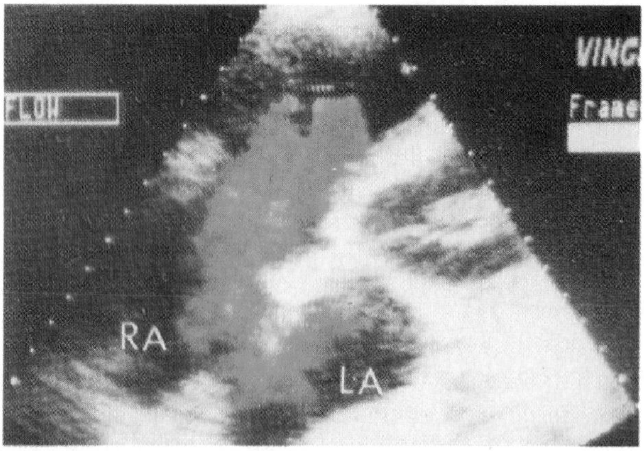

Figure 17–2. Doppler color flow image of a patient with a secundum atrial septal defect; modified four-chamber view. There is phasic flow from the left atrium (LA) into the right atrium (RA), seen as a red color signal stretching from the left into the right atrium across the area of the foramen ovale.

of the superior vena cava (Fig. 17–3). An ostium primum ASD is found at the base of the septum (Fig. 17–4).

Although this last defect can be diagnosed by 2D echocardiography using apical or low left parasternal transducer positions, CFI best defines the characteristics of its shunt flow. The flow signals through the ostium primum ASD often present a typical "butterfly" appearance that results

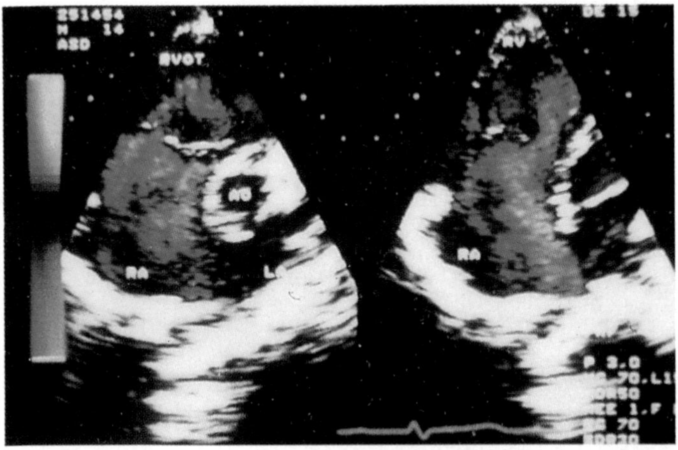

Figure 17–3. Sinus venosus atrial septal defect. Short axis (*left*) and four-chamber (*right*) views. Red signals are moving from the left atrium (LA) through the defect to the large right atrium (RA). Flow continues across the tricuspid orifice into the right ventricle (RV). AO = aorta, RVOT = right ventricular outflow tract.

Figure 17–4. Ostium primum atrial septal defect. Apical four-chamber view shows mosaic signals moving from the left atrium (LA) through a large defect (D) in the basal portion of the inter-atrial septum into the right atrium (RA). Red signals moving from both atria into the ventricles give a "butterfly" appearance typical of an ostium primum atrial septal defect. LV = left ventricle, RV = right ventricle.

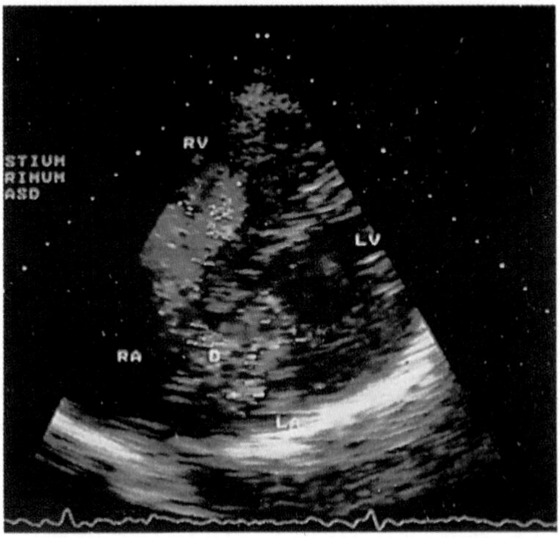

from blood moving from both atria into their respective ventricles, and from shunting from the left into the right atrium (Figs. 17–4 and 17–5).

Two-dimensional CFI helps to assess the size of the ASD and associated tricuspid regurgitation. Because of septal echo droput in 2D imaging planes, the observed width of the defect may be larger than the actual width. But the width of the flow signals observed with CFI accurately shows the size of the defect. In addition, the size of the shunt flow across the ASD that is seen in color (jet width) is directly proportional to the degree of left-to-right shunting.[9,10]

The severity of associated tricuspid regurgitation is also easily determined by CFI. The CW Doppler cursor is placed in the color flow signals representing tricuspid regurgitation in order to record accurately the peak pressure gradients; the pulmonary artery systolic pressure can then be calculated (see Chap. 13, Figs. 13–1, 13–2, and 13–3).

A color M-mode examination (conducted by placing the M-line cursor through the ASD flow signals) reveals the exact timing and direction of flow across the ASD during both systole and diastole. This examination, unlike

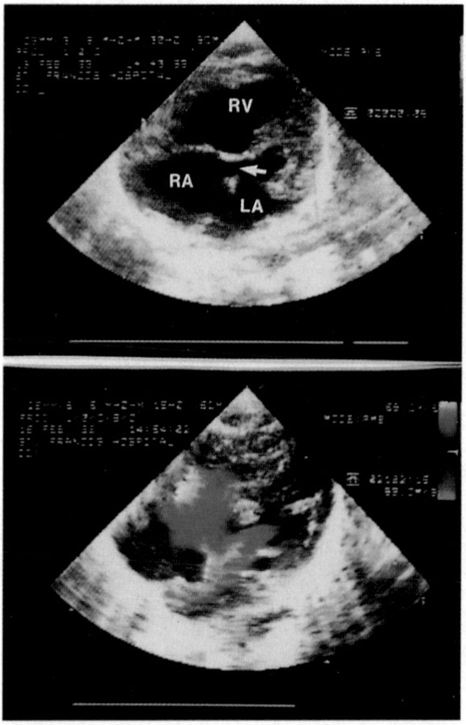

Figure 17–5. Large ostium primum atrial septal defect. *Top*: Two-dimensional four-chamber view demonstrating right ventricular (RV) enlargement and a primum atrial septal defect (arrow). LA = left atrium, RA = right atrium. *Bottom*: Color flow image showing a large volume of red flow across the atrial septal defect. Red signals moving from both atria into the ventricles give a "butterfly" appearance.

2D-CFI, can be used to time the duration of flow through the defect with respect to the cardiac cycle, because of its high frame rates. Most patients with uncomplicated ASD show left-to-right flow through the defect during both systole and diastole.

In our experience as well as in others, CFI has been extremely sensitive and specific in the diagnosis of ASD.[11] In instances where contrast echocardiography was used previously to discriminate between true septal defect and false-positive dropout, CFI has successfully replaced this more invasive diagnostic technique in our laboratory. Also, many institutions do not perform routine cardiac catheterization in patients with typical ASDs seen on CFI.

Ventricular Septal Defects

Ventricular septal defects (VSDs) are among the most common lesions in congenital heart disease; they may occur as isolated defects or as components of complex lesions. Two-dimensional echocardiography is important during both evaluation and follow-up of VSD,[12,13] but is less important diagnostically than in ASD. This is because the murmur associated with a small VSD is virtually diagnostic, and very small defects may be too small to be imaged directly. However, 2D echocardiography is a superb screening tool for other lesions that may mimic VSDs, although it may miss VSDs smaller than 4 mm in diameter.[14]

Although combined 2D echocardiography and conventional Doppler techniques are sensitive means for the detection of high-velocity signals from interventricular communications, CFI allows direct visualization of turbulent shunt flow at the ventricular level, and offers additional sensitivity and specificity in assessment of this lesion.[15–17] In addition, CFI has higher sensitivity than conventional Doppler echocardiography for multiple VSDs.[18] The direction of shunting (left to right, right to left, bidirectional), the quality of blood velocity across the defect (laminar vs. turbulent), the duration of transseptal flow (color M-mode evaluation), and the direction of the jet across the defect (for CW Doppler interrogation) are all invaluable aspects of VSD assessment provided only by CFI.

Doppler CFI indicates a VSD by showing turbulent flow signals in the right ventricle near the ventricular septum (Figs. 17–6 and 17–7) or by demonstrating a discrete high-velocity flow jet moving through an area of discontinuity in the ventricular septum during both systole and diastole. The origin of this turbulence is determined by moving and angling the transducer to obtain the best view of the signals' source. The location of their origin indicates the type of VSD—either perimembranous, muscular,

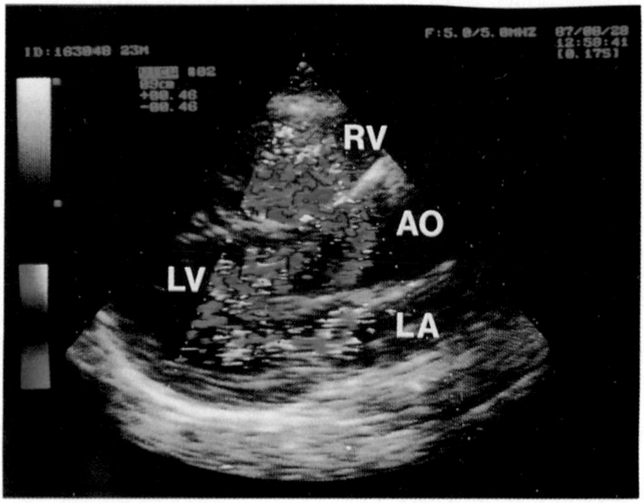

Figure 17–6. Ventricular septal defect. Parasternal long axis view. Mosaic flow in early systole, traversing the subaortic perimembranous ventricular septal defect, is seen to begin in the left ventricle (LV) and enter the right ventricle (RV). AO = aorta, LA = left atrium

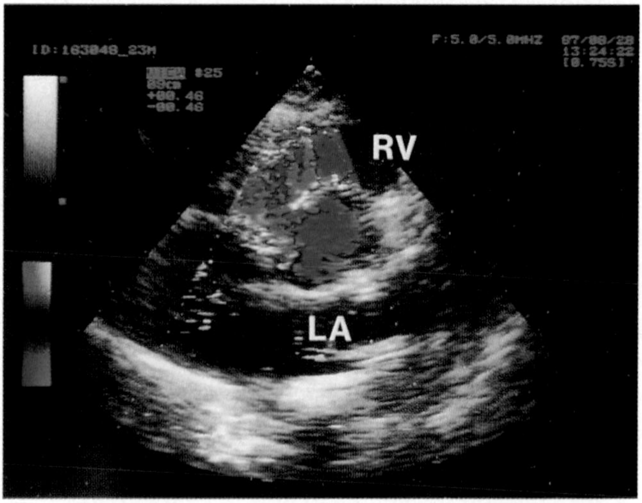

Figure 17–7. Subaortic perimembranous ventricular septal defect. Parasternal short axis view. Left-to-right shunt is seen as a mosaic pattern entering the right ventricle (RV). LA = left atrium.

or double committed. Perimembranous and muscular defects are further divided into subtypes according to their directions of flow in the right ventricle.

The size of the defect can be determined by measuring the width of the flow signals moving through the ventricular septum. This width is often easier to measure during diastole because the diastolic signals are laminar, rather than turbulent as in systole. This laminar flow, which results from the relatively low interventricular pressure gradient during diastole, may better define the anatomy and location of the defect (Fig. 17–8).

A color-guided CW Doppler examination conducted with the Doppler cursor placed parallel to the flow signals can measure the pressure difference between the two ventricles during systole. This is done using the modified Bernoulli equation ($\Delta P = 4V^2$). Left ventricular systolic pressure is assumed to be equal to right brachial artery systolic pressure obtained by cuff in the absence of aortic stenosis. The right ventricular systolic pressure can then be calculated by subtracting this measured pressure gradient from the systemic systolic blood pressure (see Chap. 13, Figs. 13–4 and 13–5). The right ventricular systolic pressure is also equal to the systolic pressure in the pulmonary artery so long as the pulmonary valve is not stenotic. In cases of aortic stenosis, the peak systolic left ventricular pressure is equal to the aortic systolic pressure plus the gradient across the left ventricular outflow tract as determined by CW Doppler echocardi-

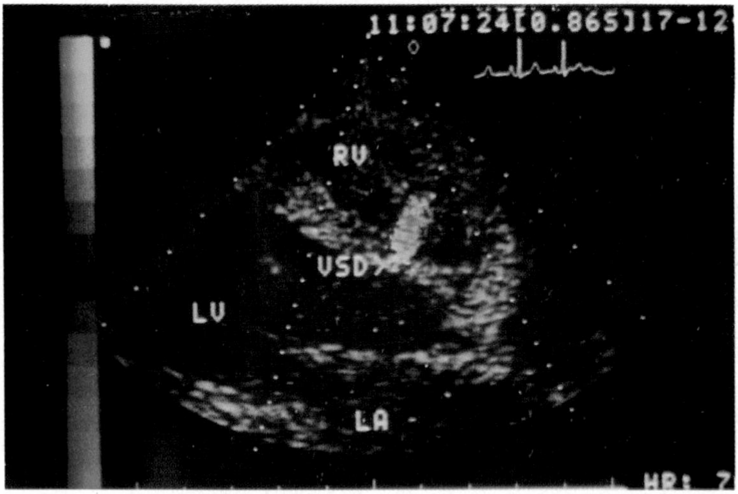

Figure 17–8. Muscular ventricular septal defect. Parasternal long axis view in diastole. The jet is displayed in orange-red (flow is toward transducer). LA = left atrium, LV = left ventricle, RV = right ventricle.

ography. In cases of pulmonic stenosis, subtracting the gradient obtained by CW Doppler imaging across the right ventricular outflow tract has resulted in a corrected pulmonary arterial pressure estimation.[11] The correlation between catheterization-measured pulmonary artery pressure and CW Doppler-estimated pulmonary artery pressure with the use of CFI to direct the CW Doppler beam has been found to be quite good, with a correlation coefficient of 0.99.[11]

A high pressure gradient across a VSD generally indicates an absence of pulmonary hypertension; a low gradient (less than 10 mmHg) indicates severe pulmonary hypertension. The degree of pulmonary hypertension determines the amount and direction of shunting through the defect.

Large VSDs may be isolated, but more commonly occur in lesion complexes such as tetralogy of Fallot, pulmonary atresia, double-outlet right ventricle, transposition complexes, and atrioventricular canal defect. Given adequate image quality, the 2D echocardiographic examination is highly sensitive and specific in diagnosis. Shunt flow is usually bidirectional, and shunt velocities are low compared to the small restrictive defects. The dynamics of shunt flows across VSDs in these patients are affected by relative left- and right-sided, intra- and extracardiac pressures and resistances. The predominant left-to-right shunting occurs during isovolumic contraction in early systole; right-to-left shunting occurs during the isovolumic relaxation period in late systole/early diastole (Fig. 17–9).

The direction and the timing of trans-VSD flow can be determined by a color M-mode examination. When the M-line cursor is placed in the VSD flow signals, the direction of flow is observed during both systole and diastole (Fig. 17–10). A small uncomplicated VSD shows predominantly left-to-right shunting during systole and diastole. As pulmonary pressure

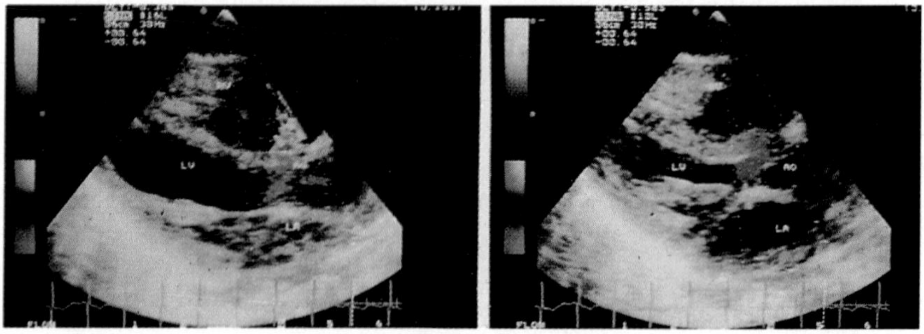

Figure 17–9. Tetralogy of Fallot. *Left*: Early systolic left-to-right flow across the ventricular septal defect is displayed in red. *Right*: Late systolic–early diastolic right-to-left flow is displayed in blue. AO = aorta, LA = left atrium, LV = left ventricle, RV = right ventricle.

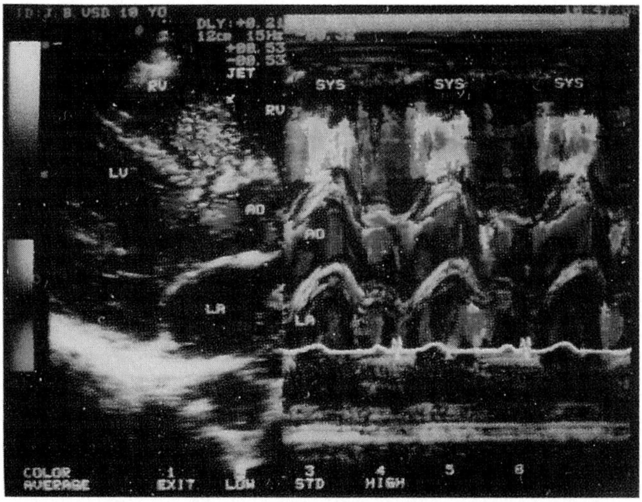

Figure 17–10. *Left*: Two-dimensional parasternal long axis view with left-to-right ventricular septal defect. The jet is visualized as a mosaic pattern traversing the subaortic perimembranous ventricular septal defect. AO = aorta, LA = left atrium, LV = left ventricle, RV = right ventricle. *Right*: Color M-mode pansystolic mosaic flow pattern across the ventricular septal defect is seen on the right ventricular side of the septum. Duration of flow is effectively demonstrated.

increases as a result of the rise in pulmonary vascular resistance, however; the duration of left-to-right flow across the defect diminishes proportionately. This is reflected on auscultation by a shortening in the length of the systolic murmur. In pulmonary hypertension, the duration of flow shortens in relation to the RR interval and is no longer pansystolic. There are preliminary data supporting a linear relationship and correlation between pulmonary artery pressure and the duration of flow across the septal defect as represented by color M-mode echocardiography.[11] Thus use of the color M-mode for temporal resolution of flow duration across the defect, by measuring duration of flow along the time axis against the electrocardiographic RR interval, can provide useful information about estimates of pulmonary artery pressure.

Patent Ductus Arteriosus

Anatomic identification of a patent ductus arteriosus (PDA), in infants and children as well as in adults, may be extremely difficult.[19] Doppler CFI is perhaps the most sensitive technique for discerning the presence of

PDA.[20–23] The best 2D-echocardiographic views for diagnosing a PDA are the high left parasternal short axis and suprasternal views. This defect can also be imaged from the standard left parasternal short axis view by angling the transducer to the left to show the main pulmonary artery and the PDA. It usually appears as a communication or gap between the bifurcation of the main pulmonary artery and the descending aorta. An enlarged left atrium and left ventricle and a dilated pulmonary artery also are observed.

Interrogation of the main pulmonary artery in parasternal short axis views gives an excellent CFI pattern in ductal patency. The flow map in this transducer position shows a characteristic red-orange mosaic pattern of the ductal jet entering the pulmonary artery along the lateral superior border of the main pulmonary artery (Figs. 17–11 and 17–12). The jet is sometimes located medially or centrally, and occasionally becomes hard to distinguish because it mixes with the flow. This jet also tends to swirl as it moves up the pulmonary artery during late diastole and systole.[24] These flow patterns differentiate PDA from surgically induced systemic pulmonary shunts that contain turbulent flow during both systole and diastole but have no discrete jet directed toward the pulmonic valve. Alternatively, the descending aorta from the suprasternal view may be used. Identification of reversal of color in diastole in the descending aorta is evidence of systemic–to–pulmonary artery shunt in the absence of aortic regurgitation. Image-directed CW Doppler echocardiography can record these high velocities and permit estimation of the presssure gradient between the pulmonary artery and the aorta.

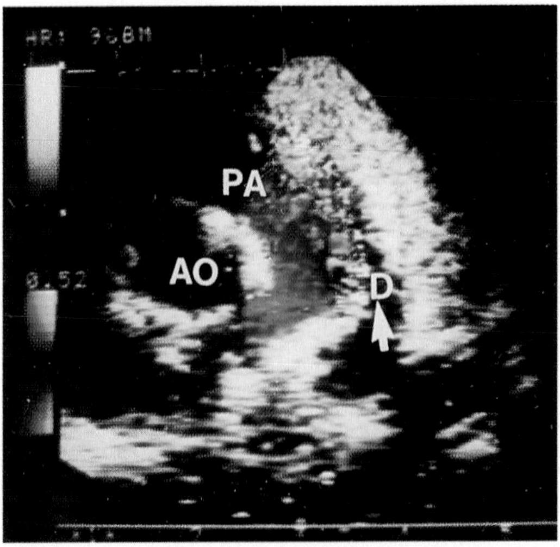

Figure 17–11. Patent ductus arteriosus. High left parasternal short axis view. Left-to-right shunt flow originates at ductus (arrow, D) and extends into main pulmonary artery (PA). Mosaic pattern is present because of high-velocity turbulent flow. AO = aorta.

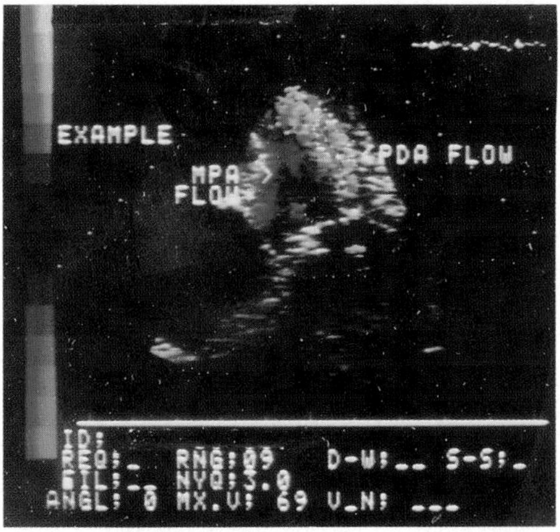

Figure 17–12. Patent ductus arteriosus. Parasternal short axis view. Systolic flow in the main pulmonary artery (MPA) is easily noted. Retrograde diastolic red/mosaic flow representing the flow from the PDA along the left superior MPA border is clearly identified.

With a PDA, Doppler CFI detects prominent turbulence in the pulmonary artery during both systole and diastole. A high-velocity continuous flow moves from the descending aorta into the pulmonary artery. With a PDA and associated pulmonary hypertension, the high-velocity flow through the PDA is not continuous. As the pulmonary hypertension increases, the flow's diastolic component disappears.

STENOTIC LESIONS

The approach and use of Doppler techniques in aortic stenosis, mitral and tricuspid stenosis, and pulmonary stenosis are discussed in Chaps. 4, 5 and 6, respectively. Obstruction to left ventricular inflow includes hypoplastic or congenitally stenotic mitral valve, parachute deformity, supravalvular mitral ring, and double orifice mitral valve. These lesions can be recognized and functionally assessed by 2D and Doppler techniques. CFI can demonstrate the spatial extent of abnormal inflow velocities and may assist in the ease of recognition and Doppler quantitation of severity. CFI is helpful in showing multiple jets when the valve leaflets are fenestrated or the orifice duplicated, as occurs with double-orifice mitral valve.[25] The apical window usually best demonstrates the jet of left ventricular inflow obstruction.

Congenital left ventricular outflow obstruction includes subvalvular (Figs. 17–13 and 17–14), valvular, and supravalvular aortic stenosis. These entities are diagnosed accurately and quantified with standard 2D/Doppler techniques. When obstruction is mild, color aliasing and/or an early systolic mosaic pattern is seen. With higher grades of obstruction, high

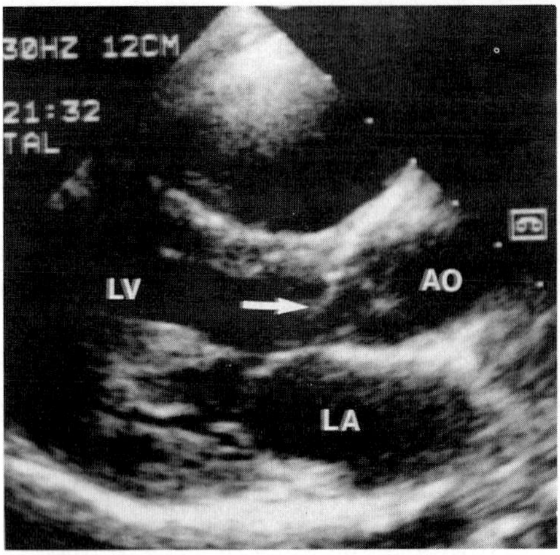

Figure 17–13. Parasternal long axis view showing a discrete subaortic membrane (arrow). AO = aorta, LA = left atrium, LV = left ventricle.

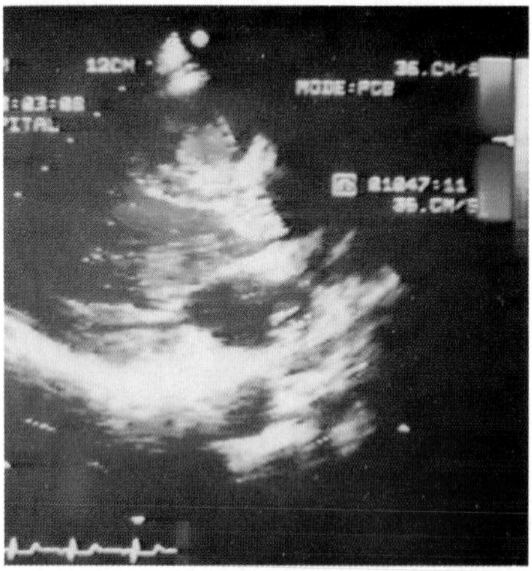

Figure 17–14. Doppler color flow image from same patient as in Fig. 17–13. There is an increase in velocity at the site of the membrane, represented as aliasing (blue-coded flow).

velocities persist throughout systole, resulting in a prolonged mosaic pattern that starts at the area of obstruction and projects distally. Examination of a left ventricular outflow lesion can be performed from apical or parasternal transducer positions. Supravalvular stenoses are best analyzed from suprasternal transducer positions.

Right ventricular outflow obstruction includes valvular and subvalvular pulmonic stenosis and branch pulmonary stenosis. The characteristics of the stenotic jet are similar to those seen with left ventricular outflow tract lesions, but with more severe obstruction resulting in a mosaic appearance. Examination is often best performed from the parasternal short axis projection of the right ventricular outflow tract, pulmonary artery, and pulmonary bifurcation. As in other stenotic lesions, direct visualization of the stenotic jet can help in alignment of the CW Doppler beam.

REGURGITANT LESIONS

Atrioventricular valve regurgitation is seen in many congenital lesion complexes. Detection and quantitation of atrioventricular and semilunar regurgitation is especially important before surgical repair of any congenital anomaly. Semilunar regurgitation occurs often in truncus arteriosus and in patients with dilated aorta, as in tetralogy of Fallot, pulmonary atresia, and ventricular septal defect. The regurgitant jet is directed variably to the right ventricle, left ventricle, or both. In general, the strategy for detection and quantitation of congenital valvular regurgitation is quite similar to that for acquired valvular lesions and is discussed in Chaps. 7, 8, and 9.

POSTOPERATIVE DOPPLER EVALUATION

Postoperative anatomy often is distorted and difficult to assess in a comprehensive manner. CFI can assist in the rapid recognition of residual shunts, valvular incompetence, and flow disturbance.

Valved conduits are subject to stenosis and regurgitation over the long term,[26] and CFI can be used to demonstrate presence of flow and degree of insufficiency. Determination of the patency of palliative systemic-to-pulmonary shunts, as well as direct visualization of shunt flow, is possible in most cases.

Detection of residual shunting following septal defect repair is a task at which CFI clearly excels. Small shunts are sensitively detected even when dehiscence is not apparent on 2D examination (Fig. 17–15). Conversely, unusual spectral patterns detected by PD/CW Doppler examination that suggest residual shunting can be confirmed or excluded as residual shunt by CFI.

After surgical correction of tetralogy of Fallot, patients routinely have a persistent, loud systolic ejection murmur along the left sternal border and pulmonic area. This murmur can be confused with residual pulmonic stenosis or a residual VSD, both of which may also be actually present following repair of tetralogy of Fallot. CFI is invaluable for assessing the murmur's significance and etiology, as well as distinguishing among residual VSD, residual pulmonic stenosis, and a functional murmur through the dilated right ventricular outflow tract.

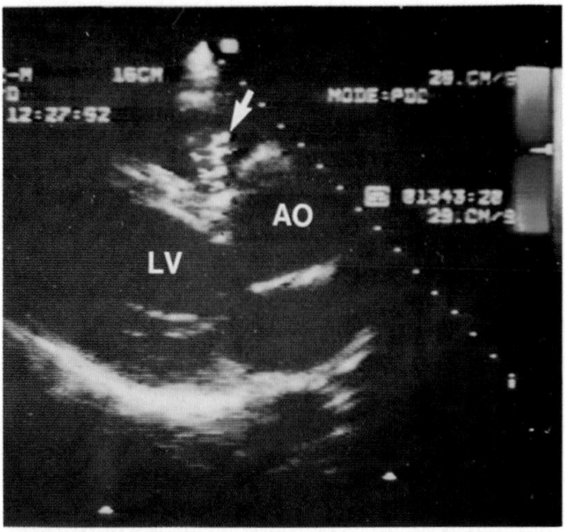

Figure 17–15. Residual ventricular septal defect following repair of tetralogy of Fallot. Parasternal long axis view. A mosaic jet is seen to cross the interventricular septum (arrow). The defect was not appreciated on the 2D image. AO = aorta, LV = left ventricle.

NEWER APPLICATIONS

Intraoperative Doppler Color Flow Imaging

Two-dimensional Doppler CFI using the epicardial and transesophageal approach is attracting wide interest (see Chap. 16). The abilities to visualize residual atrioventricular valve regurgitation after AV canal repair, residual shunts after repair of multiple VSDs, and significant mitral regurgitation after mitral valve repair are all examples of the effects of intraoperative echocardiography on clinical decision making.[27,28]

The major advantage of transesophageal CFI in comparison with the epicardial approach is that the study may be undertaken with no interference with the surgical field. This allows instantaneous feedback during the surgical procedure, which has been extremely valuable—especially in the pediatric population, where valve repair is most often preferable to valve replacement.

Fetal Cardiac Imaging

Screening for fetal congenital heart disease is being used with increased frequency in pregnant women at high risk for fetal cardiac abnormalities.[11,29] Some of the indications for intrauterine echocardiography and Doppler studies include siblings with congenital heart disease, other anomalies identified by ultrasonography associated with congenital cardiac abnormalities, arrhythmias, polyhydramnios, and maternal ingestion of drugs known to be cardiac teratogens. Fetal screening for congenital heart disease in these high-risk pregnancies can identify cardiac abnormalities and assist in the planning of delivery and follow-up. This screening evaluation can identify virtually any major cardiac abnormality.

REFERENCES

1. Armstrong W: Congenital heart disease, in Feigenbaum H (ed): *Echocardiography*, 4th ed. Philadelphia, Lea & Febiger, 1986.
2. Stevenson J: The use of Doppler echocardiography for detection and estimation of severity of patent ductus arteriosus, ventricular septal defect, and atrial septal defect. *Echocardiography* 4:321, 1987.
3. Reeder G, Currie P, Hagler D, et al: Use of Doppler techniques (continuous-wave, pulsed-wave, and color flow imaging) in the noninvasive hemodynamic assessment of congenital heart disease. *Mayo Clin Proc* 61:725, 1986.
4. Switzer D, Nanda N: Doppler echocardiography. Part II: Congenital heart disease. *Echocardiography* 2:257, 1985.
5. Missri J: *Clinical Doppler Echocardiography*. New York, Yorke Medical Books, 1986.
6. Shub C, Tajik A, Seward J, et al: Surgical repair of uncomplicated atrial septal defect without "routine" preoperative cardiac catheterization. *J Am Coll Cardiol* 6:49, 1985.
7. Lipshultz S: Are routine preoperative cardiac catheterization and angiography necessary before repair of ostium primum atrial septal defect? *J Am Coll Cardiol* 11:373, 1988.
8. Suzuki Y, Kambara H, Kadota K, et al: Detection of intracardiac shunt flow in atrial septal defect using a real-time two-dimensional color-coded Doppler flow imaging system and comparison with contrast two-dimensional echocardiography. *Am J Cardiol* 56:347, 1985.
9. Pollick C, Sullivan H, Ciyec B, Wilansky S: Doppler color-flow imaging assessment of shunt size in atrial septal defect. *Circulation* 78:522, 1988.
10. Ritter S: Application of Doppler color flow mapping in the assessment and the evaluation of congenital heart disease. *Echocardiography* 4:543, 1987.
11. Ritter S: Recent advances in color-Doppler assessment of congenital heart disease. *Echocardiography* 5:457, 1988.
12. Gutgesell H: Accuracy of two-dimensional echocardiography in the diagnosis of congenital heart disease. *Am J Cardiol* 55:514, 1985.
13. Krabill K: Echocardiographic versus cardiac catheterization diagnosis of infants with congenital heart disease requiring surgery. *Am J Cardiol* 60:351, 1987.

14. Canale J, Sahn D, Allen H, et al: Factors affecting real-time, cross-sectional echocardiographic imaging of perimembranous ventricular septal defects. *Circulation* 63:689, 1981.

15. Stevenson J, Kawabori I, Dooley T, et al: Diagnosis of ventricular septal defect by pulsed Doppler echocardiography: Sensitivity, specificity, and limitations. *Circulation* 58:322, 1978.

16. Sahn D, Swensen R, Valdes-Cruz L, et al: Two-dimensional color flow mapping for evaluation of ventricular septal defect shunts: A new diagnostic modality (abstr). *Circulation* 70(II):364, 1984.

17. Stevenson G, Kawabori I, Brandestini M: Color coded Doppler visualization of flow within ventricular septal defects: Implications for peak pulmonary artery pressure (abstr). *Am J Cardiol* 49:944, 1982.

18. Ludomirsky A, Huhta J, Vick G, et al: Color Doppler detection of multiple ventricular septal defects. *Circulation* 74:1317, 1986.

19. Ritter S, Golinko R, Cooper R: Systemic to pulmonary artery anastomoses: Pulsed Doppler evaluation of aortic flow properties (abstr). *J Ultrasound Med* 3:42, 1984.

20. Sahn D, Allen H: Real-time cross-sectional echocardiographic imaging of the patent ductus arteriosus in infants and children. *Circulation* 58:343, 1987.

21. Kyo S, Shime H, Omoto R, et al: Evaluation of intracardiac shunt flow in premature infants by color flow mapping real-time two-dimensional Doppler echocardiography. *Circulation* 70:456, 1984.

22. Swensen R, Valdes-Cruz L, Sahn D, et al: Real-time Doppler color flow mapping for detection of patent ductus arteriosus. *J Am Coll Cardiol* 8:1105, 1986.

23. Liao P, Su W, Hung J: Doppler echocardiographic flow characteristics of isolated patent ductus arteriosus: Better delineation by Doppler color flow mapping. *J Am Coll Cardiol* 12:1285, 1988.

24. Huhta J, Cohen M, Gutgesell H: Patency of the ductus arteriosus in normal neonates: Two-dimensional echocardiography versus Doppler assessment. *J Am Coll Cardiol* 4:561, 1984.

25. Reeder G, Seward J, Hagler D, Tajik A: Color flow imaging in congenital heart disease. *Echocardiography* 3:533, 1986.

26. Geha A, Laks H, Stansel H, et al: Late failure of porcine valve heterografts in children. *Thorac Cardiovasc Surg* 78:341, 1979.

27. Maurer G, Czer L, Bolger A, et al: Intraoperative color Doppler flow mapping for repair of congenital heart disease (abstr). *Circulation* 74(II):37, 1986.

28. Hillel Z, Thys D, Ritter S, et al: Two-dimensional color flow Doppler echocardiography: Intraoperative monitoring of cardiac shunt flow in patients with congenital heart disease. *J Cardiothorac Anesth* 1:42, 1987.

29. De Vore G, Hornstein J, Siassi B, et al: Doppler color flow mapping: Its use in the prenatal diagnosis of congenital heart disease in the human fetus. *Echocardiography* 2:551, 1985.

CHAPTER 18

Clinical Case Studies

The purpose of this chapter is to illustrate the usefulness of Doppler echocardiography in the format of clinical case studies. The cases selected represent a variety of cardiac pathologic conditions where combined echocardiography and Doppler techniques contributed significantly to correct diagnosis, to the estimation of the severity of the lesion, and to the clinical management of the patient. Reference is made to the specific chapter(s) relating to each case study.

CASE 1 AORTIC STENOSIS (Chapter 4)

History. A 73-year-old man was referred for cardiac catheterization to assess his aortic valve disease. He presented with a two-month history of increasing dyspnea on exertion, paroxysmal nocturnal dyspnea, and orthopnea. The patient denied chest pain and syncope.

Physical Examination. Disclosed a heart rate of 85 beats/min and blood pressure of 155/90 mmHg. Cardiac examination revealed a diffuse, heaving apical impulse in the fifth intercostal space along the midclavicular line. The first heart sound was normal. The second heart sound was single. There was a loud fourth heart sound. A grade III/VI late-peaking, crescendo-decrescendo systolic murmur was heard at the right upper sternal border. The murmur radiated to both carotid arteries and to the left lower sternal border. No diastolic murmur was heard.

Electrocardiogram. Revealed left ventricular hypertrophy with nonspecific ST-T-wave changes.

Chest X-Ray. Demonstrated moderate cardiomegaly. The lung fields were clear.

Two-Dimensional Echocardiogram. Revealed concentric left ventricular hypertrophy, dilated and moderately hypokinetic left ventricle, and thickened aortic valve leaflets with restricted aortic leaflet motion (Fig. 18–1).

Doppler Study. CFI from a high right parasternal approach was performed with the patient lying on his right side. The turbulent transaortic flow in systole was seen as aliased blue flow toward the transducer, with some red turbulent color shift at the aortic wall (Fig. 18–2). CW Doppler interrogation of this high-velocity color flow pattern produced a peak instantaneous velocity (V_{max}) of 4 m/s (Fig. 18–3), or an estimated peak gradient of 64 mmHg across the aortic valve. The aortic valve area was calculated using the continuity equation. The left ventricular outflow tract (LVOT) velocity on PD echocardiography measured 0.8 m/s. The cross-sectional area (CSA) of the aortic valve anulus was 4.4 cm^2. Aortic valve area (AVA) was calculated by the equation

$$AVA = \frac{VLVOT}{V_{max}} \times CSA = \frac{0.8}{4} \times 4.4 = 0.9\ cm^2$$

Cardiac Catheterization. The aortic valve could not be crossed despite multiple attempts with a variety of different catheters. The coronary arteries were normal.

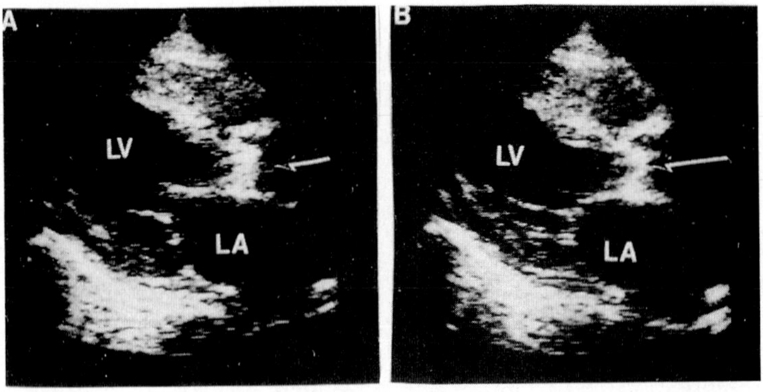

Figure 18–1. Case 1. Two-dimensional echocardiogram, parasternal long axis view. (A) Diastole. (B) Systole. The aortic leaflets are thickened and appear heavily calcified (arrow). The left ventricle (LV) is dilated and hypokinetic LA = left atrium.

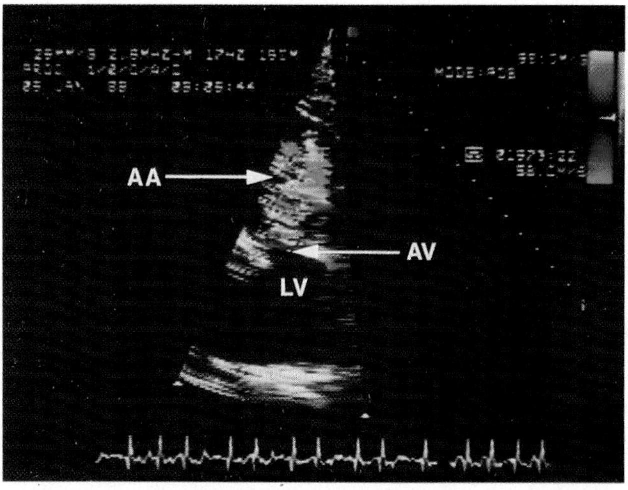

Figure 18–2. Case 1. High right parasternal view of ascending aortic flow. There is aliased blue flow toward the transducer emanating from the aortic valve (AV) into the ascending aorta (AA). LV = left ventricle.

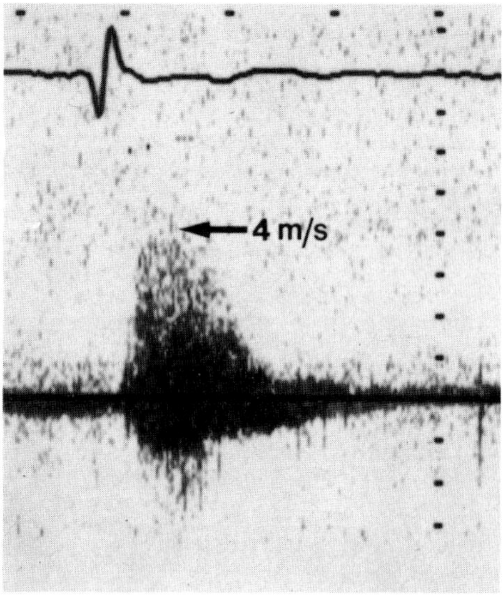

Figure 18–3. Case 1. CW Doppler interrogation of the region of blue jet imaged in Fig. 18–2 produces a high velocity of 4 m/s. On the basis of the modified Bernoulli equation ($\Delta P = 4\ V^2$), the estimated peak instantaneous gradient was 64 mmHg.

Disposition. Based on the Doppler assessment of critical aortic stenosis, the patient underwent aortic valve replacement.

On pathologic examination, the aortic valve (Fig. 18–4) contained extensive calcific deposits on the aortic surfaces of the cusps, without commissural fusion.

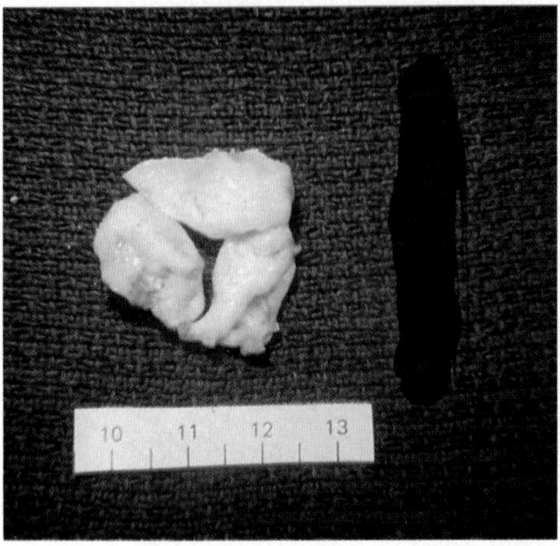

Figure 18–4. Case 1. Calcific stenosis of a trileaflet aortic valve. Thickening and calcific deposits are noted on the aortic surfaces of the cusps, without commissural fusion.

CASE 2 AORTIC STENOSIS AND REGURGITATION (Chapters 4 and 7)

History. A 65-year-old man was referred for Doppler echocardiographic evaluation of aortic stenosis and regurgitation. Over the preceding year he had developed progressive exertional angina, exertional dyspnea, and episodes of light-headedness. There was a history of hypertension. There was no history of rheumatic fever.

Physical Examination. Demonstrated blood pressure of 165/65 mmHg and a heart rate of 75 beats/min. The carotid upstroke was brisk, and the apical impulse was displaced to the sixth intercostal space at the left anterior axillary line and was hyperdynamic. There was a grade III/VI mid-peaking, crescendo-decrescendo systolic murmur at the left sternal border and right upper sternal border. The murmur radiated to both carotid arteries. There was also a grade III/VI early diastolic murmur of aortic regurgitation. The first heart sound was normal, and the second heart sound was single.

Electrocardiogram. Revealed left ventricular hypertrophy with lateral- and inferior-wall ischemic changes.

Chest X-Ray. Showed cardiomegaly and calcification of the aortic valve.

Two-Dimensional Echocardiogram. Revealed a dilated, hypertrophied left ventricle. The left ventricular systolic function was hyperdynamic. The aortic valve appeared thickened, with reduced aortic leaflet excursion. The mitral valve appeared normal.

Doppler Study. CFI from an apical five-chamber view demonstrated moderate aortic regurgitation (Fig. 18–5). The aortic regurgitant jet (red-orange) was seen to extend deep into the left ventricular cavity. CW Doppler investigation from the apex showed findings of aortic stenosis and regurgitation (Fig. 18–6). The maximal systolic velocity recorded was

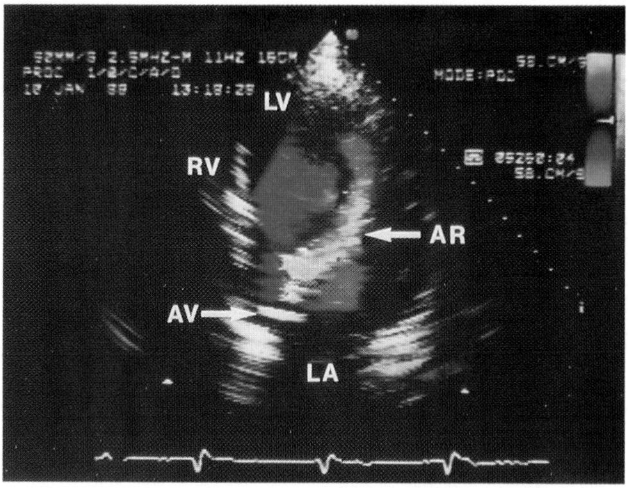

Figure 18–5. Case 2. Apical view in early diastole. The aortic regurgitation (AR) is imaged as red flow originating just below the region of the aortic valve (AV) and extending deep into the left ventricle (LV). LA = left atrium, RV = right ventricle.

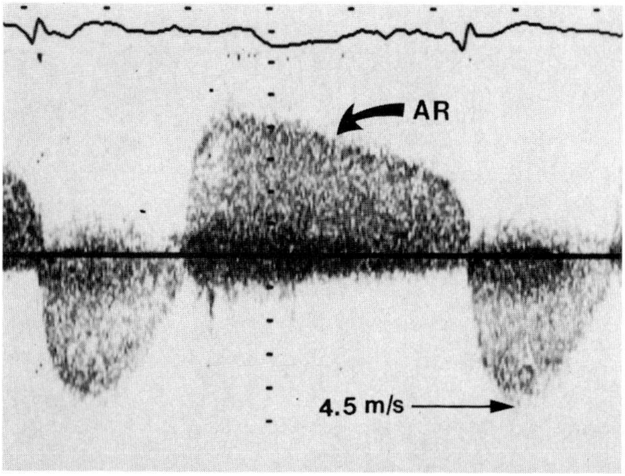

Figure 18–6. Case 2. CW Doppler echocardiogram from the apex demonstrating a peak systolic velocity of 4.5 m/s and aortic regurgitation (AR).

4.5 m/s. This equated to an estimated aortic valve pressure gradient of 81 mmHg. The slope of the aortic regurgitant jet was steep, consistent with significant valvular insufficiency. In the setting of aortic regurgitation, the aortic valve gradient is overestimated. However, the maximal velocity peaked in mid-systole, in keeping with critical aortic stenosis.

Cardiac Catheterization. Revealed extensive atherosclerotic obstructive lesions in all three major coronary arteries. The peak-to-peak aortic valve gradient was 64 mmHg, and the calculated aortic valve area was 0.6 cm^2. Moderate aortic regurgitation was seen on aortic root angiography.

Disposition. The patient underwent aortic valve replacement and coronary bypass graft surgery.

CASE 3 ACUTE AORTIC REGURGITATION (Chapters 7 and 13)

History. A 32-year-old man with a long history of intravenous drug use was admitted to hospital with a 2-week history of fever and progressive dyspnea on exertion.

Physical Examination. Revealed cachexia with mild respiratory distress. The temperature was 40°C, blood pressure 140/85 mmHg, and heart rate 110 beats/min. There were bilateral basal rales. There were an accentuated precordial apical thrust, a grade II/VI systolic ejection murmur at the left sternal border, a grade III/VI early diastolic blowing murmur of aortic regurgitation, an Austin Flint murmur, a third heart sound, Duroziez's murmur, and brisk carotid pulsations. There were no petechiae, Roth spots, Osler's nodes, or Janeway lesions. The spleen was not palpable.

Electrocardiogram. Showed sinus tachycardia and minor nonspecific T-wave changes.

Chest X-Ray. Revealed mild left ventricular enlargement and pulmonary venous congestion.

Two-Dimensional Echocardiogram. Demonstrated the presence of a large, mobile vegetation on the aortic valve (Fig. 18–7). The vegetation prolapses into the left ventricular outflow tract during diastole. The left ventricle was dilated, and the systolic function hyperdynamic in keeping with a left ventricular volume overload. The M-*mode tracing* of the mitral

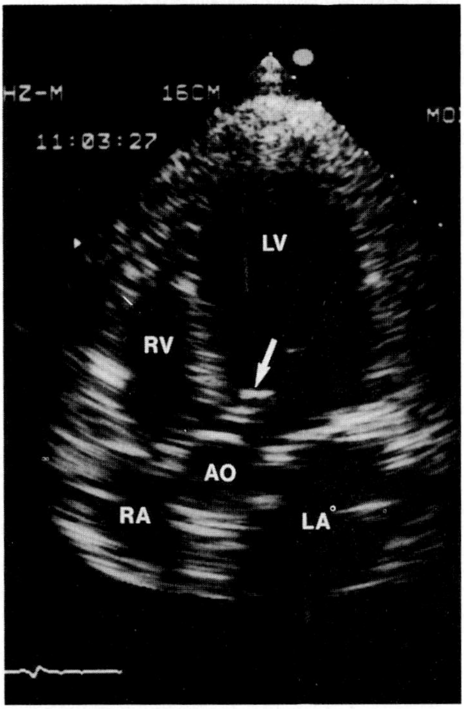

Figure 18–7. Case 3. Apical five-chamber view demonstrating a large aortic valve vegetation (arrow) prolapsing into the left ventricular (LV) outflow tract during diastole. AO = aorta, LA = left atrium, RA = right atrium, RV = right ventricle.

valve showed premature closure of the mitral valve, indicating marked elevation of left ventricular end-diastolic pressure.

Doppler Study. CFI and color M-mode studies demonstrated severe aortic regurgitation (Fig. 18–8). The regurgitant jet occupied approximately 75 percent of the left ventricular outflow tract, indicating a severe lesion. Further confirmation was obtained by CW Doppler investigation from the apical view (Fig. 18–9).

Disposition. Blood cultures grew *Staphylococcus aureus*. Therapy was initiated with intravenous antibiotics, and the patient responded well to intravenous diuretics, with resolution of left ventricular failure. On the fourth hospital day he developed progressive dyspnea and left ventricular failure. Repeat Doppler echocardiographic study was unchanged.

Based on the Doppler assessment of severe aortic regurgitation, the patient underwent emergency aortic valve replacement. Vegetations were noted in the left and noncoronary cusps. The right aortic cusp appeared flail. Six months after aortic valve replacement the patient remained asymptomatic, and the heart size and function were normal.

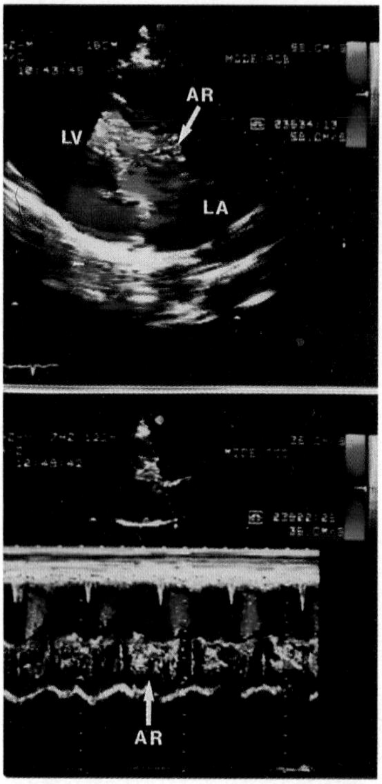

Figure 18–8. Case 3. CFI and color M-mode tracings demonstrating severe aortic regurgitation (AR). Parasternal long axis view. A mosaic pattern, representing turbulence, occupies approximately 75 percent of the left ventricular (LV) outflow tract during diastole. LA = left atrium.

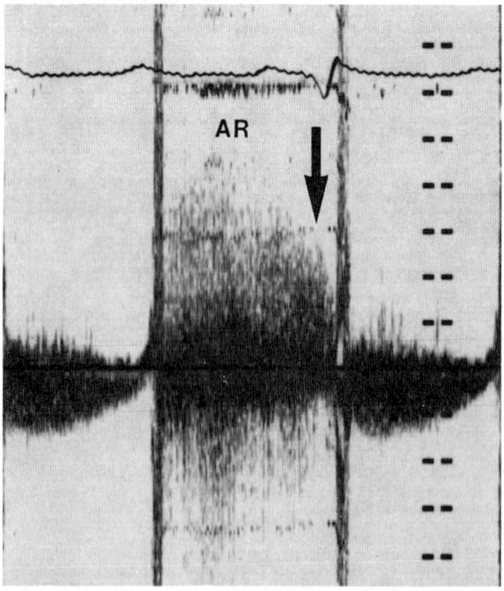

Figure 18–9. Case 3. CW wave Doppler echocardiogram recorded at an increased sweep speed to increase the accuracy of derived calculations. Aortic regurgitation (AR) is represented as flow above the baseline during diastole. The peak velocity of the AR jet at end-diastole (arrow) is 3 m/s. This predicts an aortic–to–left ventricular pressure gradient ($\Delta P = 4V^2$) of 36 mmHg. The patient's arm diastolic blood pressure was 70 mmHg. The left ventricular end-diastolic pressure is, therefore, 70 − 36, or 34 mmHg. (Scale marks = 1 m/s)

CASE 4 RHEUMATIC MITRAL VALVE DISEASE (Chapters 5 and 8)

History. A 65-year-old woman was referred for reevaluation of a previously diagnosed mitral stenosis. She had a known history of rheumatic fever in childhood and had been followed for mitral stenosis since the early 1970s. She had initially undergone cardiac catheterization in 1976, when she had been found to have a mitral valve area of 1 cm^2 and no significant mitral regurgitation. She had been clinically well from that time until symptomatic deterioration had occurred, in 1983. Repeat cardiac catheterization had revealed severe mitral stenosis, a valve area of 0.7 cm^2, and new pulmonary hypertension. The coronary arteries had been normal. An uneventful open mitral commissurotomy had been performed shortly thereafter. She had then remained asymptomatic until the 12 months preceding this referral, during which she had noted progressive dyspnea on exertion, fatigue, and several episodes of paroxysmal nocturnal dyspnea. She denied chest pain.

Physical Examination. The heart rate was 90 beats/min and regular; the blood pressure was 130/80 mmHg. The lungs were clear. The first heart sound was loud, there was an early opening snap, and there was a grade II/VI diastolic rumble with presystolic accentuation at the apex. A grade III/VI holosystolic murmur was present at the apex. The jugular venous pressure was elevated, with prominent "V" waves. The liver was not enlarged or pulsatile. There was minimal ankle edema.

Electrocardiogram. Showed normal sinus rhythm, left atrial abnormality (P mitral), and nonspecific ST-T-wave changes.

Chest X-Ray. Revealed cardiomegaly with left atrial enlargement and significant increase in the upper lobe vasculature.

Two-Dimensional Echocardiogram. Revealed a markedly enlarged left atrium and a dilated left ventricle with mild global hypokinesis. The mitral valve was thickened and demonstrated restricted motion and early diastolic doming. The right atrium and right ventricle were dilated. The tricuspid valve appeared intrinsically normal.

Doppler Study. CFI demonstrated a narrow jet made up of a central blue zone (due to aliasing from high velocities) surrounded by hues of yellow and red (representing lower-velocity turbulent flow) (Fig. 18–10). The appearance was likened to that of a candle flame. Characterization of the

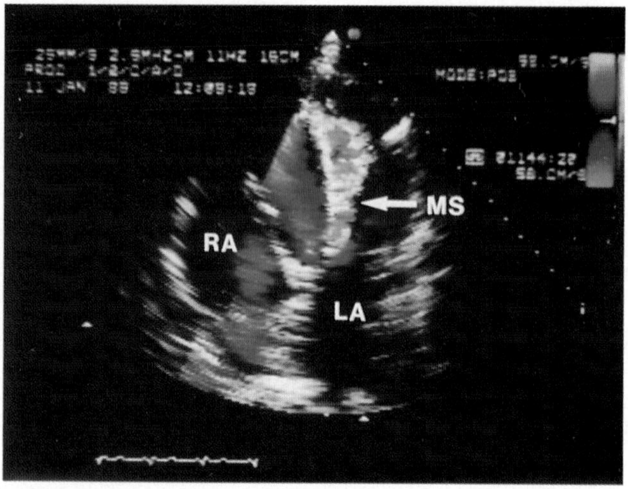

Figure 18–10. Case 4. Apical view in diastole showing the characteristic candle-flame appearance of the jet in mitral stenosis (MS). The jet has a central blue zone due to color reversal from aliasing. The peripheral zone is yellow-red, representing turbulence. LA = left atrium, RA = right atrium.

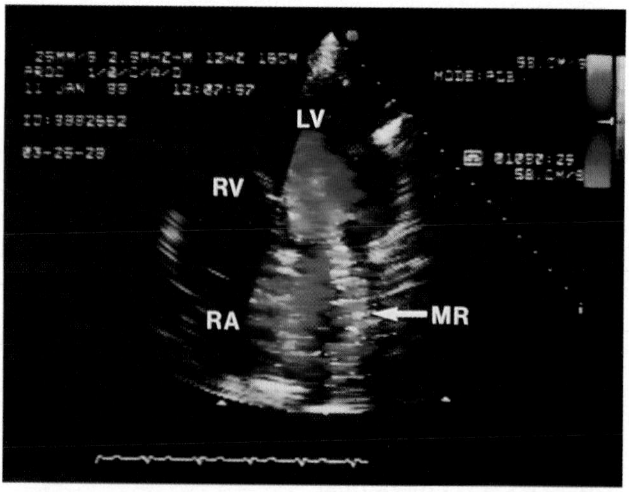

Figure 18–11. Case 4. Mitral regurgitation, from an apical four-chamber view. Mitral regurgitant (MR) jet occupies 30 to 40 percent of the left atrium, indicating moderately severe mitral regurgitation. LV = left ventricle, RA = right atrium, RV = right ventricle.

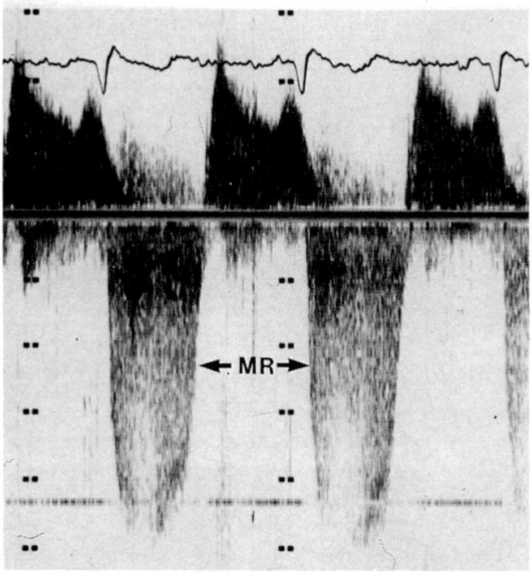

Figure 18–12. Case 4. CW Doppler tracing of combined mitral stenosis and regurgitation (MR). (Scale marks = 1 m/s)

mitral stenosis jet permitted accurate guided CW Doppler interrogation. Moderate mitral regurgitation was recorded, which measured approximately 30 to 40 percent of the left atrial area—indicating moderately severe mitral regurgitation (Fig. 18–11). CW Doppler recording from the apex (Fig. 18–12) showed a maximal velocity of 2 m/s, a pressure half-time of 200 ms, and a calculated valve area of 1.1 cm^2. Mitral regurgitation was recorded below the baseline. The pressure half-time for estimating mitral valve area is accurate in the presence of mitral regurgitation. There was significant tricuspid regurgitation, with a calculated pulmonary artery systolic pressure of 55 mmHg.

Disposition. Despite maximization of her medication regimen for congestive heart failure, the patient remained significantly symptomatic. She subsequently underwent mitral valve replacement. Repeat cardiac catheterization was not performed. At time of writing, the patient was doing well.

CASE 5 PULMONARY HYPERTENSION (Chapters 9 and 13)

History. A 34-year-old man was referred for a Doppler echocardiographic evaluation because of progressive dyspnea on exertion, chest pain, and fatigue.

Physical Examination. Revealed a heart rate of 85 beats/min and blood pressure of 115/70 mmHg. Cardiac examination showed a loud P_2, a grade

II/VI holosytolic murmur at the left sternal border that increased with inspiration, and a fourth heart sound during inspiration. The liver was not enlarged or pulsatile.

Electrocardiogram. Consistent with right ventricular hypertrophy.

Chest X-Ray. Showed right atrial and right ventricular enlargement. The lung fields were clear.

Two-Dimensional Echocardiogram. Revealed an enlarged right atrium and right ventricle (Fig. 18–13). The left atrium and left ventricle were normal in size. The interventricular septum was displaced toward the left ventricle, which is consistent with right ventricular pressure/volume overload.

Doppler Study. CFI disclosed severe tricuspid regurgitation (Fig. 18–14). CW Doppler interrogation of the regurgitant jet demonstrated peak velocities of 3.5 m/s (Fig. 18–15), indicating an approximate peak right ventricular–to–right atrial pressure gradient of 49 mmHg ($\Delta P = 4V^2$). The mean right atrial pressure was estimated at 14 mmHg. The pulmonary artery systolic pressure is, therefore, 49 + 14, or 63 mmHg.

Disposition. The patient underwent right cardiac catheterization. There was no evidence of intracardiac shunt. The pulmonary artery pressure was

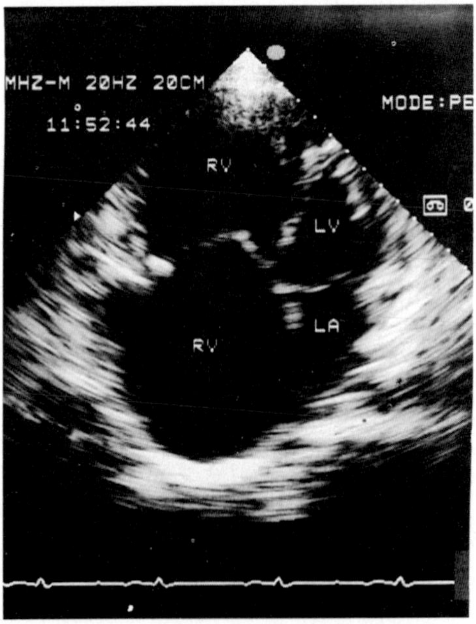

Figure 18–13. Case 5. Apical four-chamber view demonstrating a dilated right ventricle (RV) and right atrium (RA) in a patient with severe pulmonary hypertension and tricuspid regurgitation. The interventricular septum is displaced toward the left ventricle (LV). LA = left atrium.

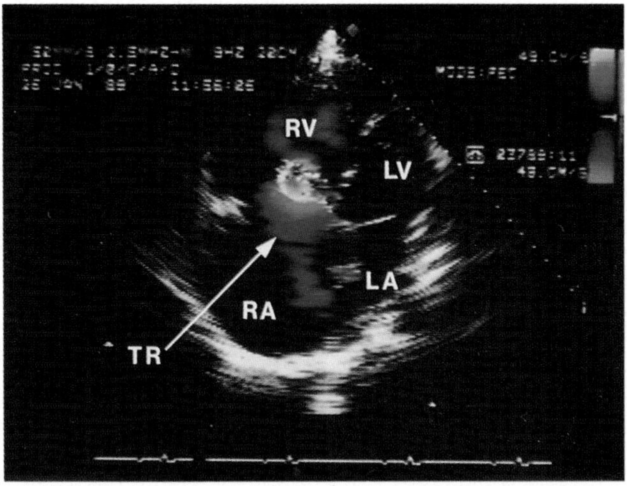

Figure 18–14. Case 5. CFI in the apical four-chamber view demonstrating tricuspid regurgitation (TR). LA = left atrium, LV = left ventricle, RA = right atrium, RV = right ventricle.

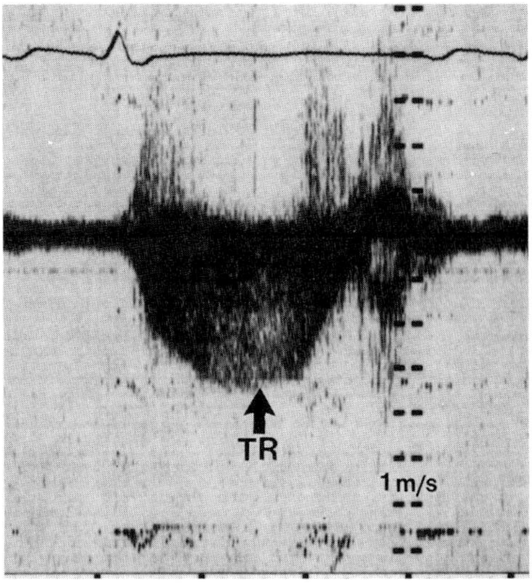

Figure 18–15. Case 5. CW Doppler tracing from the apex demonstrating the tricuspid regurgitant jet. The peak velocity is 3.5 m/s, and the calculated gradient across the tricuspid valve is 49 mmHg. The pulmonary artery systolic pressure was estimated at 63 mmHg (49 + 14).

70/25 mmHg, and the mean pulmonary capillary wedge pressure was 8 mmHg. Pulmonary angiography showed no evidence of pulmonary emboli. The patient underwent a trial of vasodilator therapy without a significant reduction in the pulmonary arterial resistance. At time of writing, he was on long-term anticoagulation therapy and was being considered for a heart-lung transplant.

CASE 6 DILATED CARDIOMYOPATHY (Chapters 7, 8, 9, and 15)

History. A 55-year-old man was referred for cardiac Doppler examination to evaluate left ventricular function. He had a one-year history of exertional dyspnea, and had recently been admitted to hospital with congestive heart failure. There was no history of chest pain, hypertension, thyroid disease, diabetes mellitus, or rheumatic fever. The patient was a known alcoholic.

Physical Examination. Revealed blood pressure of 110/85 mmHg and a heart rate of 80 beats/min, with an underlying rhythm of atrial fibrillation. There were bilateral rales at both lung bases, elevated jugular venous pressure, nonpalpable apical impulse, paradoxical splitting of the second heart sound, and a grade III/VI holosystolic murmur at the apex. A third heart sound was audible.

Electrocardiogram. Revealed atrial fibrillation, premature ventricular contractions, and left bundle branch block.

Chest X-Ray. Showed generalized cardiomegaly with pulmonary venous congestion.

Two-Dimensional Echocardiogram. Revealed enlargement of all four chambers (Fig. 18–16). There was generalized hypokinesis of the left ventricle (left ventricular fractional shortening of 12 percent). There was minimal thickening of the mitral and aortic leaflets, but no restriction of excursion.

Doppler Study. CFI demonstrated a mitral regurgitant jet that occupied approximately 30 percent of the left atrial area, indicating moderate mitral regurgitation (Figs. 18–16 and 18–17). Despite the absence of aortic regurgitant murmur, an aortic regurgitant jet was detected which was long but narrow (Fig. 18–18) and which occupied approximately 20 percent of the left ventricular outflow tract, indicating a mild lesion. Tricuspid regurgitation was also observed (Fig. 18–19).

Disposition. In light of the generalized left ventricular dysfunction, catheterization was not performed; medical therapy for congestive heart failure was administered. The presence of mitral and aortic regurgitation heightened the importance of aggressive vasodilator therapy. Doppler CFI detects and estimates the severity of multivalvular regurgitation, a frequent finding in patients with dilated cardiomyopathy.

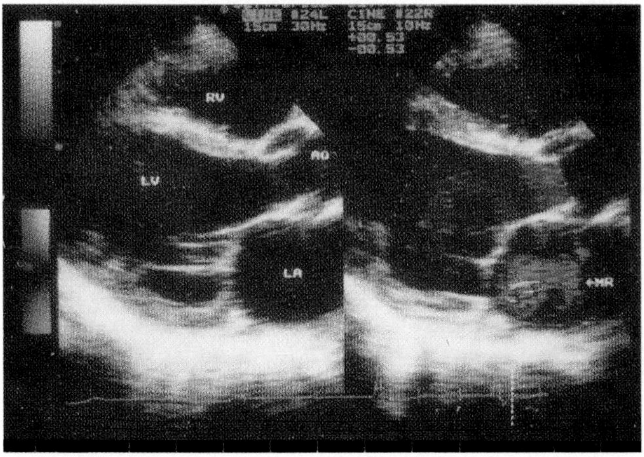

Figure 18–16. Case 6. Dual-screen (2D anatomy on left, CFI on right) echocardiography in the parasternal long axis view, demonstrating an increased end-systolic dimension and a jet of mitral regurgitation (MR). AO = aorta, LA = left atrium, LV = left ventricle, RV = right ventricle.

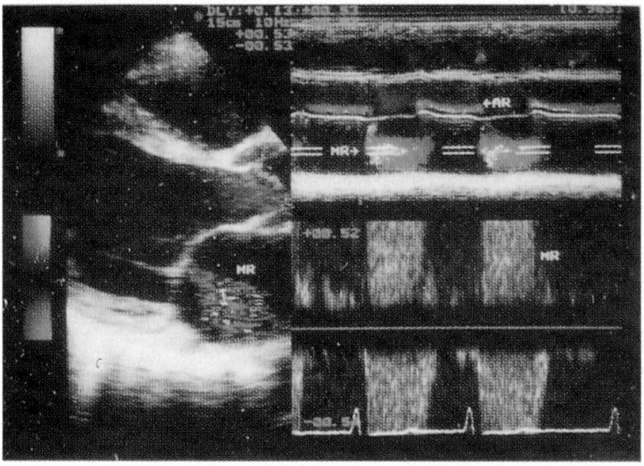

Figure 18–17. Case 6. Simultaneous Doppler CFI, color M-mode echocardiography, and PD spectral recording demonstrating mitral regurgitation (MR). Both mitral regurgitation (during systole) and aortic regurgitation (AR) (during diastole) are delineated by color M-mode echocardiography.

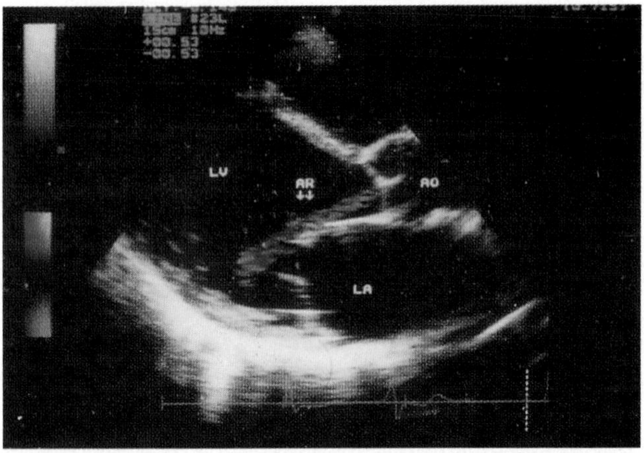

Figure 18–18. Case 6. Parasternal long axis view showing a long narrow jet of aortic regurgitation (AR) directed toward the mitral valve leaflets. AO = aorta, LA = left atrium, LV = left ventricle.

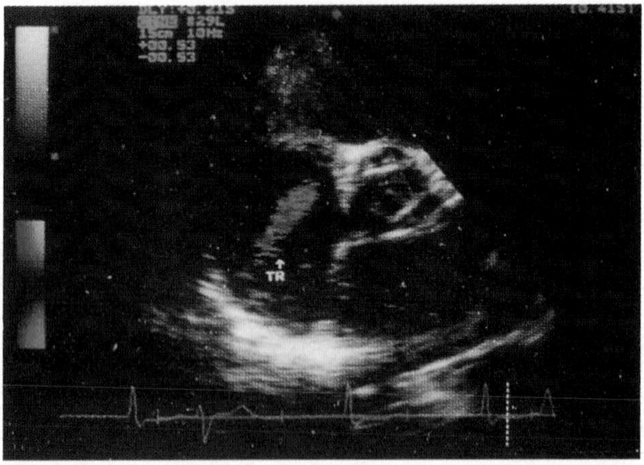

Figure 18–19. Case 6. Short axis view at the level of the aortic valve, demonstrating tricuspid regurgitation (TR).

CASE 7 PROSTHETIC MITRAL VALVE (Chapters 8 and 10)

History. A 57-year-old woman was admitted to hospital with congestive heart failure. Seven years earlier, mitral valve replacement with a porcine bioprosthesis had been performed for rheumatic mitral stenosis.

Physical Examination. On admission the heart rate was 110 beats/min, with an underlying rhythm of atrial fibrillation; blood pressure was 100/

60 mmHg, and the respiratory rate was 30/min. There was marked jugular venous distension, and there were rales over the lower halves of the lung fields. Cardiac examination showed a diffuse and displaced cardiac apex, a loud third heart sound, and a grade IV/VI holosystolic murmur audible at the apex and radiating to the axilla. No diastolic murmur was heard.

Electrocardiogram. Showed atrial fibrillation and nonspecific ST-T-wave changes.

Chest X-Ray. Revealed cardiomegaly and pulmonary edema.

Two-Dimensional Echocardiogram. Showed marked four-chamber enlargement and moderate left ventricular dysfunction. The bioprosthetic mitral leaflets appeared thickened, with findings of a flail cusp (Fig. 18–20).

Doppler Study. CFI demonstrated severe mitral valve regurgitation (Fig. 18–21). The regurgitant jet occupied approximately 40 percent of the left atrial area. The diastolic flow across the prosthesis was normal, without findings of stenosis (Fig. 18–22).

Disposition. The patient was treated for congestive heart failure; significant symptomatic and hemodynamic improvement followed. Cardiac catheteri-

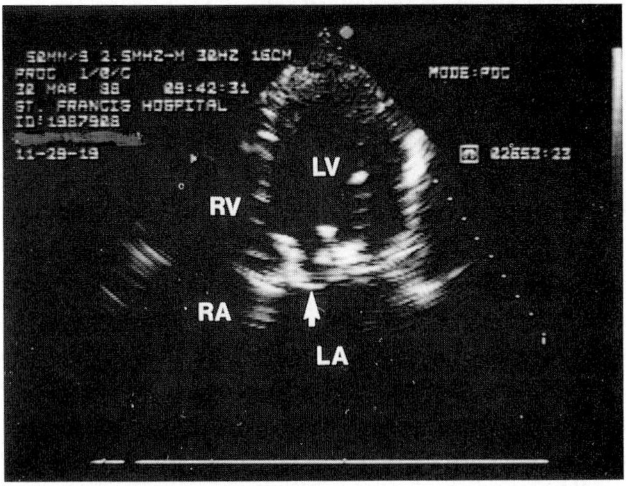

Figure 18–20. Case 7. Apical four-chamber view showing a thickened and flail bioprosthetic mitral valve leaflet (arrow). LA = left atrium, LV = left ventricle, RA = right atrium, RV = right ventricle.

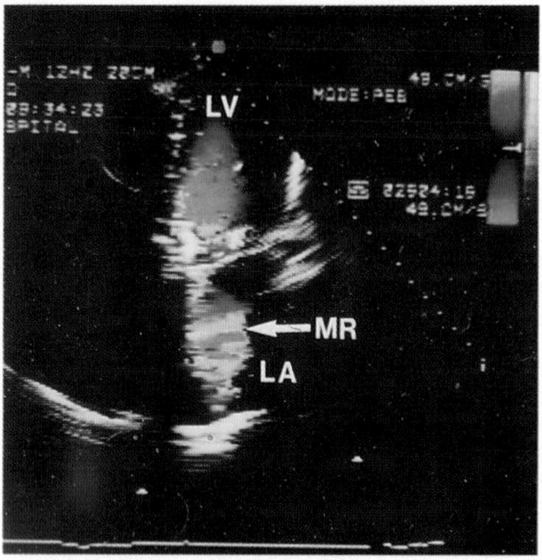

Figure 18–21. Case 7. Bioprosthetic mitral valve regurgitation (MR) from an apical four-chamber view. A mosaic pattern, representing turbulence, is demonstrated in the left atrium (LA). LV = left ventricle.

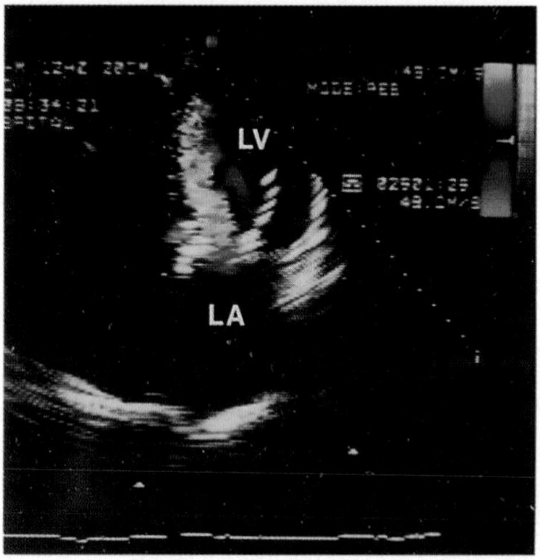

Figure 18–22. Case 7. Apical four-chamber view. A mosaic pattern, representing turbulent blood flow, is visualized in the left ventricular inflow tract of this patient with a bioprosthetic mitral valve. LA = left atrium, LV = left ventricle.

zation was performed, and showed severe prosthetic mitral valve regurgitation and normal coronary arteries. The patient underwent reoperation for replacement of the bioprosthetic mitral valve with a St. Jude Medical prosthesis. One year after surgery, the patient was asymptomatic.

CASE 8 MITRAL VALVE PROLAPSE (Chapter 8)

History. A 25-year-old woman was referred for evaluation of a systolic murmur. The patient was asymptomatic.

Physical Examination. Revealed a midsystolic click and a late apical systolic murmur. The rest of the examination was normal.

Electrocardiogram. Showed minimal nonspecific inferolateral ST-T-wave changes.

Two-Dimensional Echocardiogram. Demonstrated prolapse of the anterior and posterior mitral valve leaflets (Fig. 18–23). The cardiac chambers were normal in size, and the left ventricular function was normal.

Doppler Study. CFI in the parasternal long axis view demonstrated mild mitral regurgitation (Fig. 18–24). The eccentric regurgitant jet was directed posteriorly. Color M-mode echocardiography (Fig. 18–25) aids in the timing of cardiac events, which in this patient demonstrated mid-to-late mitral regurgitation.

Disposition. No treatment was instituted. Recommendations were given for antibiotic prophylaxis.

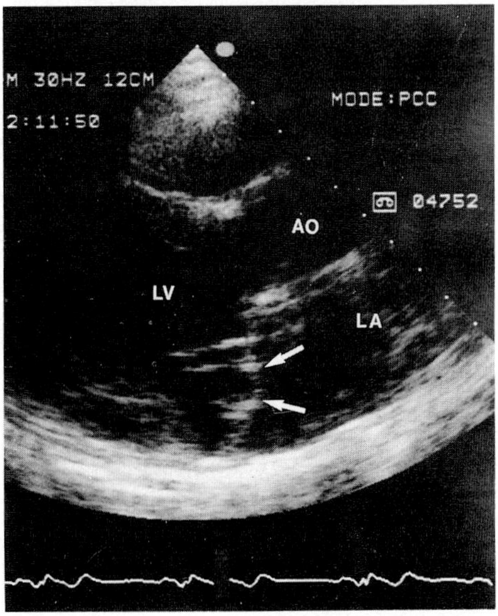

Figure 18–23. Case 8. Parasternal long axis view demonstrating mitral valve prolapse. Both anterior and posterior mitral leaflets (arrows) prolapse into the left atrium (LA). AO = aorta, LV = left ventricle.

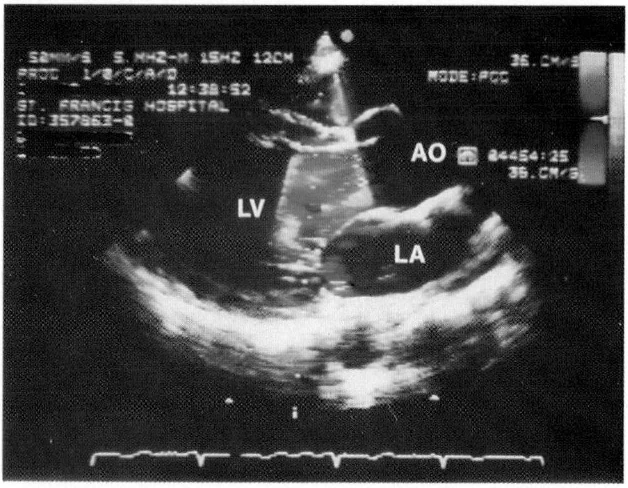

Figure 18–24. Case 8. Color flow image demonstrating an eccentric mitral regurgitant jet (blue) directed toward the posterior left atrial (LA) wall. AO = aorta, LV = left ventricle.

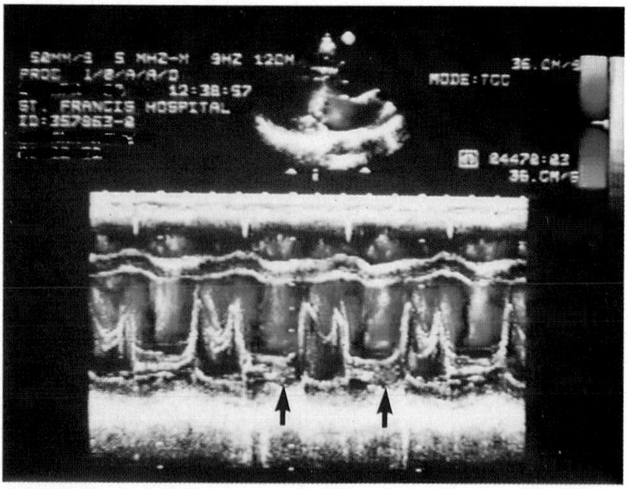

Figure 18–25. Case 8. Color flow M-mode tracing demonstrating mid-to-late mitral regurgitation (arrows).

CASE 9 ATRIAL SEPTAL DEFECT (Chapters 13 and 17)

History. A 35-year-old woman was referred for cardiac evaluation because of progressive dyspnea and a cardiac murmur. There was no prior history of rheumatic fever, ischemic heart disease, or systemic hypertension.

Physical Examination. Revealed no cyanosis or clubbing. The blood pressure was 140/85 mmHg, and the heart rate 80 beats/min. A moderate right ventricular lift was palpated. The second heart sound was persistently split with an accentuated pulmonic component. A grade II/VI midsystolic murmur was heard along the left sternal border. No diastolic murmur was noted.

Electrocardiogram. Demonstrated a frontal QRS axis of 110° with an RSR′ pattern in the right precordial leads.

Chest X-Ray. Revealed right ventricular enlargement with increased pulmonary blood flow.

Two-Dimensional Echocardiogram. Demonstrated right atrial and right ventricular enlargement. A large secundum-type atrial septal defect was seen in the subcostal four-chamber view (Fig. 18–26).

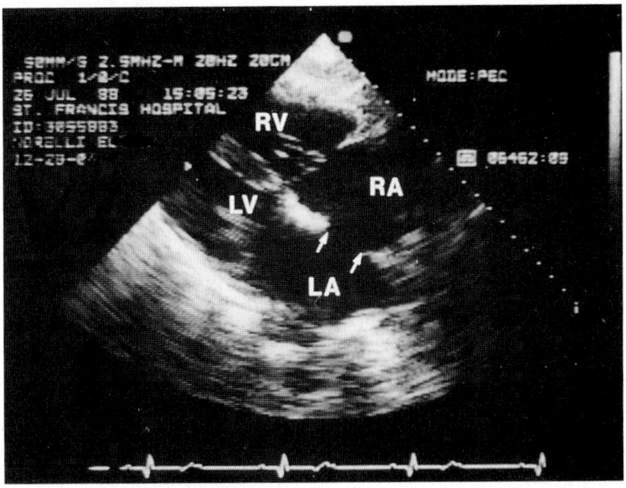

Figure 18–26. Case 9. Subcostal four-chamber view showing a large secundum atrial septal defect (arrows). The right atrium (RA) and right ventricle (RV) are enlarged.

Doppler Study. CFI from a subcostal four-chamber view indicated a large red flow arising from the left atrium and passing through the defect to the right atrium and across the tricuspid valve into the right ventricle (Fig. 18–27). There was an increase in blood flow velocity at the site of the atrial septal defect, represented as aliasing (blue-coded flow). The pulmonary artery systolic pressure was estimated from the tricuspid regurgitant jet

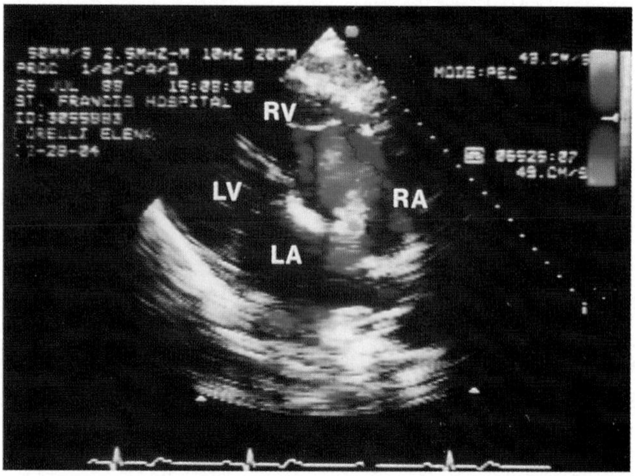

Figure 18–27. Case 9. Subcostal four-chamber view showing red flow of left (LA)–to–right (RA) shunting across a large secundum atrial septal defect. The increase in blood flow velocity at the site of the defect is represented as aliasing (blue-coded flow). LV = left ventricle, RV = right ventricle.

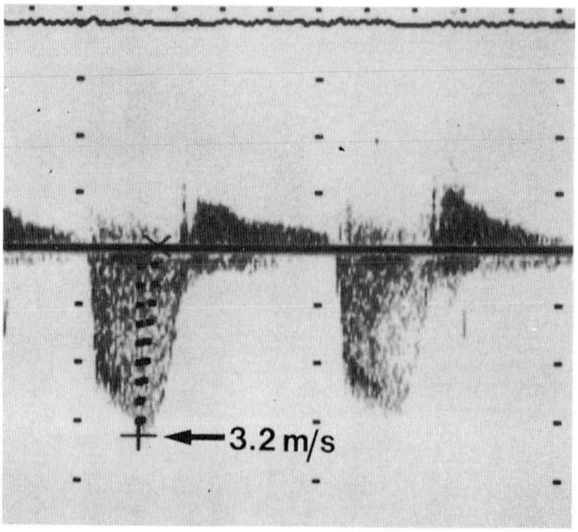

Figure 18–28. Case 9. CW Doppler recording of tricuspid regurgitation in a patient with a large secundum atrial septal defect and pulmonary hypertension. The peak tricuspid regurgitant velocity is 3.2 m/s.

(Fig. 18–28) by use of CW Doppler echocardiography from an apical view. The peak transtricuspid velocity was 3.2 m/s, translating to a peak pressure gradient of 41 mmHg. Assumption of a right atrial pressure of 14 mmHg gives a pulmonary artery systolic pressure of 55 mmHg, indicating moderate pulmonary hypertension.

Disposition. Elective surgical repair was performed, without cardiac catheterization.

CASE 10 LEFT ATRIAL MYXOMA

History. A 67-year-old woman presented with a 6-month history of fatigue, progressive exertional dyspnea, orthopnea, and paroxysmal nocturnal dyspnea, and was admitted to hospital with a syncopal episode. Three years earlier, she had sustained an inferior-wall myocardial infarction. One year before admission she had been found to be anemic and had been started on iron therapy. There was no past history of rheumatic fever, hypertension, or diabetes mellitus.

Physical Examination. Revealed a loud first heart sound, a fourth sound, and a systolic ejection murmur at the left sternal border. There was an early diastolic sound, initially confused with an opening snap, but subsequently believed to be a tumor plop. A grade II/VI diastolic rumble was heard intermittently. The rest of the examination was normal.

Two-Dimensional Echocardiogram. Showed a large tumor mass in the left atrium obstructing the mitral valve orifice during diastole (Fig. 18–29A and B).

Doppler Study. CFI demonstrated significant impairment in left ventricular diastolic inflow due to obstruction (Fig. 18–29C and D). There was minimal flow on both sides of the tumor (faint red signals).

Cardiac Catheterization. Was performed to evaluate for coronary artery disease in view of the patient's prior history of myocardial infarction. Coronary angiography showed a total right coronary artery occlusion. There was noncritical disease of the left coronary artery. A tumor "blush" was noted on selective injection of contrast medium into the left coronary artery via a left atrial branch of the circumflex coronary artery.

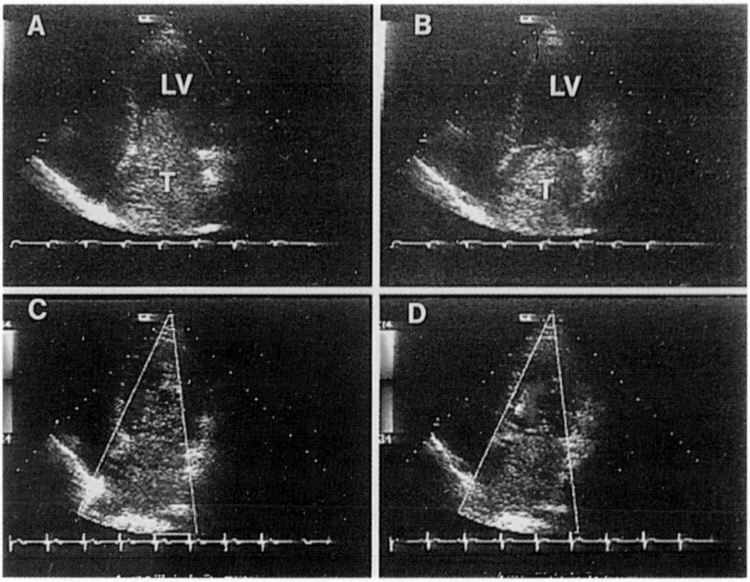

Figure 18–29. Case 10. (A) Apical four-chamber view showing a large left atrial tumor (T) prolapsing across the mitral valve during diastole. (B) Systolic frame, with tumor occupying nearly the entire left atrium. (C) CFI demonstrates a significant decrease in blood flow signals during diastole. Weak signals (red-coded flow) are seen on both sides of the tumor. (D) Normal left ventricular systolic flow (blue-coded flow). LV = left ventricle.

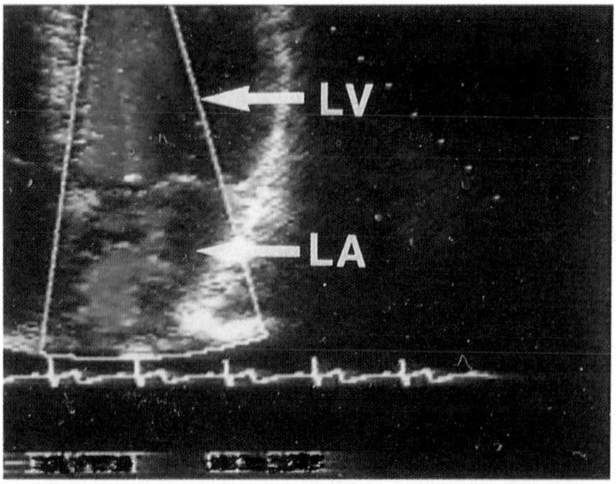

Figure 18–30. Case 10. Postoperative study. Normal left atrial filling from pulmonary veins is depicted in red, and normal left ventricular systolic flow in blue.

Disposition. The patient underwent surgical resection of a left atrial tumor. The pathologic specimen showed a large, polypoid, friable tumor. A portion of the interatrial septum was attached to a short pedicle. The histologic findings confirmed that the tumor was an atrial myxoma. A postoperative 2D color flow study was normal (Fig. 18–30).

INDEX

INDEX